FISTULA POLITICS

MEDICAL ANTHROPOLOGY: HEALTH, INEQUALITY, AND SOCIAL JUSTICE

Series editor: Lenore Manderson

Books in the Medical Anthropology series are concerned with social patterns of and social responses to ill health, disease, and suffering, and how social exclusion and social justice shape health and healing outcomes. The series is designed to reflect the diversity of contemporary medical anthropological research and writing, and will offer scholars a forum to publish work that showcases the theoretical sophistication, methodological soundness, and ethnographic richness of the field.

Books in the series may include studies on the organization and movement of peoples, technologies, and treatments, how inequalities pattern access to these, and how individuals, communities and states respond to various assaults on well-being, including from illness, disaster, and violence.

Jessica Hardin, *Faith and the Pursuit of Health: Cardiometabolic Disorders in Samoa*
Carina Heckert, *Fault Lines of Care: Gender, HIV, and Global Health in Bolivia*
Alison Heller, *Fistula Politics: Birthing Injuries and the Quest for Continence in Niger*
Joel Christian Reed, *Landscapes of Activism: Civil Society, HIV and AIDS Care in Northern Mozambique*
Beatriz M. Reyes-Foster, *Psychiatric Encounters: Madness and Modernity in Yucatan, Mexico*
Sonja van Wichelen, *Legitimating Life: Adoption in the Age of Globalization and Biotechnology*
Lesley Jo Weaver, *Sugar and Tension: Diabetes and Gender in Modern India*
Andrea Whittaker, *International Surrogacy as Disruptive Industry in Southeast Asia*

FISTULA POLITICS

Birthing Injuries and the Quest for Continence in Niger

ALISON HELLER

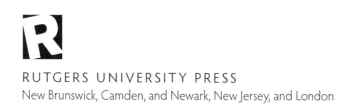

RUTGERS UNIVERSITY PRESS

New Brunswick, Camden, and Newark, New Jersey, and London

Library of Congress Cataloging-in-Publication Data

Names: Heller, Alison (Alison W.), author.
Title: Fistula politics : birthing injuries and the quest for continence in Niger / Alison
   Heller.
Other titles: Medical anthropology (New Brunswick, N.J.)
Description: New Brunswick : Rutgers University Press, 2018. | Series: Medical
   anthropology: health, inequality, and social justice | Includes bibliographical
   references and index.
Identifiers: LCCN 2018012992| ISBN 9781978800373 (cloth) | ISBN 9781978800366
   (pbk.)
Subjects: LCSH: Women—Health and hygiene—Niger. | Fistula—Treatment—
   Niger. | Reproductive health—Niger. | Women—Niger—Social
   conditions—21st century.
Classification: LCC RA552.N55 H45 2018 | DDC 362.1082096626—dc23
LC record available at https://lccn.loc.gov/2018012992

A British Cataloging-in-Publication record for this book is available from the
British Library.

All photos by the author

♾ The paper used in this publication meets the requirements of the American
National Standard for Information Sciences—Permanence of Paper for Printed
Library Materials, ANSI Z39.48-1992.

www.rutgersuniversitypress.org

Manufactured in the United States of America

While so many relationships proved unreliable in the face of illness, my research revealed the steadfast and unwavering bond between mother and daughter. Women lucky enough to have their mothers were protected from the worst social consequences. They were advocated for and rarely alone.

This work is part of my story with my own mother. When her diagnosis came, days before I boarded my plane to Niger, she wouldn't let me stay. When her treatments failed, she wouldn't let me stop. She was a seeker of knowledge, a fighter for justice, and my strongest supporter. She, an immovable force, always at my side.

This is for her.

CONTENTS

FOREWORD

LENORE MANDERSON

Medical Anthropology: Health, Inequality, Social Justice is a new series from Rutgers University Press designed to capture the diversity of contemporary medical anthropological research and writing. The beauty of ethnography is its capacity, through storytelling, to make sense of suffering as a social experience and to set it in context. Central to our focus in this series on health, illness, and social justice, therefore, is the way in which social structures and ideologies shape the likelihood and impact of infections, injuries, bodily ruptures, and disease as well as chronic conditions and disability, treatment and care, and social repair and death.

The brief for this series is broad. The books are concerned with health and illness, healing practices, and access to care, but the authors illustrate too the importance of context—of geography, physical condition, service availability, and income. Health and illness are social facts; the circumstances of the maintenance and loss of health are always and everywhere shaped by structural, global, and local relations. Society, culture, economy, and political organization as much as ecology shape the variance of illness, disability, and disadvantage. But as medical anthropologists have long illustrated, the relationships of social context and health status are complex. In addressing these questions, the authors in this series showcase the theoretical sophistication, methodological rigor, and empirical richness of the field while expanding a map of illness and social and institutional life to illustrate the effects of material conditions and social meanings in troubling and surprising ways.

The books in the series move across social circumstances, health conditions, and geography, and their intersections and interactions to demonstrate how individuals, communities, and states manage assaults on well-being. The books reflect medical anthropology as a constantly changing field of scholarship, drawing on research diversely in residential and virtual communities, clinics, and laboratories, in emergency care and public health settings, with service providers, individual healers, and households, with social bodies, human bodies, and biologies. Medical anthropology once concentrated on systems of healing, particular diseases, and embodied experiences, but today the field has expanded to include environmental disaster and war, science, technology and faith, gender-based violence, and forced migration. Curiosity about the body and its vicissitudes remains a pivot for our work, but our concerns are with the location of bodies in social life and with how social structures, temporal imperatives, and shifting exigencies shape life courses. This dynamic field reflects an ethics of the discipline to address these pressing issues of our time.

Globalization has contributed to and adds to the complexity of influences on health outcomes; it (re)produces social and economic relations that institution- alize poverty, unequal conditions of everyday life and work, and environments in which diseases increase or subside. Globalization patterns the movement and relations of peoples, technologies, and knowledge as well as programs and treat- ments; it shapes differences in health experience and outcomes across space; and it informs and amplifies inequalities at individual and country levels. Global forces and local inequalities compound and constantly load on individuals to impact on their physical and mental health, and on their households and communities. At the same time, as the subtitle of this series indicates, we are concerned with ques- tions of social exclusion and inclusion, and social justice and repair—again both globally and in local settings. The books will challenge readers not only to reflect on sickness and suffering, deficit and despair, but also on resistance and restitu- tion—on how people respond to injustices and evade the fault lines that might seem to predetermine life outcomes. Although not all the books take this direc- tion, the aim is to widen the frame within which we conceptualize embodiment and suffering.

Alison Heller takes us to the heart of suffering. The setting is Niger, and, in par- ticular, the four institutions in which women of all ages, married and single, with and without children, place their faith in the promises of doctors, donors, wom- en's health advocates, and the media that their condition—the "sickness of leak- ing urine"—can readily be cured. Women with vaginal fistulas—holes from their vagina to their bladder or rectum from traumatic childbirth and poor obstetric care, which leak urine and feces—wait for months and years until their number comes up and a surgeon is on hand to effect repair. Many return for more surger- ies; yet with each repeat surgery and further scar tissue, repair is less likely to occur. Others wait for surgery that turns out to be inappropriate: they may have recur- rent bladder infections, or pelvic organ prolapse, or pelvic floor weakness, and do not, after all, have fistula.

Fistula Politics instantiates the embodiment of gender, certainly. But as Heller illustrates, familiar accounts of rejection and divorce, nasty co-wives and jealous in-laws, abandonment by kin, social exclusion, depression, and suicide overshadow other stories of women's resilience, pragmatism, and making do. Nigérien religious and kinship systems, gender, politics, and economics intersect to influence whether, when, and if women seek care when they are in labor, and from whom they receive care. These circumstances pattern women's risk of fistula, their expe- rience of the condition, and their access to medical care.

Most of the women who end up in Niger's centers for fistula repair are desper- ately poor, rural women, who are often illiterate. Heller's interlocutors traveled across the country, often at great personal risk, far from their husbands and kin, in search of a cure. In their absence from home, their husbands bring in co-wives, their families reconstitute, and their children grow up. Meanwhile, at the centers, women forge new ties, brought together by their faith and the everyday rituals of workshop, and by ethnic identity and language.

In this superbly illustrated book, drawing on her work with one hundred of the women who had chosen a pilgrimage of repair, Heller illustrates how popular narratives about fistula serve the interests of humanitarian organizations and their supporters, donors, surgeons, and the media, far more so than the interests and life chances of the women with fistula.

ABBREVIATIONS

AQIM	al-Qaeda in the Islamic Maghreb
CNRFO	Centre National de Reference des Fistules Obstétricales (National Reference Center for Obstetric Fistula)
CSL-Danja	Centre de Santé Léprologie de Danja (Danja Leprosy Health Center)
CSLF-Danja	Centre de Santé, Léprologie et Fistule (Danja Leprosy and Fistula Health Center)
DFC	Danja Fistula Center
DHS	Demographic and Health Surveys (Enquête Démographique et de Santé et à Indicateurs Multiples)
FGC	Female genital cutting
FGM	Female genital mutilation
Lamordé	National Hospital of Lamordé
NGO	nongovernmental organization
MMR	Maternal mortality ratio
RVF	Rectovaginal fistula
SIM	Serving in Mission (formally known as Soudan Interior Mission [since 1893], then Society for International Ministries [since 1980s])
UNFPA	United Nations Population Fund
VVF	Vesicovaginal fistula
WFF	Worldwide Fistula Fund

ABBREVIATIONS

NOTE ON TERMINOLOGY

The condition: Obstetric fistula is a birthing injury caused by prolonged obstructed labor that results in chronic incontinence. Although *fistula* technically denotes any abnormal pathway in the body, throughout this book, I use the term as shorthand to denote obstetric fistula.

The place: The country officially titled the Republic of Niger, I refer simply to Niger. Its citizens are Nigériens (or Nigeriens), not to be confused with their neighbors to the south, Nigerians.

The women: To protect individual identities and respect confidentiality, I use pseudonyms for all of my interlocutors (and identify them by age and ethnicity). In some cases, I recognize that the use of pseudonyms is more for effect—to uphold a principle—than it is effective. In the two quotes from media pieces (where women's real names are used by journalists), I substitute pseudonyms as a nod to women's privacy while recognizing that their identities can still be easily uncovered through an internet search. I have considered this in my decisions regarding what to reveal and conceal.

FISTULA POLITICS

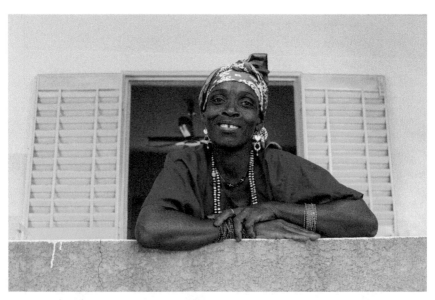

Portrait of a Fulani woman in Niamey, Niger

1 · INCONTINENCE AND INEQUALITIES

I came to know Fana, a 42-year-old Tuareg woman originally from Mali, at an obstetric fistula center in Niger's capital city, Niamey. Twenty-six years before we met, she had developed a birthing injury following complications during her first childbirth. Although the internal damage had been repaired seven years prior, the deep social, economic, and emotional scars continued to mark her everyday existence.

Fana was married at the age of 15 and soon after became pregnant. When her contractions began, she refused to acquiesce to the supplications of her family to deliver in the neighboring village's health center, its reputation tarnished by a string of recent maternal mortalities. Fana, who more than 25 years later remained just as stubborn, remembered how her resistance never wavered, even as her labor failed to progress for two days, then four, and finally seven full days. With each sunset, the quiet concern of her family swelled. Still, Fana reasoned that her chances of survival were better if she just stayed home.

After a full week of labor, Fana delivered a stillborn baby boy. Five days later, a persistent trickle of urine began to leak from her vagina. It did not stop for two decades.

Like many women who develop fistula, neither Fana nor her family had ever heard of the condition. Yet for the next 19 years much of Fana's life was dedicated to managing her incontinence and looking for treatment. Her quest for corporeal and social "normalcy" spanned five pregnancies, four husbands, three decades, two living and two stillborn children, one failed surgery, and—finally—a success: Fana was healed seven years before we met. But most women's pursuit of normalcy does not end with continence. Nor did Fana's. Long after the hole was sewn shut and the perpetual wetness had dried, her life was shaped by fistula and her tortuous quest for a cure.

Fana's story is one of economic deprivation, only exacerbated by the political turmoil in northern Mali, where the rise to power of the militant organization al-Qaeda in the Islamic Maghreb (AQIM) worsened her ill health and pushed her to cross the border into Niger. Her experiences with fistula were shaped by conditions of poverty and structural violence. Fana's fistula was both caused by and resulted in poverty. Yet her story is also one of unlikely empowerment within a context of major constraints. Through necessity, Fana learned to advocate for her own health care, fight for the custody of her daughter Safi, and negotiate new rules with her latest husband and co-wife. Her story extends across decades, borders, and marriages. The causal connections are complicated. And contrary to many media and humanitarian portrayals of women suffering from fistula in sub-Saharan Africa, Fana is anything but passive. In the pages that follow, Fana's words, and the words of 99 other women with fistula in Niger, bring to life how this birthing injury is experienced, lived with, treated, hidden, resisted, capitalized upon, and integrated into everyday life.

In a world of one-percenters and the "bottom billion," where the space that separates people within and between countries is ever expanding, the consequences of inequality and the concentration of power pervade everyday life. Maternal health is a particularly powerful area for thinking about the winners and the losers of global exchanges and local connections. Global disparities in maternal mortality rates—that is, the deaths of women due to childbirth or pregnancy—between resource-rich countries and resource-poor countries are astonishing. They are among the largest of any vital indicator.

In sub-Saharan Africa, one in 36 women will eventually die from pregnancy-related complications. In the often overlooked West African country of Niger, the number is even higher. One in 23 Nigérien women will die from maternal causes. This begins to make sense in the low-level clinics of rural Niger: nurses and midwives may have purchased their degrees without hands-on training, and a practice called "abdominal expression"—physical force applied to the woman's abdomen by a practitioner's knees, elbows, or an external object during labor—is common. Poor access to often poor quality health services produces poor outcomes. To give some perspective, following the perilous route many West African migrants attempt every day to the north of Niger through the Sahara, across Libya and the Mediterranean Sea in Greece, the lifetime risk of maternal death for women is more than one thousand times lower: 1 in 23,700 (World Bank 2018).

Despite the high rates of maternal mortality, for every woman who dies from obstetric complications in Niger approximately 10 more suffer from severe acute maternal morbidity (Prual et al. 1998). These women experience severe complications in pregnancy, labor, or the postpartum period. Counted as "near misses," on the threshold of life and death, they survive—yet this survival comes at a cost. As a result of obstetric complications or poor management, an estimated 10 to 20 million women develop obstetric-related disabilities each year (Filippi et al. 2006). Some injuries are common; for instance, in the Gambia, nearly half (46 percent) of all reproductive-age women sustain pelvic damage from childbirth (Walraven et al. 2001). And some of the injuries are uncommon but life altering, as is the case with obstetric fistula. Although hemorrhage, hypertensive disorders, and sepsis are all important contributors, obstructed labor—the cause of obstetric fistula—is the leading cause of maternal morbidity in Niger (Prual et al. 1998).

Fistula might be imagined as a physical manifestation of global inequity, local disempowerment, spatial precarity, and economic vulnerability. Although between 1 and 2 million women live with fistula in the Global South, predominantly in sub-Saharan Africa, it is nearly nonexistent in the Global North (Adler et al. 2013; Lewis, De Bernis, and WHO 2006). The last fistula hospital in the United States closed its doors over one hundred years ago, when biomedical obstetric care became widely accessible. And while globally anywhere from 6,000 to 100,000 women develop fistula each year, very few come from cities, in Africa or elsewhere.[1]

Fistula is often referred to as a condition of poverty, but it is also a condition of rurality. No matter how destitute, a woman living in a city like Lagos, Abidjan, or Niamey is unlikely to labor at home for a week as Fana did before making her way across town to a hospital. Even a woman of relative means deep in the Sahelian grasslands cannot move a health center closer, improve the conditions of the roads, or ensure that a qualified practitioner equipped with necessary materials can be found when she eventually arrives.

Fistula can more accurately be called a condition of *regional* rather than *individual* poverty, although the two are tightly entangled. It is a consequence of power differentials between multiple actors at multiple scales, ranging from the local to the global—between, for example, husbands and wives, practitioners and patients, and multinational trade organizations and Nigérien government officials. Fistula results from vulnerabilities to global, regional, and household-level poverty, to gender inequalities, and to reproductive demands.

Relegated to far corners of the rural Global South, obstetric fistula has until recently been shrouded in relative obscurity. But an increase in international attention to the condition has spawned a proliferation of organizations and institutions focusing on fistula prevention and surgical repair across sub-Saharan Africa.[2] Fistula is no longer thought of as a lifelong condition of incontinence; biomedicine now offers hope for a full recovery. However, despite media and humanitarian accounts of fistula surgery as a relatively straightforward and highly effective intervention, for Nigérien women the pursuit of surgery often involves disappointment—long waits and frequent surgical failures. As a result, the lives of many women in Niger are transformed twice: once by a delivery gone awry, and again by the quest for continence, which can take them away from their families, husbands, and their social, productive, and reproductive lives for months, years, and sometimes decades. These absences are socially and emotionally (and sometimes financially) costly. Yet, despite the high price of treatment, women remain tethered to fistula centers by their hope for a cure and their faith in the power of biomedicine. This often misplaced confidence in surgery's promise to reestablish bodily and social integrity is fueled by the clinics and their financial interests in holding women.

By engaging with the women whose lives have been transformed by the condition, in this book I read through fistula to illuminate many larger questions about power, biomedicine, stigma, resilience, care, kinship, commodification, and representation within the context of illness and treatment-seeking in sub-Saharan Africa. This exploration of the lives of women with fistula enables us to better understand how women whose agency is constrained—by rurality, age, ethnicity, poverty, and parity—navigate the West African health care systems that have been privatized and decentralized by half a century of neoliberal policies.

This book's title, *Fistula Politics,* reflects not only the fraught and contested struggle over limited resources and the power to define and diagnose that play out in the public health sector, but also alludes to the broader politics of gender, Islam, biomedicine, humanitarianism, and a postcolonial global order. Throughout this book, I explore the manifold competing and collaborative power dynamics that shape women's social worlds, expose them to stigma, and determine their access to and outcomes of care.

Countless stakeholders have something to gain or lose when working with women with fistula. Competing for limited pots of funding and fleeting public interest, international nonprofit organizations are invested in highly choreographed narrative control. Niger's underresourced, weak public health infrastructure depends on funding from these same multinational nonprofit organizations. Fistula surgeons and their staff gain international visibility, prestige, paychecks, and per diems through often exploitative and frequently harmful biomedical encounters from which women struggle to disengage.

But it is not just the biomedical and public health establishment that has a stake in fistula politics. Husbands fear fistula's implications for their wives' fertility and their own social status. For co-wives, fistula changes the balance of power in the endless competition over scarce emotional and material household resources. In-laws may see fistula as the point to cut and run from a failed investment. Local religious leaders grapple with questions of purity, piety, and obligation after reproductive failure. And, ultimately, fistula marks a bodily, social, and perceptual rupture for the women it affects, requiring their skillful navigation of their own corporeal boundaries while remaining both socially visible to those back home and ontologically recognizable to themselves. These multileveled patterns of cooperation and contest where a panoply of actors have a stake in fistula and its outcome determine Nigérien women's experiences, helping to explain their vulnerability to fistula and mediating their success or failure in treatment-seeking.

These intersecting macro and micro politics actively shape a woman's vulnerability to fistula stigma and her power to resist it. Fistula politics help us to understand whose interests are served by the application of fistula stigma, and how that stigma manifests and transforms throughout a woman's life. When we under-stand the politics at play, we can ask whether surgically repaired bodies lead to repaired conceptions of self and ultimately repaired social relationships. How is social stigma negotiated in the face of illness and treatment-seeking? How does the stigma of fistula grow out of and illuminate attenuated structures of support? How do local networks of care expand or contract in times of illness? How can co-wives be both integral parts of and the greatest threats to women's conjugal health? How might treatment-seeking be paradoxically harmful, and how might that be a result of the media and humanitarian organizations that aim to help? These questions—how, why, and when women's identities are reconfigured fol-lowing fistula—undergird this book.

REPRESENTATION

Fistula is a lens that allows us to better understand how distant forms of suffering are represented, commodified, and medicalized, and why this matters. Because fistula spares the whiter and wealthier bodies of urban women—it is a condition almost unimaginable in Western bodies—it has come to be seen in the Global North as an archaic disorder of "traditional" Africa, affecting poor, brown-bod-ied women in the "deepest" parts of the continent.[3] Often conceptually coupled with female genital cutting (a spurious link), fistula has captured the imagina-tion of the West, where damaged genitals become a synecdoche for the oppres-sion of African women who are rendered invisible and silenced by culture and religion.

Recognizable representations of fistula and the women who suffer from it are most visible in Western media and humanitarian donor fistula narratives. Recall the story of Fana that opened this chapter: a narrative of frustration, hope, loss, resilience, and chronicity. In contrast, Jamila's story is similar to many popular and humanitarian portrayals of fistula's passive victims. In his *New York Times* edito-rial, "Where Young Women Find Healing and Hope," Nicholas Kristof (2013) introduces Jamila as a patient at Niger's Danja Fistula Center, drawing from and reproducing the familiar narrative tropes of fistula:

> DANJA NIGER—They straggle in by foot, donkey cart or bus: humiliated women and girls with their heads downcast, feeling ashamed and cursed, trailing stink and urine . . .
>
> The first patient we met is [Jamila Garba]; with an impish smile, she still seems a child . . . Her family married her off at about 11 or 12 . . . She was not consulted but became the second wife of her own uncle.
>
> A year later, she was pregnant . . . She suffered three days of obstructed labor . . . The baby was dead and she had suffered internal injuries including a hole, or fis-tula, between her bladder and vagina . . .

Jamila found herself shunned. Her husband ejected her from the house, and other villagers regarded her as unclean so that no one would eat food that she prepared or allow her to fetch water from the well when others were around . . . She endured several years of this ostracism . . .

A few months ago, Jamila heard about the Danja Fistula Center and showed up to see if someone could help. Dr. Steve Arrowsmith, a urologist from Michigan . . . operated on Jamila and repaired the damage . . .

Women who have suffered for years find hope here . . . They are courageous and indomitable, and now full of hope as well.

I knew Jamila. I met her in February 2013 while I was in Niger researching women with obstetric fistula, six months before Nicholas Kristof's visit to the Danja Fistula Center. This was not how I would have told her story. Kristof's take is an exemplar of how fistula is often presented by a global media—worst-case scenarios, lurid tales in which girls are victimized by African men: abused, neglected, broken, dismissed, and discarded. Tales in which brown-skinned girls must be saved, and Westerners—their goodwill, their dollars, their surgeons, and their scalpels—must save them. In these tales, through Western humanitarian efforts and technological solutions, women are transformed physically, emotionally, socially, and sometimes religiously.

Over long chats, leisurely meals, and in-depth interviews with Jamila at the Danja Fistula Center, I heard a multifaceted story highlighting her impressive resilience and her negotiation of constraints. Jamila was married when she was around 14 years old to an adopted son of her grandmother. He was young too, and in Niger family marriages are considered the best kind of matches. At the beginning of their marriage they were happy. They were in love. Jamila told me that although she was married, they waited years before consummating their marriage—as was custom for young brides in her village. And when she eventually got pregnant, they were joyous. But her labor went badly, and she was left with a fistula. Her husband did not divorce her, and he certainly did not throw her out. After all, she had grown up in her grandmother's house, where he lived as well—when she married, she changed rooms, not houses. His home was her home.

But his behavior changed, and his love faded. He began to ignore and neglect her. After a year, as is common in Niger he took another wife as permitted by Islam.[4] He married again before he could afford to construct another hut for her, despite Islam's requirement that husbands provide for wives equally. No longer having a space of her own, Jamila packed up her few things and moved across the courtyard, returning to her grandmother's room.

Jamila was not married to her uncle, she had not been ejected from her home when she developed fistula, and biomedicine did not heal her. Although Kristof suggests that Jamila had begun her search for treatment only months before, during our long talks she explained that her quest for cure had begun years ago. When

I met her, she had already undergone six unsuccessful surgeries. When we last spoke, that number had climbed to eight, and there was little hope that she would go home dry.[5]

The attitude toward women with fistula displayed by Nicholas Kristof, who has referred to these women as "lepers of the 21st century," "pariahs," and "the most wretched people on this planet" (2009, 2016), suffuses Western media. For example, *The Guardian* also has portrayed women with fistula as the world's "modern-day lepers," and both CNN and al Jazeera have positioned fistula as "a fate worse than death" (Grant 2016; Munir 2014; Winsor 2013). In the discourse of donors, media, and some scholarly works, obstetric fistula is presented as profoundly stigmatizing, a condition that results in divorce by husbands, abandonment by kin, exile from communities, and high rates of depression and suicide.[6] Often with good intentions—to bring attention and resources to a previously invisible population of women—donor agencies and the global media generate and circulate a narrative of an iconic sufferer: young, stigmatized, and redeemable through surgical intervention. However, during the many months I spent in Niger with women with fistula, I found few archetypical stories of suffering or sufferers. Rather, I discovered impressive accounts of women's resourcefulness, resilience, and agency as well as great variability in their clinical encounters.

The monolithic narrative of fistula, crafted at a distance in the newsrooms of New York and the offices of nongovernmental organizations (NGOs) in Washington, D.C., offers a compelling account of how women are devastated by the condition. The humanitarian and media industries have been deeply influential in how fistula care is envisioned and provisioned, but paradoxically often in ways that are counterproductive for the women's goal of returning to their prefistula conjugal and social lives. Critiquing humanitarianism or the media is not a goal in or of itself of this work, both because I agree with their good intentions—to better the lives of millions of women—and because it is neither conceptually novel nor practically useful. However, carefully tracking how good intentions combine with long-standing colonial preconceptions offers not only a powerful counternarrative for social marginalization but hope for its reduction. Critical examination of the humanitarian and media fistula narrative offers some insight into why, even when healed, fistula continued to mark Fana's everyday life and why Jamila was still waiting for her ninth surgery.

The stories of women like Fana and Jamila open up the lived realities and the social construction of obstetric fistula, neither of which can be examined without the other. The realities of treatment-seeking are influenced by the humanitarian and media formulations of fistula, which become reified social facts that are imbricated with clinical practice and everyday life. The critique of these narratives is thus instrumental, as it shapes available avenues of care, social perceptions, and embodied experiences.

"BROKEN VAGINAS" AND THE SICKNESS OF URINE

Seven years before I came to know her, Satima lay unconscious in her brother's arms. He carried her into the small emergency and triage room at Maternité Issaka Gabozy—Niger's top reference hospital for obstetric complications. Satima's labor had begun six days before in a rural village approximately 450 kilometers north-east of Niamey, which had no access to quality emergency obstetric care. Her labor did not progress normally, and when she was wheeled into the operation block for an emergency cesarean section, she was no longer conscious. Although Satima survived, her child did not, and her body was permanently marked by the strug-gle. When she finally awoke in the maternity ward, she found herself in a shallow pool of her own urine. She had developed what is referred to locally in Hausa as *ciwon yoyo fitsare,* the sickness of leaking urine.

Obstetric fistula results from prolonged and obstructed labor whereby pro-tracted pressure of the fetal head against the vagina, bladder, or rectum damages soft tissue, starving it of blood and eventually producing pressure necrosis. If this process is not interrupted by delivery, which in the case of obstructed labor usu-ally requires biomedical intervention such as cesarean or forceps delivery, the labor (and the resultant pressure) can last several days.[7] In around 90 percent of cases, the fetus does not survive (Ahmed and Holtz 2007; Delamou et al. 2016; Wall 2012). The ischemic tissues die, and depending on how the fetal head was posi-tioned during the labor, an abnormal pathway between the vagina and bladder (vesicovaginal fistula) and/or vagina and rectum (rectovaginal fistula) is produced. The result is persistent incontinence of urine and/or feces through the vagina.[8] Fistula severity and symptoms can vary dramatically, as can the effects on a woman's psychosocial and physical health.

It is useful to think of fistula as the result of a "field injury" to a broad area, or as part of the "obstructed labor injury complex" as described by Arrowsmith, Hamlin, and Wall (1996). Fistulas are complex, and they are regularly accompanied by multiple birth-related urologic, gynecologic, gastrointestinal, musculoskele-tal, neurological, or dermatological injuries. Women with fistula may suffer from perineal nerve damage (causing leg weakness and foot drop), stress inconti-nence, vaginal scarring, secondary infertility, renal failure, tissue loss, urethral loss, cervical destruction, amenorrhea, or pelvic inflammatory disease, among other problems. Women often arrive to fistula centers unable to walk due to nerve damage. Some have persistent infections, excoriated thighs, and constant pain. Others have undergone emergency hysterectomies, although they often do not know it. Women arrive consumed with anxiety—their bodies leak, and they are immobile, infertile, or inelastic. Fistula may be only one of their many health concerns.

Although fistula can cause long-term problems with physical health, includ-ing local infections, skin conditions, and kidney damage from attempts to manage the condition by limiting fluid intake, a woman with fistula can, after an initial period of recovery from her traumatic labor, live a long and largely healthy life. Thus, the consequences of chronic fistula are often considered predominantly social and emotional: social isolation, marital disruption, and worsening poverty, anxiety, and depression may all be associated with fistula in addition to the related health problems (see Ahmed and Holtz 2007; Barageine et al. 2015; Lavender et al. 2016; Mselle and Kohi 2015; Wall 2012; Yeakey et al. 2009). But these outcomes can vary dramatically depending on the individual woman, her social context, and her treatment-seeking experience.

Small, fresh fistulas are sometimes closed with catheterization alone, but surgical intervention is the most effective treatment. Under ideal conditions, first-time operations on women with small fistulas that do not involve the bladder base or urethra offer women the best chance of success. However, after undergoing catastrophic labors, most women in Niger do not have straightforward injuries. Some 65 to 80 percent of Nigérien cases are "complex" and thus difficult to repair (Cam et al. 2010; Falandry 2000; Karateke et al. 2010). Fistula surgeries frequently fail. Even when they "succeed," they do not necessarily restore continence; in some women the hole may be closed, but the leaking persists. Repaired injuries often break down; after the first operation scarring accumulates, delicate tissues harden, and repeated repairs become less and less likely to succeed (Wall 2006). Yet women in Niger were rarely counseled about the likelihood of surgical success or failure. When catheters are removed after surgeries and urine begins to pool, surgeons and nurses usually tell women to be patient and to wait for another operation. There is no agreed-upon standard by which women may be categorized as "incurable" or "inoperable"; many women who have undergone double-digit surgeries, with almost no chance of repair, cling to hope at the fistula centers. The surgical backlogs grow as these women pass their days and months waiting for operations that rarely materialize and that seem doomed to fail.

DUSTY SKIES AND UNCERTAIN HORIZONS

Niger is the largest country in West Africa; occupying about 1.3 million square kilometers, it is the combined size of France, Spain, Portugal, and Belgium (figure 1). Yet few people—particularly North Americans—have heard of it. It is regularly mistaken for Nigeria. Microsoft Word programs do not even recognize its people, "Nigériens" or "Nigeriens" (pronounced nē-ˈzher-ē-ən, as distinct from their southern neighbors—nī-ˈjir-ē-ən) in its dictionaries. Niger's invisibility confers the risk of ill-fitting parallels to better known, but very different, African contexts.

The experience of fistula in Niger is often mapped onto the experience of fistula in better-studied countries such as Ethiopia, home of the celebrated, long-established, and well-funded Hamlin Fistula Hospitals. Anita Hannig's ethnography on fistula (2017) in largely Orthodox Christian Ethiopia highlights some

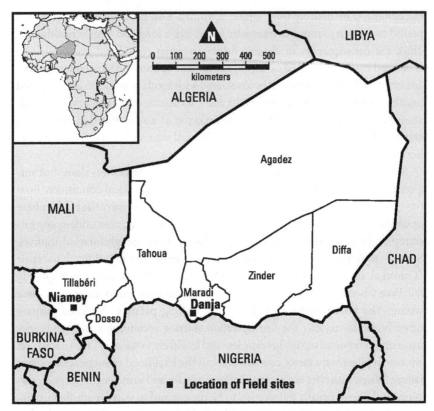

FIGURE 1. Map of Niger and its eight regions, with the Niamey and Danja field sites indicated (map by Eureka Cartography)

of these differences. For example, among Christians in Ethiopia, who practice monogamy, women with fistula are commonly divorced after the onset of their incontinence. In polygynous Islamic Niger, husbands are more likely to add another wife than to subtract one. These sustained, but drastically transformed, marital relationships result in very different lived realities of the same condition.

The process of treatment-seeking in Niger also has little in common with that in Ethiopia. At the Hamlin Fistula Hospitals, admittance, triage, physiotherapy, hospital life, and surgical intervention are streamlined, efficient, active, and promise good chances for successful outcomes (Hannig 2017). In the Bahir Dar fistula center in northwestern Ethiopia, Hannig (2017) found that a woman's entire stay, from admittance to release, averaged only 18 days, significantly less than the 32-day average in the fistula center in Ethiopia's capital. During their time at Ethiopian centers, women's daily schedules are highly structured; they are seen by practitioners, attend courses, and watch educational films. In contrast, the women at the fistula centers in Niger had, at the time I met them, already been waiting almost six months (an average of 180 days—10 times longer than in Ethiopia); their waiting times ranged from two weeks to six years, and some had already undergone up to 11 failed surgeries. After we first met, most of these women continued to wait, and many were still waiting at centers for operations when I left Niger at the end of 2013.

Ethiopia's fistula hospitals teem with outside researchers and visiting surgeons, internal audits, and media coverage. By contrast, the fistula centers in Niger, particularly in the capital city Niamey, were often places of marked inactivity, with few if any staff on duty and remarkably little medical care, where women filled their days with waiting. This opacity of management can breed inefficiency, invisibility, and corruption. I make this comparison between Ethiopia and Niger to highlight the fact that illness and treatment-seeking are highly context dependent. Women's experiences and narratives of fistula in Niger—an Islamic, polygynous, poor country with insufficient health infrastructure—are unique.

Niger became independent from France in 1960, but its transition from colonialism to democracy was challenging. Over the years since independence, the landlocked Sahelian nation of 20.7 million people has grappled with single-party authoritarianism, Tuareg insurgencies, and military coups (Idrissa and Decalo 2012). Presently Niger contends with concurrent natural disasters of droughts, desertification, and floods; increasing threats of terrorism and violence along the border regions of Mali, Nigeria, and Libya; and a fertility rate that effectively doubles the population every 20 years. Given these barriers to peace and prosperity, Niger's economic struggles are unsurprising.

Niger does have vast wealth in natural resources—it holds the fifth largest deposits of uranium in the world. Uranium revenues led to a period of relative affluence in the mid-1970s, but by the early 1980s a profusion of petroleum in the global market and a decline in uranium demand due to the antinuclear movement led to the uranium market's collapse; Niger's brief era of prosperity came to a sudden end. The nation's borrowing continued, and debt amassed. After the bust of the uranium boom, Niger could no longer support its newly expanded bureaucratic sector and fell into bankruptcy. Structural adjustment programs designed and implemented by the World Bank and International Monetary Fund (IMF) were intended to radically cut government expenditures, decentralize service provision, transfer costs from the state to citizens, and minimize the role of the state to address economic crises; in countries such as Niger, the former structures were viewed as both overly interventionist and inefficient.

The neoliberal policies of austerity, structural adjustment, and increasing marketization that affected so many African countries in the 1990s resulted in years of unpaid salaries, shrinking public services, decreased wages and educational scholarships, pervasive corruption, and increased dependence on external aid. Investment in the health and education sectors slowed—few health centers were built, and few students were trained to eventually provide quality care within the remaining clinics' crumbling walls. In 1994, the local currency was devalued by

50 percent, catalyzing political instability and accelerating the decline into poverty for most Nigériens. In 1995, as part of a larger neoliberal movement in cost recovery, Niger's Ministry of Health followed guidelines set by the Bamako Initiative and instituted user fees in their health systems, resulting in a 30 to 40 percent reduction in consultations (Ridde 2015). In the absence of qualified practitioners or accessible public health centers, rural Nigériens were forced to rely heavily on unpaid village health workers and the intermittent care provided by charities and Christian missionaries.

Although the policies of structural adjustment have since fallen out of favor, the harm they caused has been long-lasting; since the 1990s, Niger's economy has seen little improvement, and most economic sectors have remained at a virtual standstill. By 2016, almost half the population lived on less than US$2 a day, and the country's gross national income was among the world's lowest (World Bank 2018). Outside of the subsistence agriculture and animal husbandry on which the majority of Nigériens rely, the people's economic prospects are extremely limited. Many are involved in small-scale trading, transport, and informal markets; the few formal sector jobs has discouraged formalized education. As a result, Niger has the lowest rate of youth literacy in the world, at only 24 percent; the rate is lower still among adult women at 9 percent (World Bank 2018). Due to the low levels of secondary education, Niger has been unable to train enough qualified health care workers to meet its growing demands.

With few economic or educational opportunities, many Nigériens have redoubled their religious practice, finding moral purpose through religion.[9] Piety in practice is not only a reflection of deeply held religious conviction, but also a means to demonstrate power, status, and wealth (or *arziki,* prosperity and well-being) when other means to do so are limited. In Niger, religious practice, modernity, and aesthetics are tightly entwined. Women with some money often invest in woven prayer mats, multiple strings of shiny prayer beads, and the Arab-inspired *abaya*—black robes set in stark relief to the colorful local garments.

Along with elaborately embroidered robes and traditional prayer beads, female staff at the Niamey fistula centers often wore tally counters on their hands, reminding me of the mechanical hand-clickers used by the school bus drivers and librarians of my childhood. Serving both as a visible display of moral worth and a fashion statement, these pedometers of prayer reflected the deeply material and highly performative side of piety (and social class) in Niger. But poor, rural women can enact piety only in the ways available to them: visible prayer, modesty, and increasingly conservative dress.[10]

Religion in the context of weak governmental institutions and few employment options has also led to a growing threat of radicalization. Affiliates linked to al-Qaeda in the Islamic Maghreb (AQIM) and the Islamic State (ISIS) pledged group Boko Haram are active in Niger, and they have become increasing threats to the population and the country's stability. Although these groups are largely held in contempt by the majority of Nigériens, in an era of globalized Islam, what it means to be Muslim is being actively contested and redefined.

Such environmental, historical, political, and economic precarity has resulted in regularly dismal evaluations by the United Nations. As Claire Wendland reminds us, "Health indicators, like poverty statistics, tend to be most uncertain where life (and record keeping) is most precarious" (2012, 111). So, it is with care and a critical eye that we place Niger in a decontextualized global competition to be rated, ordered, and otherwise classified. Still, when considered with a healthy dose of skepticism, these numbers do indicate that lives of contemporary Nigériens are defined by widespread insecurity.

Niger is ranked last on the United Nations Human Development Index and is considered the least developed country in the world (United Nations Development Programme 2014). It also has the world's highest total fertility rate, 7.6 births per woman, which far surpasses the second highest, Somalia, which has 6.5 births per woman (DHS Program 2018).[11] This confluence of extreme poverty and population-level pronatalism leaves Nigérien women particularly vulnerable to poor maternal outcomes. The maternal mortality ratio (MMR), defined as the number of deaths due to pregnancy, childbirth, or postpartum complications per 100,000 live births, is often used as a proxy for the general quality of a country's health care system. The MMR for Niger was estimated by the World Bank in 2015 as 553 per 100,000. This was a marked improvement over 2005, when the MMR was measured at 760, and 2000 when it was 850, though these numbers, like all figures regarding women's obstetric health in Niger, should be viewed with some skepticism (see Wendland 2016).

Niger is also said to have one of the highest rates of obstetric fistula in the world. Given that the incidence and prevalence numbers for fistula in Niger are not definitive (the data are often the result of opaque methodologies and guesstimates), Johns Hopkins epidemiologist Saifuddin Ahmed has estimated the incidence to be between 700 and 800 new cases a year (Ahmed and Genadry 2013). At their current capacity, Niger's fistula centers only operate on a combined total of 500 to 600 cases a year. Ahmed estimates that if all 500 to 600 currently performed operations were successful (unlikely), and if no more fistula patients arrived at the centers (even more unlikely), it would take more than 26 years to clear Niger's backlog of current fistula patients.

GATHERING DATA

I conducted ethnographic research in three urban fistula centers in Niger's capital, Niamey, and one rural fistula center outside of Maradi (see figure 1). I spent the year 2013 and the summers of 2010 and 2014 in Niger. I observed 100 women with fistula from six ethnic groups over time. I also spent time with and inter-viewed nine family members and five husbands of women with fistula as well as 23 fistula experts.

I adopted a mixed-methods approach to data collection to address gaps in the existing fistula research—specifically, the lack of women's voices regarding their experiences of the condition and the treatment process, the absence of studies engaged with women over the long term, and the need for studies that integrate both qualitative and quantitative methods. I worked with these hundred women to gather data including their demographic profile, reproductive history, life events leading up to fistula, subjective experiences of living with fistula, internal and external fistula-related stigma, ruptures in social relationships, experiences seeking treatment, and perisurgical and postsurgical experiences (specifically social, economic, and emotional changes). To do this, I triangulated, using in-depth inter-views, participant observation, and structured surveys. All the interviews were conducted in Hausa or French (both of which I speak) or Zarma (which I do not speak—I relied on my research assistants for translation). The Tuareg, Fulani, Kanuri, and Mossinke women who were also included in the research were multilingual, so I was able to interview them and chat informally in either Hausa or Zarma.

I conducted participant observation in the clinics and the women's home vil-lages during all phases of this research project. The observational data enriched and often contradicted what the interlocutors said during interviews and surveys. Because these contradictions reveal life's messiness, particularly in regard to the subjects that cause us the most pain—such as crumbling relationships, bodily shame, reproductive failures, and futures of uncertainty—an approach of trian-gulation was integral to understanding the nuanced manifestations of fistula's lived experience. I spoke with women. I watched them. I talked with their fami-lies and husbands. I read their charts (when I was granted their permission to do so). I administered surveys. Then I interviewed them again.

When interviewed three times over the course of a year, a woman might respond first that she is married, then divorced, and finally conclude, "I really don't know." Her chart might document her conjugal state as married, while her mother might assert that she is certainly divorced. Although this lack of cohesion presents challenges for quantification, it reveals the fluidity of experience, the women's uncertainty about the future, and the care they exhibited in their self-representation. These ambiguities themselves are essential data about the discontinuities, rup-tures, and anxieties at the heart of living with and seeking treatment for obstetric fistula. Understanding the lived experience of fistula is highly interpretive work, requiring a certain amount of translation, deduction, and even supposition and guesstimation.[12]

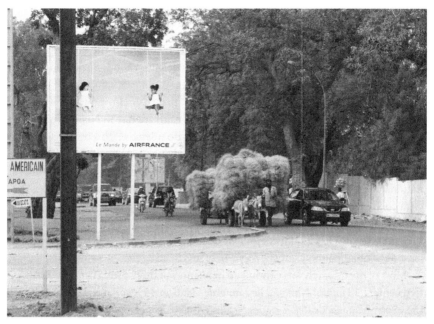

FIGURE 2. On a main thoroughfare in Niamey, donkey carts sharing the road with SUVs, taxis, motorcycles, and luxury vehicles

Niamey

Niger's capital city of Niamey is relatively tranquil compared to other West African capitals, which seem to vibrate with the constant motion of too many taxis on too few roads (figure 2). In Niamey, men congregate on benches and prayer mats, drinking strong tea under acacia trees. Commuters on bicycles pass by boys on overburdened donkey carts; in turn, the carts are passed by foreigners and Nigérien elite in white Land Rovers, the quintessential symbol of Western aid organizations. Camels advertise the newest cell phone or internet promotion as they languidly traverse the city—ambulatory billboards, branded without the least bit of irony.

Compared with other cities in Niger, Niamey is relatively liberal and westernized. Women weave through the city on motorcycles. Some do not veil or cover their hair, although most do. Conference rooms are evenly populated with tailored Western suits and *boubous,* local garments with flowing tops made of waxed *bazin* (hand-dyed polished cotton). Like many large cities of the Global South, in Niamey parallel worlds exist side by side. On the city's busiest roads, pack animals burdened with towering stacks of firewood share lanes with hulking military caravans. Girls in floor-length *hijabai* (tailored veils) with elaborate patterns of facial scarification share sodas with young women whose uncovered hair and heavy makeup compliments Western-style, Chinese-produced jeans and blouses. Hausa and Kanuri peoples from the central and eastern regions, Zarma from the west, Tuareg from the north, and Fulani from throughout the country come together here, settling in ethnically homogenous neighborhoods but sharing work, economic hardships, prayers, and opportunities.

Yet, unlike many other large African cities, these synchronous realities feel somehow convergent. Conspicuous forms of wealth are rare in Niamey, and skyscrapers, freeways, and lavish shopping centers do not exist. This impression of a kind of flattening of economic inequality is borne out by the numbers. The Gini coefficient, which measures income distribution (and thus inequality) within a nation, ranges from 0 (perfect equality) to 1.0 (maximal inequality). In Niger, the Gini coefficient is 0.34—among Africa's lowest. For comparison, the continent's greatest inequality is found in South Africa, which has a Gini coefficient of 0.63; the United States has a Gini coefficient of 0.41 (World Bank 2018). In the world's least developed country, most everyone seems to struggle.

Most of my research was conducted in Niamey at three fistula centers. The first two centers, *l'Hôpital National de Lamordé* (National Hospital of Lamordé) and the *Centre National de Reference des Fistules Obstétricales* or CNRFO (National Reference Center for Obstetric Fistula), were operated by the Nigérien state as one semi-integrated unit. Located in the Sonuci neighborhood of Niamey, along the Tillabéri road, the CNRFO received both simple cases and referrals for complex fistulas from across Niger. My third Niamey research site, located just across the street from CNRFO, was run by the NGO *Dimol-Niger*. The organization Dimol was one of the first NGOs in Niger to become involved in fistula prevention, treatment, and reintegration work. However, when I was there, the organization had lost its capacity to provide surgical interventions, and it served only as a kind of hostel for women with fistula. Many women who spent months at the center, as we will see, did not know that they would never be operated on at Dimol.

Although the Niamey centers attracted women from all over the country (and sometimes from beyond Niger's borders), the women at the centers usually spent their time in ethnically homogenous "neighborhoods" on center grounds. In the Tuareg districts, light-skinned women lounged under makeshift tents of fabric, tree branches, and cinder blocks. More comfortable outside, the women braided each other's hair, wove baskets, constructed leather bags, and chatted in Tamasheq. Also clustered outdoors, napping, chatting, or praying, the Fulani women were easily recognizable: brightly colored fabrics, intricately beaded jewelry, "whiskered" patterns of facial scarification, tattooed bottom lips, and distinctively braided hair. In the Hausa *zongo* (a term used for settlements across West Africa populated by Hausa-speaking immigrants), Hausaphone women typically crowded together indoors or on shaded patios, reading from a Qur'an, listening to static-wrapped clips of music or sermons from a Nokia phone, or resting under a rare working fan. The rest of the indoor space belonged to the

Zarma women, who had demographic dominance in Niamey and within the centers (although not within Niger as a whole). With sufficient numbers, the Zarma women often subdivided themselves based on age.

Although these three centers in the country's capital were tucked into typical urban neighborhoods, the lives of the largely rural patient population of women at Niamey centers were not particularly urban. Women rarely left the centers' suburban confines or even the centers themselves, as most women had no money to spend, nowhere to go, and no one to take them there. Despite the promise and excitement of life in the capital, for rural women lacking money, know-how, and male protection, city life was unexplorable, so it was left largely unexplored.

Danja, Maradi State

I landed in Niger for my year of research in January 2013, on the day that French forces intervened in the neighboring country of Mali to fight groups affiliated with al-Qaeda in the Islamic Maghreb (AQIM), who had taken over the northern regions. Instability and fear spilled across the border. Due to a string of recent events—prison breaks, kidnappings, terrorist threats, suicide bombings—and growing instability in the south from Nigeria's terrorist organization Boko Haram, the Nigérien government restricted the movement of Westerners. At the beginning of my research, Westerners reportedly could no longer leave the capital without military escorts or U.S. embassy approval (although reports conflicted). Despite the warnings about volatile neighbors and travel restrictions, I spent a total of five months in the rural town of Danja, 700 kilometers east of the capital.

To skirt the overland travel restrictions, in February 2013 I took a United Nations Humanitarian Air Service flight to Niger's third largest city (a step up from my usual ride: a three-seater missionary bush plane that shook, hummed, and flew too low to the ground for my comfort). Maradi is often considered the country's economic and religious capital. Of its 175,000 people, the majority are ethnically Hausa, although it also has large ethnic Fulani and Kanuri minority populations. Maradi is around an hour's drive from Niger's very porous border with Nigeria, and money, commerce, people, and religious conservatism flow in from the south.

Fifteen kilometers south of Maradi, and 30 kilometers north of the Nigerian border (70 kilometers from the Nigerian metropolis of Katsina) is the *Centre de Santé, Leprologie et de Fistule Danja* (Danja Center for Health, Leprosy, and Fistula, or CSLF-Danja). Established in the 1950s as the Centre de Santé Léprologie de Danja (Danja Leprosy Health Center) by SIM (Serving In Mission, formally Soudan Interior Mission), the hospital originally operated as a mission hospital for leprosy patients.[13] SIM converted long-term leprosy patients to Christianity; the patients then settled and built lives and families in Danja village, two kilometers from the hospital, establishing a small pocket of practicing Christians (Cooper 2006).[14] The hospital eventually expanded to offer health services beyond leprosy care.

In 2012, a new set of buildings housing the Danja Fistula and Training Center officially opened on the hospital campus. The center was run by Worldwide Fistula Fund, an international secular nonprofit based in Illinois, in cooperation with SIM. Here, women could receive free repair surgeries, postoperative care, and a suite of capacity- and skill-building classes. To house the women through the sometimes very lengthy process of care (which can include months of waiting, recuperation, rehabilitation, and sometimes additional surgeries), women stayed in "the village," six small houses built behind the hospital. Because fistula occurs largely in rural populations with very little economic capital, most women had spent two or more days traveling to the clinic. Many had left their homes on foot, walking for several hours before reaching a place where mule carts or taxis could be found. None spoke French, Niger's official language. The vast majority were decorated with elaborate patterns of facial scarification marking their ethnic and regional provenance.[15]

Although the providers of care at the Danja Fistula Center were largely Christian, the patient population was not; nearly all women were faithful adherents of Islam. But in intimate spaces, strict practices of piety loosen. I spent much time with women behind the mud walls of compounds, shielded from the male gaze and protected from strict norms of coverage, silence, and invisibility. Behind the bricks, women spoke unguardedly of the intimate details of their bodies, their marriages, and their sexual lives. Although Maradi is known as the heart of religious conservatism in Niger, a stronghold of the Izala movement pushing for greater adherence to Islamic law,[16] within these walls women wore skimpy tanktops and thin, hastily tucked wraps. Their heads were bare. Their knees peeked through their skirts as they painted their feet with henna swirls. As time passed, my hair tumbled from my loose head scarf. Women pulled on the collar of my shirt to compare our undergarments. My notions of "appropriate dress" morphed, and as my comfort level with the women grew, my sleeves shortened.

I forgot how conservative their world outside of the intimacy of our shared space continued to be. In a Christian hospital, surrounded by women, the strict religious practice of Maradi seemed immaterial. But of course it was not. Frequently I would run into a group of women with whom I had become close, near the improvised market along the road. If they had not grabbed me, I would not have recognized them. No part of their skin would be visible. They would be covered from head to toe in synthetic black fabric. Long *hijabai*, tailored veils that covered their heads, permitted a kind of mobile seclusion, allowing them to move freely in public space. Dark socks were worn with their flip-flops, black gloves were donned despite the heat, and *niqabi*—layered face veils—were tied around their foreheads, some allowing for eyes to peek through, others meeting onlookers with a solid black panel (figure 3). While I was at first disoriented by the public/private divide, the women at Danja expertly navigated the expectations of piety.

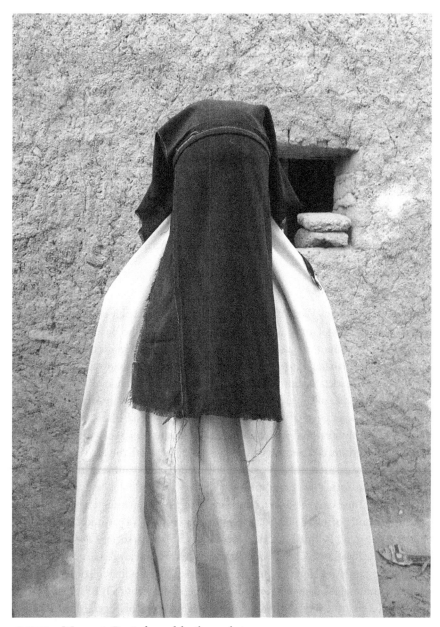

FIGURE 3. Woman in Danja dressed for the market

But it was not without conflict that pious Muslim women came to seek care at a Christian hospital. In Maradi and surrounding villages, rumors circulated of proselytization at Danja (these rumors were not entirely unfounded, as I show in chapter 7). Although Danja arguably offered women the best opportunity for care in the country (Heller 2017), many women's families discouraged them from seeking care there, preferring that they remain in the state system. The state fistula centers around the country were overburdened and understaffed, while the only thing lacking at Danja was patients.

Without the benefit of ethnographic texture, Danja appears to be the best choice for women seeking treatment, but context matters—and women and their families regularly chose against the center. Just as the experience of fistula in Niger is highly dependent on local context and cultural expectations of marriage, womanhood, and fertility, the experience of treatment-seeking cannot be disentangled from the highly charged and profoundly localized social, religious, and political environments within which fistula care exists. From a distance, the forces—political, economic, socioreligious, and highly personal—that shape realities are blurred. Local conflicts, constraints, and controls are rendered invisible, replaced by generalities—assumptions of a pan-African (or even pan-Global South) experience of fistula.

The Women

Compared with many West African countries, Niger is relatively ethnically homogenous, composed of only eight main ethnic groups. According to the 2010 Nigérien government census, the largest ethnic group in Niger is the Hausa, constituting more than half (56 percent) of Niger's population, followed by the Zarma and its closely associated ethnic group, the Songhai (21 percent of the population). The Hausa are one of the largest ethnic groups in sub-Saharan Africa, with over 40 million people, most of whom live in Niger and Nigeria. The Zarma-Songhai, a highly socially stratified society historically reliant on slavery, are a relatively small ethnic group, concentrated in southwest Niger. Both the Hausa and Zarma are sedentary farmers, living primarily in the arable southern tier of Niger (although the Zarma live predominantly in the west while the Hausa regions are in the central and east of Niger). Hausa and Zarma-Songhai societies are Islamic (predominantly of the Maliki-Sunni school), patrilineal and patrifocal, and widely practice polygyny. Within both Hausa and Zarma-Songhai society, divorce is common and easily attained, but women are expected to quickly remarry.

The remainder of Nigérien people are nomadic, seminomadic, or historically nomadic pastoralists. The seminomadic, Islamic, and traditionally stratified Tuareg live predominantly in the Saharan and Sahelian regions of Niger, Mali, Burkina Faso, Libya, and Algeria and speak a Berber language, Tamasheq. Found primarily in the north of Niger, the Tuareg constitute 9 percent of Niger's population. The Tuareg follow bilateral descent and inheritance patterns and practice oasis gardening, caravan trading, and livestock herding. Tuareg practices have been undergoing significant transformation due to the forces of Islamization and sedentarization, as many Tuareg now live at least part time in villages, resulting in the decline of women's historically high status and relative autonomy (Rasmussen 2004). The Tuareg are underrepresented in government, are often resented by sedentary ethnic groups like the Hausa and Zarma-Songhai, and are thus polit- ically marginalized. These tensions have led to repeated Tuareg rebellions in attempts to form an independent Tuareg nation-state.

Fulani, also known as Peul, Fula, and Fulbe, are a broad ethnic category of nomadic and seminomadic pastoralists and agro-pastoralists who live predomi- nantly in the semiarid Sahel across West Africa and speak Fulfulde. Dispersed throughout Niger, Fulani comprise 9 percent of the population. Fulani are patri- lineal, patrilocal, and moderately polygynous. Much of Fulani identity, tradition, and economic stability revolves around cattle. However, decreases in livestock holdings and increased household economic demands have pushed many Fulani pastoralists to agro-pastoralism, diversifying their livelihoods to reduce risk and increase resilience to environmental and social conditions (Ducrotoy et al. 2017). As with most mobile pastoralists, Fulani still tend to live in geographically mar- ginal, particularly disadvantaged areas.

The remaining ethnic groups of Niger are the Kanuri (found in the far east of the country), who constitute 5 percent of the population, and the Toubou, Gurma, Diffa Arabs and smaller minority groups, who together make up the remainder of Niger's population.

Of the hundred women included in this research, 41 were Hausa, 31 were Zarma or Songhai, 14 were Tuareg, 8 were Fulani, 5 were Kanuri, and 1 was Mossinke from Mali. Although the women's ethnic identities were not considered in developing the research sample, the 100 women are ethnically representative of the popula- tion. Hausa women were slightly underrepresented and Zarma women slightly overrepresented in the sample, likely because three of the four fistula centers were located in the capital of Niamey, which is Zarma territory. Although women come to the capital from all over the country to seek care, Hausa women in the east and central regions of the country often first seek treatment in regional hospitals or in Nigeria or Chad. The ethnic composition of the women interviewed at the fis- tula center outside of Maradi was far less ethnically diverse; 23 of 25 women (92 percent) identified as Hausa.[17]

Niger—like so many sub-Saharan African states—is defined by *brassage,* a cultural and ethnic blending or hybridity. Although for ease of quantification I categorize women by their self-identified primary ethnicity (typically that of their father), such labels distort Niger's historical and ethnocultural realities (Alidou 2005). Not only are families often ethnically mixed (ethnically complex family formations are particularly common in the context of polygyny), but in a more abstract sense, ethnic groups are not discrete: they have blended with neighboring groups for centuries. As Ousseina Alidou (2005) has explained, "pure" ethnic groups are a relatively new construct in Niger, reflecting Western conceptions of fixed African identities and emerging from colonial and postcolo- nial opportunistic politics of division. Nigériens often embody ethnic compos- ites, with synchronous multiethnic and multilingual identities. Many women I came to know were raised bilingual or trilingual, practiced customs with roots in multiple ethnic traditions, and came from mixed families in historically mixed regions.

In their educational attainment, the women I came to know were a lot like rural Nigérien women generally. According to the Demographic and Health Surveys (INS and ICF International 2013), 80 percent of women in Niger (and 88 percent of rural women) have no public or Western-style education and less than one percent (0.1 percent of rural women) have any education above secondary school. No woman in my sample attended more than eight years of schooling and 89 percent had no primary education at all (although most had some Qur'anic instruction). Even among women who had attended public school and were taught in French, the national language of instruction, none were literate in the language, nor could any woman comfortably navigate more than basic French greetings.

However, women who do not attend French-speaking government schools are not necessarily poorly educated. In 2001, there were more than 51,000 Qur'anic schools in Niger, educating 560,000 students, 35 percent of whom were simultaneously attending Western-style schooling (Alidou 2005). Qur'anic schooling begins when children are around four or five years old, and pupils are taught the basics of reading and writing in Arabic, proper pronunciation of suras (verses of the Qur'an), and the five pillars of Islam. Qur'anic schooling culminates in the memorization (and recitation) of the Qur'an. Secondary Islamic education in Niger takes place in the madarasa (*makarantar ilimi*), is taught in Arabic, and involves in-depth study of the Qur'an, Islamic law, classical Arabic, the *hadith* (the sayings of the Prophet Muhammed), and *sunnah* (the tradition of Muhammed). Although the women at centers could not read or speak French, many could recognize and replicate Arabic letters, others could read select Arabic prayers, and nearly all learned from and taught one another what they knew in an effort to become better Muslims.

As is the case with much of the western Sudanic belt (a region which covers much of Niger, Mali, Senegal, and Burkina Faso), approximately 95 to 98 percent of the population of Niger is Muslim (INS and ICF International 2013; Meyer et al. 2007). Around 95 percent of Nigérien Muslims are Sunni, the majority linked to Sufi brotherhoods; the remaining 5 percent are Shi'a. All 100 women I interviewed, all their family members, and all but three of the experts identified as Muslim.

Yet, these 100 women were markedly diverse. They were young and old, with an average (estimated) age of 31 years old, ranging from 15 to 70. They had developed fistula at a variety of points in their reproductive lifespans, from their first to their twelfth pregnancies, ranging from the ages of 13 to 54 (with an estimated average age of 23 years old). They also had a vast range of experience. For some, fistula was an acute condition developed late in life. For others it was a chronic, and lifelong injury. The average amount of time a woman had lived with fistula before I spoke with her was nearly seven years, but the length of time she had lived with the condition ranged between one month and 50 years. (See the appendix for demographic data.)

Studying Incontinence

Worldwide, around thirty percent of women are affected by female urinary incontinence, a phenomenon that is largely caused by aging, menopause, and childbirth; the incidence increases for women who have had more pregnancies (Al-Badr 2012; Avery and Stocks 2016; Diokno et al. 2004; Li, Low, and Lee 2007).[18] With the highest total fertility rate in the world, Nigérien women are thus quite familiar with some uncontrollable leaking. However, because women cannot see the interior of their bodies, they do not always understand that an abnormal anatomical connection is causing their incontinence.

The Hausa term for fistula, *ciwon yoyo fitsare,* or "the sickness of leaking urine," highlights effect rather than cause. Locally, researching fistula is not a study of an anomalous condition but of incontinence out of place, a study of degree—a common female malady that has become unmanageable, irregular, "too much." Women may arrive at fistula centers leaking, with stories of mistreatment, concealment, or social isolation, only to be diagnosed not with fistula but an infection. Although in this book I approach women's experiences through the frame of fistula—a condition unseen, accessible only through the diagnosis of specialists—the women themselves do not. "Fistula" is a Western, biomedical frame of cause superimposed on women's experience of effect. It will become clear that this frame does not fit perfectly.

As a doctoral student from the United States with little personal religion and living alone, on the face of it I had seemingly little common ground with the deeply pious, communalist, pronatalist women who populated fistula centers across Niger. Yet, I came to appreciate what connected us, what set us apart from other Nigérien women. Because being under 150-centimeters tall increases a woman's risk of obstructed labor (and thus her risk of obstetric fistula), fistula centers often house smaller-than-average women. At 4 feet 11 inches (<150 centimeters) and nearly 30 years old with no children; my size, presumed infertility, and apparent lack of familial connection made me seem slightly less alien, slightly more relatable in clinics full of unrepresentatively short, largely childless, often socially isolated women. In time, I forged deep relationships of care and reciprocity with many women at the centers. They came to rely on me for information about their bodies, etiologies of their conditions, hospital timelines, and clinical prognoses. In turn, I relied on them for everything: data, friendship, and essential knowledge on how to be in their world. We bonded over our loneliness, our fears for the health of those we loved for whom we could do nothing, and the disempowering distance. We bonded over music videos played on old Nokia phones, snacks, and monotony. Building rapport across cultural, economic, linguistic, and health divides took time, openness, and humor.

On very hot days, when the prospect of conducting another interview felt particularly onerous, languid afternoons often degenerated into play—or rather, something approximating play but probably closer to a theater of the absurd. When I am in the United States, surrounded by people who understand my cultural references, who value a dash of irony, and who can appreciate the art of self-deprecation, I do all right for myself—I can get by at a cocktail party. But in Niger, lacking the necessary linguistic and cultural sophistication, my sense of humor morphed into that of the stereotypical uncle: trite, somewhat awkward, and often unseemly.

As my relationships with women at centers grew closer, they came to expect and participate in my often intentionally odd and sometimes unintentionally inappropriate behaviors. I began dancing without rhythm. In turn, women would dress me up in their clothing and have me perform "Nigérien" tasks like walking around the yard with stuff balanced precariously on my head. I would tickle adult women. They would pose elaborate photoshoots. I would ask them about orgasms and pornography and draw diagrams of vaginas in the dirt, indelicately explaining the mechanics of use for the tampons they would find in my bag. They would guess my age (usually in the ballpark of pubescent years) and call me *tsofuwa,* or old woman, when they found out that I was 30 (and childless). I have a man's name (Ali) and sometimes wore pants, so they would tease me, asking about my wife and calling me by male pronouns. I admit, I was mostly a bizarre oddity. Still, it seemed to work for me, particularly in fistula centers where women's days were typically filled with little but the existential weight of waiting. Play filled our afternoons, deepened our laugh lines, and provided relief from interviews in which women revisited their trauma, exploitation, and loss.

Like many anthropologists, I spent my months in the field navigating the flaws and challenges of the anthropological endeavor—attempting to balance objectivity and self-reflexivity within the ever-shifting political realities of field sites and global currents of power. Anthropology is defined by fieldwork. Our intimate knowledge of a place and its people, and the method by which we choose to engage with our site—ethnography—can, ideally, circumvent the systems that control the flow of information. Ethnography allows our subjects to speak in their own voices. As anthropologists, our job is to amplify those voices, in all their complexity and moral ambiguity.

I take seriously the feminist concern with empathy—an exploration of ethical intersubjective practices and modes of knowing. Yet empathy, as Clare Hemmings writes, "does little to challenge the temporal grammar of the Western feminist subject" (2011, 203). As close as we became, I tried to never forget how different our realities were. Women's pain, uncertainty, and structural constraints were inescapable and life-defining. As I diligently recorded their suffering, translating their trauma into publications that would advance my career, I was painfully aware that their loss was my gain. Conflicted, I hoped that this process and the words that I eventually wrote would transcend the theoretical, affecting Nigérien women directly by altering perceptions and shifting interventions. I strove to practice what Nancy Scheper-Hughes calls "good enough" ethnography: within the limits imposed both by outside forces and by my internal struggles to reconcile the cultural self I brought with me to the field, I carefully and compassionately listened, observed, and recorded (1992, 28). What follows are the words of the women, their families, and practitioners in Niger as I heard them.

ORGANIZATION OF THE BOOK

In this book, I examine how a group of Nigérien women navigate physical constraints and reproductive expectations within a postcolonial, neoliberal humanitarian marketplace. I complicate concepts of stigma often tied to fistula and examine how the condition fits into local notions of the body and local structures of support in times of illness. I examine what it means for these women, and their husbands, families, kin, and communities, to seek treatment. I tease out notions of surgical success and examine the clinical encounter between these vulnerable populations and the biomedical establishment in the market-oriented, philanthrocapitalistic, neoliberal terrain to which health care in the Global South has been relegated.[19] Finally, I explore the harmful, though unintended, consequences of humanitarian representation and intervention, which permeate the ways in which fistula prevention, treatment, and postsurgical reintegration efforts are conceptualized and implemented.

I have organized this book around three main themes: the lived experience of incontinence; clinical encounters; and humanitarian and media representation. As much as this work is about global forces and international exchanges, at its core *Fistula Politics* is an exploration of the intimate—sexuality, love, care, kinship, identity, and emotion. In part I, "Living Incontinence," I use rich, in-depth, and extended ethnographic research to expose and explore the complexities of fistula's lived experience. I examine how women and their husbands, kin, and communities conceptualize, talk about, and treat fistula bodies. I look specifically at the ways in which the "sickness of urine" fits into local notions of the body and local structures of caretaking and support in times of illness. I draw from and build upon previous work on incontinence, chronic illness, postsurgical subjectivities, and rehabilitation by Lenore Manderson (2011) and Lenore Manderson and Carolyn Smith-Morris (2010). I explore the links between intimate others, corporeality, identity, and shame among women who have undergone reparative surgeries, and examine their resultant altered self-conceptions. I critically engage with local understandings of aberrant bodies and genitals, shame, and pain. I examine what it means to be a woman who must negotiate reproductive constraints within pronatalist terrains with a body that is perceived as damaged or disabled.

In chapter 2, "Fistula Stigma," I illustrate the ways that fistula-related social stigma affect women internally and externally, altering their perceptions of self and their relationships with their spouses and co-wives, families, and communities. I unravel popular understandings of stigma and offer new ways to think about the concept. I argue that whether a woman is stigmatized by fistula, and in what circumstances, almost entirely depends on her preexisting social relationships. I demonstrate that, while fistula results in experiences of shame and embarrassment for the majority of women, very few women perceived or experienced mistreatment or social distancing. This contradicts the previous narratives of fistula. I find that the few who experienced social rejection were already socially vulnerable before their fistulas began—they were exceptionally poor, in unstable marriages, or, most importantly, living without the protection of their mothers.

In chapter 3, "Liminal Wives," I explore the diverse, dynamic, fluid, and complex ways in which fistula and treatment-seeking affect women's marital lives. Because of the complicated dynamics of polygyny in Niger, fistula offers a unique lens through which the impacts of chronic illness on family life can be explored. Co-wives, who compete for often scarce resources for themselves and their children, can both undermine and prove essential to the ability of wives with fistula to maintain healthy marital relationships.

In part II of the book, "Clinical Encounters," I use a political economy approach to focus on the clinical encounter between the disempowered woman and the biomedical establishment. I explore the interplay between gender, circumscribed agency, poverty, structural violence, and the biomedical apparatus in sub-Saharan Africa.

In chapter 4, "The 'Worst Place to be a Mother,'" I examine women's engagement with health services during labor, demonstrating how organizational failure, pride, corruption, and regional poverty result in delays, deaths, and disability. I offer a counternarrative to the dominant explanatory structures of public health, which too often place the blame for poor maternal health outcomes on the women themselves, their families, and the "traditional" cultures to which they are thought to belong.

In chapter 5, "The Indeterminable Wait," I look critically at how women engage with the health system once they develop birthing injuries. Drawing from previous research on the history of global capitalism, colonial and postcolonial health services, and clinical encounters in African contexts, I explore how the selective invisibility of certain afflictions (particularly chronic conditions) affects women's pursuit of care. I investigate the ways in which biomedicine, particularly surgery, is positioned as a "magic bullet." Yet, I argue, it falls short of treatment objectives— failing to heal the majority of women—and the processes of treatment itself results in increased social marginalization and stigma. And while fistulas may signify bodily, social, and emotional rupture for the women who have them, for those who treat them, fistulas represent economic gain. Women seeking surgeries are continuously exploited by both private and state-affiliated actors, for whom potential fistula funds from development and humanitarian agencies represent their best opportunity to get ahead.

In the third and final part of this book, "The Marketplace of Victimhood," I examine how humanitarian organizations represent the bodies of women in the Global South. I challenge, deconstruct, and decenter the archetypical fistula narrative that is circulated and reproduced in the global media and through humanitarian agencies' appeals to donors. This part of the book offers a critique of methodology, of hasty investigation, and of partial representations—of the ready-made template, the mad-libs of fistula, where a name and an adjective are swapped out but the story is essentially the same. And it is a critique of those of us who perpetuate these fictions—of the media, of humanitarian organizations, of scholars, and of readers who uncritically accept these timeworn narratives about Africa and Africans, particularly those about women who are victims of being African.

In chapter 6, "Superlative Sufferers," I historically situate humanitarianism in Africa, arguing that representations of women with fistula follow a formulaic and long-standing pattern of engagement with women's bodies in the Global South, and in Africa particularly. This chapter is heavily influenced by a tradition of anthropological critiques of development, humanitarian aid, global health initiatives, and colonial and postcolonial Western engagement with African bodies.[20] I critique the ways in which distant, gendered suffering is passively viewed and consumed, and ultimately commodified and medicalized, by the Global North.

In chapter 7, "Costs and Consequences," I turn to the conceptual and concrete effects of the humanitarian and media narrative around fistula. I examine the rhetorical links that are frequently drawn between the woman with fistula and the iconic leper, essentializing women and perpetuating a global media and donor narrative of stigma. When the fistula centers assume that women with fistula are the "new lepers," and treat them as such by physically isolating and segregating them, I show how, like the leprosaria before them, centers may unintentionally cause the social stigma, marital rifts, and declining health that these organizations aim to address. The implicit assumptions created by the dominant fistula narrative about women's quality of life back home has concrete consequences on fistula prevention, treatment, and rehabilitation programming—consequences that are evident in long wait times at centers, a singular focus on surgery rather than improved management of chronic fistula, flawed reintegration programs, an undermining of women's concealment strategies, and a disregard for women's confidentiality. I briefly sketch some policy solutions for these problems in chapter 8, the book's conclusion.

PART 1   LIVING INCONTINENCE

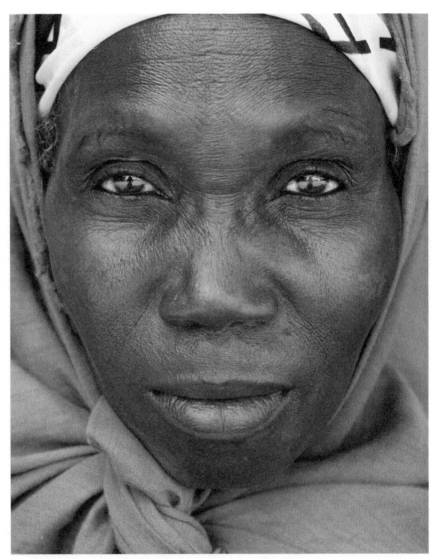

Portrait of a Zarma woman in Niamey, Niger

LARABA'S STORY
Rejection, Resistance, Refusal

Although she rarely left the confines of the fistula center, Laraba spent hours staring at her own reflection in a palm-sized mirror. Carefully tending to her makeup, she drew dark lines around her lips, above her eyebrows, and down the center of her forehead to the tip of her nose, darkening the distinctive facial scars that mark many Kanuri women from southeastern Niger. Not infrequently, Laraba would find me engrossed in conversation with another woman. She would open my bag, take my camera, grab me by the wrist, and pull me to her room, demanding yet another portrait to capture her modernity. The photograph was always the same: Laraba on her prayer mat, with her pink prayer beads and cell phone in hand—perfectly posed modernity.

At 27 years old, Laraba had lived with fistula for over a decade. She was loud and outspoken, and even (some might say) occasionally abrasive; I often found myself wondering how the formative years of Laraba's young adulthood, spent on the grounds of fistula centers across Niger, had shaped her—how they had hardened her. We all learn to adapt.

When I first met Laraba, she was harsh, quick to issue insults and uninterested in being interviewed. But I suppose I grew on her because after several months she pulled me aside and questioned why I had not asked again to interview her. "We are friends, aren't we?" She was reclining on her bed, attached through a catheter to a bag that was slowly filling with her urine. A week before, she had undergone her eighth surgery. On this day, 10 months after she had arrived at this particular fistula center, she was full of hope and wanted to tell me about her life.

At the age of 14, Laraba was married to an older man—the first cousin of her father. She did not know him; she had not even seen him until she was already his wife. "A young girl's opinion isn't asked. Sometimes, like in my case, she won't even know that she's to be married until the marriage has finished and she has moved to her husband's house," she explained.[1] But Laraba—headstrong even then—did not want to be married and refused to accept her fate. For one year after her marriage, she resisted her husband and would not pass the night at his home, enacting the same ritual of resistance each evening as soon as the sun set. Yet her intransigence was matched by that of her father. Every night, she fled her marital home. Every night, her father dragged her back to her husband. And every night, she sprinted right back to her parents' home as refuge. Furious at her disobedience and humiliated by her impertinence, her father became violent: "He'd hit me until my blood would redden his hand, but still, I wouldn't go back."

Her mother did not agree with her father's brutality, and she had not wanted Laraba to marry the man in the first place, but, as Laraba said, "wives have no power compared to their husbands." Her mother eventually separated from her father over this, returning to her natal village in northern Nigeria. Laraba was left behind, both because she was already married and because in Niger's patrilocal society a woman may divorce her husband but all her weaned children with him must stay behind. Laraba was left without an advocate—no community elders, no one with sway or say to speak on her behalf. It was Laraba, powerless, young, and female, against her father and her husband, both religious scholars and respected men within the community. Without support, her campaign of resistance did not last long.

What finally made Laraba accept her marriage was neither threat nor physical violence, but, according to her, the nefarious forces of the occult. Laraba's father and husband commissioned a potion from a local sorcerer that was poured over her head while she slept. When she awoke, she had a terrible headache that worsened over the following week. The pain was paralyzing; eventually she had no choice but to submit to her husband. Once she did, the throbbing stopped as abruptly as it had begun.

Although her husband was not unkind, life with him was difficult. Laraba hated him and refused to acquiesce to his demands. When he would ask her to do something, she would refuse. When he told her to fetch water or run errands, she would run into the fields and sit there all day, emboldened by her own defiance.

Laraba miscarried both her first and second pregnancies, which worsened tensions at home. She was resolute that she would not spend her third pregnancy in her husband's home. But when Laraba went back to her father's home, he exploded in anger. He was furious that she continued to disobey his wishes, and he refused to let her stay. So Laraba quietly sold what she owned, cobbling together the necessary funds to cross the porous Niger-Nigeria border. She made her way to the villages surrounding the Nigerian city of Maiduguri in hopes of finding her mother. After a long, arduous, and risky journey, she found her mother's natal village only to learn that her mother had already returned to her father in hopes of reconciliation. But Laraba's maternal extended kin had opposed Laraba's marriage—they had had their eyes on another young man for her to marry—so they let her stay.

She had been in labor for two days when her aunt noticed that the fetus had changed positions. All the women agreed that this could be dangerous, and eventually they decided to take her to a health clinic. There, Laraba spent three days waiting for care, shuttled between two similarly ill-equipped low-level clinics. On her fifth day of labor, she was no longer conscious. When she awoke, she found herself in a different hospital, lying in a different bed, soaked in a deep puddle of her own urine. She learned that the body of her dead baby had been cut out, and what remained was a hole—a fistula.

Laraba returned to her father's home, but she found life unlivable. She leaked. She had nerve damage sustained from her long labor, and she could not walk as a result. Wet and immobile, she was mistreated. Her father interpreted her fistula as comeuppance for her repeated defiance. Laraba told me how daily life was a struggle: "I cried until I had no more tears left. My father's other wives and their children, they wouldn't eat with me or sit with me. My mother was kind to me, but since she had left my father, even though she came back to him, she had no more power against her co-wives . . . My family didn't care if I was dead or alive, sick or well. They didn't worry about what was happening to me."

Eventually, she made her way to a hospital in Niger's eastern city of Diffa, on the border of Nigeria. After nine months of sleeping on a plastic mat in the hospital courtyard, she was told that they could not operate on her there. She was instead referred to Zinder, a city 500 kilometers to the west. But the doctor at Zinder's maternity hospital would not operate on her fistula until her feet and legs had healed from the nerve damage. Given how difficult her life was at home, Laraba decided to wait at the hospital in Zinder. Without any physical therapy, it took four full years for her legs to regain their function and strength. She was far from her aunt's home in Nigeria, and no one came to visit her during her years in the hospital. In her fifth and sixth year at the center in Zinder, she underwent five operations. None was successful, and with each failed operation her chances for success shrank. "I leaked every day. I leaked all of the time. The operations did nothing," she remembered.

Her father refused to come to see her, and he never sent money. Laraba's husband visited her twice when she was at the center in Diffa, but never again after that. He never sent money either. He married three other women, and the year before I met Laraba he officially divorced her so that he could marry his newest girlfriend and remain within the Islam's limitations of four wives.

The center in Zinder lost its only fistula surgeon, a government employee who had been ordered to move to Niamey, likely due to political rivalries and competition over fistula cases. Eventually, a year later, the center filled a bus with leaking women and shuttled them 900 kilometers west to Niamey. Laraba remained in Niamey for nearly a year.

At this point in the interview, Laraba became upset and began mindlessly playing with the ringtones on her new cellphone—a gift from one of the many nongovernmental organizations (NGOs) that had passed through over the years. When she looked up, she continued: "We aren't here because we like it, we are here because we don't have a choice. Who would bring me back home? With what money? If it wasn't paid for me to come here to Niamey, I would never have come."

A week after Laraba told me her story, her catheter was removed. One afternoon I found her curled up on her cot. Through her tears, she told me that the operation had not worked. She was still leaking.

Soon after, Laraba left the center to stay with a distantly related family member in a neighboring town, just outside of the capital. A few months later, I was surprised to see her at an international fistula conference held in Niamey. To open the conference, local representatives had brought along two women to give personal testimonies. Laraba stood in front of the large crowd, looking particularly cosmopolitan in her heavy makeup and shiny pink *hijabi* that shimmered in the light. Through a translator, she told the crowd that because of fistula, her life had been filled with sorrow and problems, but thanks to the doctors and donors she was now dry, and she would have another chance at life. The United Nations Population Fund (UNFPA) reported on Laraba's testimony in the article "Taking Stock: Ten Years Fighting Fistula in Niger":

> "I wish to launch an appeal to our parents to stop marrying their girls so young.[2] For me, under the age of 18, a girl should not be married," said [Laraba Oussman], fistula survivor, 26, after telling her story at the opening of the workshop. She was married at the age of 14. Her fistula, developed during her first childbirth, was repaired only after eight surgeries. "I will now return home and continue testifying. Some women hide. They don't know what they have and that they can be treated," concluded Ms. [Oussman]. (Campaign to End Fistula 2013)

At the break, I found Laraba reapplying her makeup in the bathroom. "You're dry!" I exclaimed as I swung my arms around her, ecstatic about the news. Gazing down, she muttered, "No. I am still wet, but no one wants to hear that story."

I never understood why Laraba told a room full of fistula experts from across the globe that she was dry. Perhaps she had crafted and deployed her testimony for her own purposes.[3] Perhaps clinic staff had asked her to tell the room that she was dry. I often stumble across Laraba's face on the websites of various NGOs, or in photographs in international news articles on fistula in Niger. Having spent approximately nine out of the last 10 years in various fistula centers, Laraba had become somewhat of a professional patient. After so many years, she knew how to work within the fistula system.

When I left Niger, Laraba was still waiting at the Niamey center for her ninth surgery. Her family had told her to stay there until she was healed. "Maybe that's forever," she said with a shrug. Forever did not seem far off. Years later, when I last saw Laraba, she had not left the center. By then, she was waiting for her seventeenth surgery.

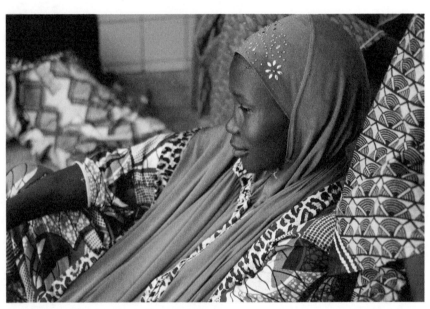

Portrait of a Hausa woman in Niamey, Niger

2 · FISTULA STIGMA

In popular narratives, fistula is characterized by profound stigma. Women like Laraba—rejected and adrift—populate our imaginations. Because they leak, smell, and may be infertile, women with fistula are assumed to transgress patriarchal expectations, losing value and social standing. When I began spending time at fistula centers, I expected to meet heavily stigmatized and largely abandoned young women who were finding corporeal and social redemption through surgery. The reality was far more complicated.

As I immersed myself in women's stories, I discovered a vast diversity in women's experiences of stigma. Laraba—unsupported, alone, and abused—was not the norm. When we expect to find a monolithic experience of rejection, we tend not to interrogate the when, why, how much, and to whom of fistula stigma. We often fail to ask in whose interest is its application. How does it manifest, and how does it transform throughout a woman's life? Why are some women able to resist "spoiled identities," but others are not? And how does social context—the quantity and quality of a woman's social ties *before* she developed fistula—alter her vulnerability to stigma? As I explored these questions, it became clear that it takes power to stigmatize and structural disempowerment to be stigmatized.

According to most women I came to know, occurrences of abuse were rare and were experienced overwhelmingly by women who had already been in precarious social situations—women like Laraba. These women were in unstable marriages, and they had lacked familial advocates well before their catastrophic labors. Although most women did not experience mistreatment, shunning, or abuse (what we might call *external* fistula stigma), most women did shoulder a heavy weight of shame, loss, and shattered identities (or *internal* fistula stigma). Pervasive, deeply individual emotional and psychological burdens—these were the defining consequences of fistula.

THINKING THROUGH STIGMA

Over the years, social scientists have used the concept of stigma to explain why some individuals are perceived as abnormal and how they are socially discredited. According to sociologist Erving Goffman (1963), *stigma* is a socially undesirable difference, discrediting attribute, behavior, or reputation resulting from a process whereby one's identity is "spoiled" by the reactions of others; stigma acts as a social regulatory mechanism. According to Goffman, its effects can be devastating, exerting its influence over the lives of the stigmatized through social and psychological processes and everyday acts of exclusion, rejection, devaluation, structural discrimination, and limited opportunities.[1]

Stigma helps elucidate why some people are valued while others are discounted or considered with disgust. But not all difference is socially discrediting, and a difference that may lead to discreditation or discrimination in one community may be rather unremarkable in another. To understand why stigma occurs in some contexts but not others, Lawrence Yang and his colleagues (2007) suggested that we need to ask "what is most at stake?" at a particular place and time. They situate stigma as a fundamentally moral issue—arising, as Arthur Kleinman (2006) puts it, when "what really matters" in someone's local world is jeopardized. By framing stigma as intersubjective and embedded in local moral contexts, we can understand it as a highly pragmatic response—a psychological defense when one's moral experience is threatened. Through discredit, stigmatizers (and to some extent, those who are stigmatized) uphold the status quo; they defend their moral worlds.

When a woman's full transition into adulthood is predicated on her role as wife and mother, when her social value is a function of her reproductive success, and when her moral worth is based on her purity, fistula arguably threatens "what matters most." Contextualized within the highly patriarchal and pronatalist context of rural Niger, stigma is then an unsurprising response to women's reproductive failure, potential future infertility, bodily and spiritual impurity, and reduced sexual availability to their husbands.

Yet, not all Nigérien women with fistula experience stigma. Why not? Does the failure to embody the idealized Nigérien woman matter less in some communities than in others? For some women, is less at stake? To understand when, why, and to whom stigma is applied, we must move beyond the question of what matters most and look instead to what Richard Parker and Peter Aggleton (2003) call the "political economy of social exclusion." They argue that stigmatization takes place within a larger context of power and domination. It results from the *social interaction* between those with a perceived difference and those who both negatively evaluate that difference and have the social power to exert their cognitions. Such dynamics reinforce mechanisms of exclusion and strengthen social inequities of class, race, gender, and sexuality.[2]

In other words, the powerful exert stigma, and the powerless are vulnerable to it. But what does it mean to be "powerless" in a place where potentially disempowering circumstances—poverty, lack of education, and rurality—are the norm? In this chapter, I explore the lived experience of fistula, and examine what sets apart women like Laraba who endured high rates of social abuse and mistreatment. The experiences of these few women show us that fistula exploits and exacerbates other preexisting social vulnerabilities.

Is "Fistula Stigma" the Right Frame?

In Niger, the social consequences of fistula are not directly linked to the condition's physiology. It is not the physical hole itself (which may or may not exist) that matters to women or that shapes their illness experiences, identities, or treatment within their communities. Hidden deep within the body, most women I met did not understand exactly what a fistula was, or which anatomical mechanisms had failed. For these women, their leaking was indistinct from other forms of incontinence—various conditions conceptually co-categorized as *ciwon yoyo fitsare,* or the sickness of leaking urine.[3]

For example, Samira (55, Fulani), whom I spoke with at a Niamey fistula center, had developed a fistula following a long and complicated labor 27 years prior. Fortunately, after a year of treatment from a local herbalist, her leaking had diminished and ultimately disappeared. Samira was dry for nearly a quarter-century, but two years before we met, her incontinence returned. The consequences were devastating: "Many people will not eat with a woman who leaks urine. Many gossip about me—*fitsare gare ta,* she has urine, they say. The urine, it smells. People cover their noses when I am around. When they do this, it is as though they are asking me to leave. Some say that Allah is punishing me. Some insult me, calling me worthless . . . [This mistreatment] only started with the sickness. I feel ashamed, but what can I do? I am not well. I am leaking." When I asked Samira how her illness affected her gendered identity, self-conception, and sexuality, she scoffed, "With fistula, I can't think about being a woman, I am not even a human anymore." The malignant social repercussions of incontinence that Samira experienced were among the most severe I had recorded.

One afternoon, Samira was visibly upset and confused; she had just learned that she would not be operated on—neither that day nor any day in the future. Bewildered, sitting outside on a dusty mat, with an intravenous catheter still taped to her hand, she explained: "When I was in the operating room, the doctor said he couldn't find the hole. So he told me he couldn't operate. I don't know what I am to do now." When I later asked her surgeon what went wrong, he shrugged: "She doesn't have a fistula. Maybe it is an infection?"

No one but a surgical specialist knows if women are leaking urine due to a hole in their birth canal or, like Samira, for some other reason—an infection, urethral weakness due to high parity, reduced bladder size, obstetric-related damage, or aging.[4] Many women suffer the social consequences associated with fistula if they visibly leak urine, whether or not they have the abnormal anatomical connection that defines the condition. This becomes an issue for the 22 to 55 percent of women who, even after their fistulas have been stitched shut, experience persistent incontinence because of lasting damage to the bladder, urethra, or urethral sphincter (Arrowsmith, Barone, and Ruminjo 2013; Murray et al. 2002; Siddle, Vieren, and Fiander 2014).[5] These women technically no longer have fistula, but they may not perceive, comprehend, or experience a difference in their condition following surgery. They continue to leak, so by local logics they still have the sickness of leaking urine.

When we discuss fistula stigma, we sometimes use it as a proxy for what might be more accurately described as heavy incontinence-related stigma or infertility-related stigma. There is no local understanding of fistula that transcends its symptoms. The vast majority of women who develop fistula—86 of the 100 women I came to know—knew nothing about fistula before they developed it themselves. Neither women nor their families, kin, or communities had a preexisting framework about fistula or its accompanying stigma within which to place their experience. In Nigérien villages, fistula has no lore, no personality of its own—no symbolic meaning like that attached to human immunodeficiency virus (HIV), epilepsy, or cancer. So although in this chapter I discuss "fistula stigma," I urge caution against its reification; this is a biomedical, Western frame superimposed onto a local Nigérien context where, strictly speaking, neither "fistula" nor "stigma" are locally significant concepts.

MEASURING FISTULA STIGMA

Measuring stigma was a complicated undertaking. The concept has no clear translation in any of Niger's local languages, and thus no precise local meaning. I eventually operationalized fistula stigma as an umbrella concept encompassing interconnected attitudinal and behavioral components that could be measured using proxies (Fife and Wright 2000; Link et al. 2004).[6] Stigma can be separated into external stigma (actual experiences of discrimination) and internal stigma (shame and internalization of stereotypes). For me, fistula stigma came to mean external components of social isolation, physical exclusion, verbal and nonverbal mistreatment, and financial insecurity, *and* internalized or subjective components of shame, uselessness, fear, impurity, and identity loss.

Studying fistula stigma proved difficult. Higher evidentiary value is accorded to what we researchers can observe rather than what our interlocutors only recount. External stigma, or mistreatment and avoidance, we can identify primarily through our interlocutors' memories, sometimes of the past few decades. Observation is more complicated. Although we can watch women interact with family or community members, just being there introduces bias (for example, when observed, people tend to behave how they believe they ought to rather than how they otherwise would). And the hurt born from fistula, from mistreatment or verbal abuse, is often unobservable to an outsider. It can be subtle. It happens in private moments—sexual rejection behind the closed doors of a bedroom, cruel words quietly exchanged between co-wives, a disgusted glance from a trusted friend. So I relied on triangulation, synthesizing data derived from in-depth interviews with multiple stakeholders, participant observation (when available and ethical), and standardized surveys.[7]

To corroborate ethnographic data, I quantitatively measured the intensity and frequency of internal and external fistula stigma using a standardized survey of 18 questions, which I adapted from the HIV/AIDS Stigma Instrument (HASI-P; Holzemer et al. 2007). The first 11 questions focused on perceived *external* stigma—experiences of everyday conduct by others, such as mistreatment, abuse, and shunning. I asked women to recall incidents of verbal abuse (including ridicule, insults, or blame: five questions), fears of contagion (apprehension by others to making contact: three questions), and social shunning (deliberate limitation or halting of social interaction: three questions). The last seven questions focused on the *internal* experience of stigma—shifts in women's understanding of self, such as shame, identity loss, embarrassment, and fears of judgment and mistreatment.

Popular discussions of stigma focus heavily on external dynamics, but the survey revealed that for women with fistula, internal stigma was far more relevant (table 1). Women reported limited mistreatment, with verbal abuse averaging 0.74 per question response out of 3 possible points, social shunning 0.37, and fear of contagion 0.28 (zero points were assigned to responses of never, one point for once or twice, two points for several times, and three points for almost always). In contrast, women underscored the emotional and psychological burden of the condition, with the category of negative self-perception averaging 1.78 per question response out of 3 possible points.[8]

This trend is clearer when we look at the distribution of survey responses (figures 4 and 5). When questions regarding verbal abuse, social shunning, and fear of contagion are aggregated into the meta category of external stigma, only seven of the 100 women reported high or very high rates, while 76 women reported none or low. In contrast, for questions categorized as negative self-perception, which I call internal stigma, 66 women reported high or very high rates, and only 15 women reported none or low.[9] Given these data, fistula stigma for Nigérien women was primarily defined by internal processes, not the reactions of others.

Learning from the Extremes

The majority of surveyed women—76 percent—perceived no or low external fistula stigma. For many, fistula caused anxiety (in the way any illness might) and shame (in the way a similarly out of control body would), but it largely left their social lives unscathed and their support systems intact. Yet for some women, the consequences of fistula were profound. For a handful of women, the condition affected every aspect of their lives: eroding social bonds and community status, enhancing precarity within households, exacerbating poverty, causing profound emotional distress, and diminishing chances of keeping or finding an intimate

TABLE 1 Self-reported results from the standardized stigma survey of 100 women with fistula

Question Because of fistula, how often have the following things happened?	Category	Score (0–3)
I feared that others would look at me to see if I was wet.	Negative Self-Perception	2.23
I felt shame.	Negative Self-Perception	2.01
I felt useless.	Negative Self-Perception	1.85
I felt as though I brought many problems to my family.	Negative Self-Perception	1.78
I felt like I am no longer a woman.	Negative Self-Perception	1.77
I was afraid someone would judge me or gossip about me.	Negative Self-Perception	1.43
I felt that I could no longer go to ceremonies.	Negative Self-Perception	1.38
Someone told me that I had no future.	Verbal abuse	0.85
Someone mocked me when I passed by.	Verbal abuse	0.8
Someone told me that Allah was punishing me.	Verbal abuse	0.53
Someone refused to eat from the same plate as me.	Fear of contagion	0.49
People avoided me.	Social shunning	0.49
People visited me less often.	Social shunning	0.45
Someone said I was responsible for my sickness.	Verbal abuse	0.4
Someone asked me to leave because of my smell.	Verbal abuse	0.39
Someone refused to share the same drinking cup with me.	Fear of contagion	0.28
A friend of mine refused to speak with me.	Social shunning	0.16
I was asked not to touch someone's child.	Fear of contagion	0.08

NOTE: Survey adapted from the HASI-P (Holzemer et al. 2007). Average scores demonstrate that women experienced higher internal stigma (negative self-perception) than external stigma (verbal abuse, fear of contagion, and social shunning).

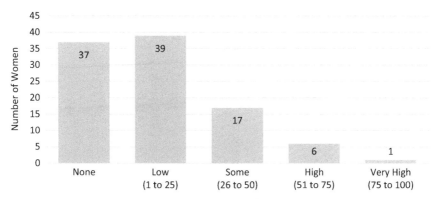

FIGURE 4. Perceived external fistula stigma measured among 100 women with fistula, as measured through a standardized 18 question survey, normalized and aggregated into categories of none, low, some, high, and very high

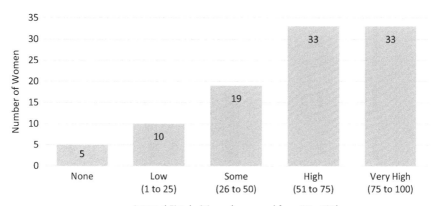

FIGURE 5. Internal fistula stigma among 100 women with fistula, as measured through a standardized 18 question survey, normalized and aggregated into categories of none, low, some, high, and very high

partner. Such was the experience of the seven women who reported high or very high rates of external fistula stigma on the survey.[10] Although these women are the minority, they help us to understand who are most vulnerable to fistula stigma, particularly the kind of external stigma emphasized in most media and donor accounts.

Who were these women with histories of abject abuse and devastating marginalization? In most ways, these seven women were not significantly different than the remaining 93 women. They did not markedly diverge in age at marriage, ethnicity, age at interview, years of living with fistula, number of living children, number of pregnancies, or even marital status (Table 2).

TABLE 2 Selected characteristics of the seven women who reported high or very high rates of external stigma as compared with the remaining 93 women

Characteristic	Saouda	Rabi	Kaltumi	Bibata	Hasana	Salamatou	Sadata	Average of all seven women	Average of remaining sample (N = 93)	P value*
Perceived external fistula stigma (scale: 1–100)	85	70	67	58	55	55	52	63	11	**.0001**
Internal fistula stigma (scale: 1–100)	52	76	71	62	100	95	48	72	58	.22
Ethnicity	Zarma	Zarma	Songhai	Hausa	Mossi	Kanuri	Fulani			
Age at interview	26	32	45	28	20	41	45	33.9	30.7	.45
Years living with fistula	1	0.5	4	5	2	25	10	6.8	6.7	.97
Mother present in life at time of fistula	No	No	Yes	Yes	No	Yes	No	57%	15%	**.005**
No. of living children	0	3	4	0	0	0	3	1.4	1.1	.59
Total no. of pregnancies	3	6	7	2	1	1	8	4.0	3.7	.80
Marital status**	D	S	D	M	D	D	S	14% M; 29% S; 57% D	40% M; 34% S; 23% D	.12
Age at first marriage	21	15	16	14	13	13	16	15.4	15.5	.97
Number of co-wives	1	2	2	1	0	Doesn't know	2	1.33	0.72	**.03**
Family marriage	No	Yes	Yes	Yes	Yes	No	Yes	71%	62%	.59
Forced marriage	No	No	Yes	No	Yes	No	No	29%	38%	.64
Months at fistula center	8	0.5	3	36	18	72	3	21	4.4	**.0001**

* P value indicating level of statistical significance of difference between groups. Bolded values indicate a significant difference at Alpha =.05. **D = divorced; M = married; S = separated.

But there were three notable (and statistically significant) differences. These seven women had an average of 1.3 co-wives each, nearly double the average of the remaining women (0.72).[11] Admittedly, reducing marital descriptions to quantifiable data (such as conjugal status, number of co-wives, and rank) is highly problematic given the fluidity of marriage in Niger (discussed in detail in chapter 3). Numbers cannot reflect when or why a husband takes a new wife or divorces another, nor women's multiple marriages over a lifetime. Still, the relationship merits our attention. Because women often compete for scarce material, social, and emotional resources when they share a household, co-wives may work to undermine each other and elevate their own position. For example, Baraka (37, Hausa) believed that because of her visible leaking, poor health, and the associated financial costs, her two co-wives had come to resent and despise her. They had waged a campaign of defamation, gossiping about her at home and throughout their community. They insulted her smell, her apparent infertility, and her worthlessness, urging their husband, "It is we who do all of her work because she is always sick. She should leave this house!" Yet the causal relationship may be reversed. Instead of co-wives resulting in greater stigma, greater stigma might result in more co-wives. It is plausible that a husband is more likely to take additional wives when a first wife has fewer community ties, lower social status within the community, and less familial protection—in other words, when she is more stigmatized. Women's life narratives suggested that greater fistula stigma is likely both a cause and an effect of more co-wives.

Additionally, the seven women with the highest external stigma had been waiting at fistula centers significantly longer than their peers. When I initially interviewed them, these seven women had waited an average of 21 months—nearly two years—compared to an average of four months among the remaining 93 women. The difference was startling, but again the quantitative data do not indicate causality. It is possible that, like Laraba, these heavily stigmatized women sought refuge at centers from particularly hostile living environments. But perhaps the long waits were unavoidable, due to fistula severity, surgical failure, and toxic politics (to which I return in chapter 5). Because long absences from home can attenuate women's social connections back home, reduce the number of their advocates, and alienate them from their husbands and households, it is plausible that these prolonged waits could be a cause, rather than a reflection, of fistula stigma.

Without the Protection of a Mother

The power of one social fact to predict external fistula stigma exceeded that of any other indicator: the presence of a mother as a protective figure (figure 6). In rural Niger, a woman's mother (but not necessarily her family) proves to be her greatest defender and advocate. Women with fistula who lived with or near their mothers tended to experience shame but little to no mistreatment. Motherless girls

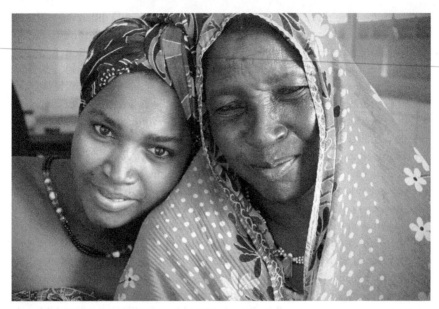

FIGURE 6. Portrait of a Tuareg woman with her mother

and women, however, were married significantly earlier than their peers and suffered from more negligence and withholding of medical care once pregnant. Women who birthed without the protection and advocacy of their mothers labored significantly longer at home before they were taken to a health clinic, which increased their risk of devastating obstetric consequences. When they developed fistula, without the support of a strong ally and gatekeeper, motherless women were particularly vulnerable to destructive intrahousehold and community politics.

From both a quantitative and qualitative perspective, the women who had lost their mothers (due to untimely death, migration, abandonment, or sometimes divorce) experienced the greatest degree of social stigma.[12] Of the seven women with the highest rates of external fistula stigma, four (more than 57 percent) did not have a mother active in their lives. Of the remaining 93 women, who experienced moderate to low or no external stigma, only 14 (15 percent) had faced fistula without their mothers.

The women believed that mothers are bound by an unbreakable love and commitment to protect their children. Regardless of circumstance, a mother would never turn her back on her daughter, women told me, and most of the mothers I spoke with agreed. Tchaibou, who had accompanied her 34-year-old daughter to the fistula center, explained, "In our village and almost all of the villages, a mother is the only one who will never be disgusted by her daughter—never!"

Women who did not experience mistreatment in the wake of fistula often credited the both literal and figurative shelter provided by their mothers. For example, Maimouna (52, Zarma) explained, "No one treated me badly. You understand, since I had gotten the sickness I was with my mother . . . If you have a mother, you can't suffer . . . But really, if you don't have a mother and you get this sickness, you will suffer greatly." The women who lived beyond the watch of their mothers did have very different relationships with their families and their wider communities, and they often recounted stories of mistreatment and the lack of financial support.[13] Rabi (32, Zarma) whose mother had passed away when she was a child, agreed that in the case of fistula it was only the public respect for a woman's mother that moderated people's bad behavior: "If your mother is there, people won't talk about you. But if she's not there, they have no shame; they will say anything."

In explaining how motherless girls and women are unprotected from gossip, community mistreatment, and suffering, Rabi and Maimouna perfectly described the experience of Hasana, one of the seven women who reported the most severe external stigma. When I first met her, Hasana—then in her early twenties—had been living at a fistula center for the previous two years. She had lost her mother to complications in childbirth: "My mom died during the delivery of the child she had after me. It was Allah's destiny for her. It happened during a long labor, and she wasn't taken to a hospital quickly enough . . . Four days had passed that she was in labor at home. She still hadn't delivered, but she began hemorrhaging. It was only when she started losing blood that they decided to take her to the hospital . . . But they hadn't even arrived at the hospital when she died. She died on the road."

Hasana and her twin sister, who were just toddlers at the time, were left alone and unprotected. The girls were split up, shuttled between households of their paternal kin. Hasana spent most of her childhood living with her father's younger sister. But her childhood did not last long. Hasana believed that her aunt resented her presence and considered her a drain on resources; finding her a husband was an easy way to be rid of her. When Hasana was only 13 years old, her aunt pushed her into an unwanted marriage. She lamented, "Because my mom was dead, I was married too young. It would never have happened if she was there."

Hasana was not exceptional; many women who were raised away from their mothers were married earlier than their peers. The 18 women who had no mother at the time of their marriage were married at an average age of 14.3 years old, which was significantly younger than the remaining 79 women, who were married at an average age of 15.7 years old.[14]

Married early, often in unsupportive partnerships (from which they may have tried to flee, breeding more hostility), the motherless girls and women may have actually been at increased risk for developing a fistula. Most women in Niger return to their natal homes to give birth, where their mothers will lobby to rapidly evacuate them to a health center in the case of apparent complications. But motherless women seldom have an advocate in the household, and so they tend to endure longer labors at home. Reluctant to spend the money (or time), less risk-averse household members or female neighbors are more likely to wait to see if the complications will simply resolve.

Eighteen women had no mothers at the time of their labors that caused fistula. These women labored at home for an average of 2.3 days before accessing care at a health clinic (laboring for an average of 3.1 total days) compared with the remaining women who labored for an average of 1.6 days at home (while also laboring for an average of 3.1 total days). There was no difference in the total time in labor, but women without mothers were kept at home for an average of 15 hours longer than other women (P=.016, statistically significant). They were also significantly more likely to labor entirely at home, with 32 percent of motherless women—compared to 13 percent of the women with mothers—never seeking or receiving care at a biomedical health center (P=.031, statistically significant).[15] Although, as I describe in chapter 4, birthing at a clinic is not necessarily safer than birthing at home, the motherless women had a lower chance of receiving necessary—and potentially lifesaving—interventions such as cesarean deliveries.

This was the case for Hasana, who was left to labor at home for three days and was taken to a health center only on the fourth day. By then, she was barely conscious and the internal damage was already done. Hasana's twin sister, Nayé, who had grown up with their paternal grandmother, had a similar experience. Nayé was also married particularly young and lived in heightened poverty. Like their mother and like Hasana, no one pressed to evacuate her to a health center; everyone thought they could wait a little longer. After a full week of laboring at home, Nayé began to hemorrhage. Just like their mother, Hasana's twin sister died on the road, en route to the health clinic. She left behind two girls under the age of five who were sent to live with paternal aunts. So it is that the cycle of maternal mortality and morbidity perpetuates.

Following early pregnancies, prolonged labors, the denial of healthcare, and eventually the development of fistula, motherless women were more vulnerable to community and familial mistreatment due to their conditions. Once debilitated by a catastrophic labor and the development of a fistula, Hasana believed that her aunt considered her a loathsome burden and undeserving of care:

> She was disgusted by me. She didn't take care of me. But it was my aunt who raised me, so I couldn't leave her house. I spent one year with fistula before going to the hospital . . . because my mother was dead. If my mother were there, she would have brought me to the hospital. But my aunt refused to accompany me to the hospital. My aunt said that she wouldn't give me money for transportation. Before I got sick, I did everything at my aunt's house, but when I got sick, I couldn't cook or clean, and my aunt didn't want me around anymore . . . Even others knew how my aunt treated me, so they did it too. So my friends were disgusted, and they ran from me.

Hasana returned to her father's home, but her natal household became a place of ridicule and cruelty. The worst came from her father and stepmother: "The father doesn't take care of [the children]. He's just a father. And if the mom is not alive, he doesn't care for them . . . If my mom were alive, even with the sickness that I had, she would be with me, accompany me to the hospital . . . Whatever the situation, a mother does not throw out her children, but a father will . . . Some people in the village say, 'It's because your mother is not alive that your father and stepmother treat you like this.'"[16]

Like Hasana, Saouda—one of the seven women who experienced profound social stigma—was left unprotected after her mother had died in childbirth. As a young child, she was left in the care of her resentful stepmother. Just like Hasana, she was isolated at home and treated with distain:

> Even as a child, my mother's co-wife hated me. She'd tell me that every bite of food I took was a bite taken from her own children's mouths. When I got [fistula], things were much worse. She was very happy that I became ill. When she prepared food, she'd never give me any. I was always hungry. She ridiculed me. She told everyone in the village about my condition. She wanted me gone . . . Often the people in my house would say that I did it on purpose—that I peed on purpose. They'd cover their noses when I was near . . . People in my house were the only ones who did this—people outside of the house would even advise my family to take better care of me.

Hasana's and Saouda's narratives underscore the overlooked costs of maternal mortality—the children left behind, motherless, vulnerable, and without advocates. Often raised by duty-bound stepmothers or aunts, motherless girls are considered competition for scarce household resources, seen to be taking food from their stepsiblings' or cousins' bowls and clothing from their backs, and thus are married off earlier. In turn, these girls are themselves more vulnerable to risky and unassisted deliveries, and resulting poor outcomes like fistula. Finally, left leaking and often ill, unprotected motherless women are often subject to the worst social abuse. As Hasana explained to me: "Without the protection of a mother, who would protect me?" Not waiting for an answer, she whispered, "No one. No one would protect me."

POVERTY AND POWER

I visited Fana a few times at her father's home in Niamey. She lived in a shed-like structure in the corner of a large lot where the carcasses of ravaged semitrucks were sent to rust away (figure 7). The walls of her house were made from a handful of wooden beams and interwoven plastic bags that had once held cement and

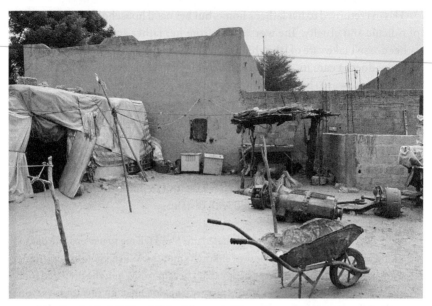

FIGURE 7. On the far left, Fana's father's house in Niamey, on a lot where he worked as a guard of old semitrucks

rice. The ground was sand, and the roof was a single sheet of corrugated tin covered with a tarp. Pieces of plastic were balled up and stuck in the holes where the metal had rusted through. Fana lived there with her father, her stepmother, and their children. About 10 of them called this place home.

Fana's father was employed as the guard of this lot, but he had recently fallen ill (a symptom of which, incidentally, was incontinence). Although there was tension between Fana and her stepmother, particularly because money was tighter than usual due to her father's illness, Fana managed to make ends meet and fill her daughter's belly. "When your parents are separated, it is hard to find a place for yourself to be. In Mali, I would go two days without eating anything. And then, I might only eat the chaff of millet. Here, there is enough food for my daughter. We eat once or twice a day. So I stay here and make do." But with her father's deteriorating health, she spent her days worrying about where they would go and how they would eat if he lost his job, or worse.

Fana had endured the multiple burdens of poverty, ethnic discrimination, illness, and a health care system crippled by the recent political instability in northern Mali. Fistula was not the determining factor in her life narrative of struggle and mistreatment:

> Even before I had fistula, people mocked me. I was very poor, and for people who are very poor, even if you don't do anything, even if you aren't sick, people mock you. But if you are rich, people want to be close to you . . . A rich woman can get a

fistula, but as soon as she's at the hospital, she'd be seen; she'd be fixed. If a woman is rich and she gets fistula, people won't run away from her. They wouldn't dare mock her. They'd come to her as soon as she called. No, they wouldn't mistreat her. They would say, "Allah has his reasons." But when a poor woman gets fistula, they will mock her and say that she got fistula because she is poor or because she has behaved badly. With poverty, if you fall ill and you have no money, it is so hard to get better. Getting medicine, getting enough to eat—sometimes it is impossible. You sometimes have a hard time getting one meal a day, and almost never more than that. So, if someone by the kindness of Allah gives you 500 Franc CFA [approximately $0.80 USD], you can buy some *gari* [manioc flour] and eat. But that's all. And if you are sick, you can't get better like that.

I asked Fana if it was hard to be a woman in Niger. Invoking the concept of intersectionality, she explained, "Being a woman or a man, it doesn't matter if you are poor—being poor is hard on both. But poverty brings more helplessness to a woman than to a man. If you are rich, then as a woman you can be a man's equal." Fana fingered a coin she had been holding on to, and she reflected, "Before I got this sickness I was a poor woman. But when the sickness came, I became poorer."

Even if they share many dimensions of inequality, not all women experience the same degrees of powerlessness in the event of fistula. The intersections of culture, power, and difference, or what Parker and Aggleton (2003) call the "political economy of social exclusion," help explain why some women with fistula experience intense social stigma while others do not. Young women, women without mothers, women living outside the protective boundaries of familial advocates, and women who were otherwise already engaged in unequal power relationships were especially vulnerable to social exclusion and marginalization in the wake of fistula. Fana—without a mother, away from her country of origin and her community, an ethnic minority, destitute, divorced, and a single mother—experienced multiple and concurrent interrelated, intersecting forms of marginalization and social discrimination. Her fistula exposed and potentially exacerbated but did not create the power differentials and intersecting burdens of gender, poverty, and familial vulnerability under which she lived.[17]

Conversely, women with strong familial advocates, postmenopausal women, women successfully engaged in market activities, or women with living children—women whose social status was less precariously moored in local relationships of power—were largely able to resist external (and often also internal) fistula stigma. Obstetric fistula does not necessarily cause negative social consequences; it often only intensifies existing precarity and unequal power relationships.

STIGMA AND THE SISTERHOOD

When we hear these stories of rejection, the "stigmatizers" are usually husbands, co-wives, families, and communities; we do not think of other women with fistula—other "victims"—as complicit. Yet fistula centers are not always safe spaces, and just because another woman also leaks does not mean she will provide empathy, compassion, or care. There is no guarantee that women will find an environment of camaraderie and fellowship—an imagined "sisterhood of suffering" (Browning, Fentahun, Goh 2007; Wall 2002). I found that hierarchies were quickly established at the centers. Who leaked more? Whose wetness was visible? Who smelled? Who could not afford perfume? Who had living children? Who received regular visitors? Among women at the centers, external fistula stigma was not tied to fistula per se, but rather to its severity, a woman's social status, and her ability or willingness to manage it—to remain "clean." As Nana (56, Hausa) explained, "Every day I wash and I wash. So, for me, women who smell, women whose feet are always wet, women who don't keep themselves clean—well, they were dirty to start."

While some women at centers did feel liberated from the daily pressures of bodily regulation, particularly the demands of secrecy and concealment, the women who struggled to meet the tacitly agreed-upon standards of fistula management were often mistreated. Due to a very large and complex fistula, Hadiza (33, Hausa) leaked noticeably more than other women at the centers. Unable to control her visible incontinence, she did not experience a "sisterhood of suffering"—admitting that she felt more socially isolated and judged by other women with fistula than she had at home: "Women here mistreat each other. They tell each other that they smell bad. The other women here always tell me that I smell bad, they tell me to leave . . . Even women here, they will look at my wrapper to see if I am wet. They are very unkind to me."

After a long and emotionally painful conversation, Hadiza seemed reluctant to leave the sweltering room where we had been sitting. Inattentive to the implications of her hesitance or my request, I asked Hadiza for a contact phone number. She had not memorized the number, but her neighbor had written it on a scrap of paper that was tucked into her bag in the next room. She whispered a barely audible apology and slowly stood up. Within seconds, as though a bowl of water had been overturned, urine splashed against the concrete floor and flooded in all directions. Ashamed, Hadiza stared at her feet.

Not all fistulas are identical; not all incontinence is the same. Even among the women at the centers, all with some degree of leaking, Hadiza's incontinence was notable. It could not be concealed or easily managed with a fabric pad or an extra skirt wrapper. Unlike most other women, Hadiza was often wet, and the smell of urine clung to her, engendering poor treatment, gossip, and to some extent, contempt from the other women. In the many months that followed, I never again saw Hadiza sit. In an attempt to avoid the mistreatment from the other women, she stood, leaned, or perched.

INTERNALIZING STIGMA: LEAKAGE, LIMINALITY, AND LOSS

Hadiza was clearly ashamed of—had very high internal stigma about—the severity of her condition, a feeling reinforced by the other women's treatment of her. Internal stigma such as that displayed by Hadiza is highly characteristic of fistula sufferers, and this makes sense when we think about stigma as, in part, a moral issue, and we presuppose that stigmatized conditions are those that threaten what matters most for sufferers. With "broken vaginas," "incompetent cervixes," or "cursed uteruses," fistula threatens Nigérien women's primary role and the source of their social value: as wife and mother. And because they have "open vaginas" or "vaginas that pour," fistula also defiles women, rendering them impure both physically and religiously. Constantly wet, out of control, and incapable of performing daily activities, women like Hadiza were perpetually overcome by the indignities of incontinence. In coping with the condition, often through shunning their social commitments and rejecting tenets of relational reciprocity, women are also perceived as impolite and unreliable—as bad community members (which is discussed further in chapter 7). In the wake of transformed relationships with their husbands and their sexuality, personal identity, religious practice, and social contacts, many women's primary experience of fistula is a profound sense of shame.

Ashamed

Shame (*kunya* in Hausa, *haawi* in Zarma, or *semteende* in Fulfulde) mediates most interactions Nigérien women have. It is a central component to social life, particularly for young people, women, and anyone else in society's lower rungs. Shame structures daily relationships, and causes many Nigérien women to avoid making direct eye contact with elders, saying the names of their husbands, in-laws, or first-born child, or broaching inappropriate topics (Smith 1954; Pierce 2007). The never-ending quest to avoid *kunya* (shame) affects women's speech, dress, sexuality, and reproductive health. Binta (26, Hausa) explained that shame was an integral part of rural people's behavior: "It is the character of people of the bush to have shame . . . Every day, every day, they always feel shame."

Given the deeply engrained nature of *kunya*, it is not surprising that the women's most significant experience of fistula was a profound sense of shame. They expressed feeling shame due to their inability to attend important ceremonies within their communities such as marriages and baptisms (although some women, who were adept at concealing their incontinence, did continue to attend these events). They felt shame because of their visible lack of control over their basic bodily functions, and shame that those to whom they ought to be social seniors (such as children) could see the wetness that would run down their legs and pool at their feet. They felt shame, too, that their most intimate— their most shameful—body parts were so visibly broken.

Jamila (16, Hausa) explained, "No one treats me poorly, but still, I feel shame. I feel *kunya* because of the urine. *Kunya* in knowing that people will notice my wetness." Zina (37, Hausa) explained, "My husband didn't say anything about my condition. But even if he didn't react, as a sick person, you know that you've changed. You don't feel the same. You don't have health there [in your vagina], and you feel ashamed."

Shame is entrenched in these women's identities; it is embodied. In the survey that I conducted with all 100 women, only 24 claimed not to feel shame because of their fistula. These women, like Zuera (26, Hausa), often explained, "I did not buy this illness at the market. Illness comes from Allah, so why feel shame?" However, the survey question on personal shame elicited the most adamant and consistent responses; the majority of women (53 of 100) felt ashamed "most of the time."

Without Use, without Value

Women frequently lamented that because of their fistulas they were no longer productive members of their households or communities—they were no longer "useful." Many women felt their usefulness was constrained by the exigencies of managing their incontinence or by the social implications of their "broken vaginas." Some women suffered physical weakness due to infections, nerve damage, or prolonged fasting to regulate their leakage. Many were limited in their ability to contribute to their households through farming, the preparation of meals or foodstuff, or the collections of water or wood. They felt unable to satisfy either the material or sexual needs of their husbands.

Ade (26, Zarma) was a skilled farmer before she developed fistula, but she abandoned her fields after she became ill. "I don't do anything. I am in the house," she complained. Her finances were affected, leaving her with no money to take care of her own needs or the needs of those close to her. Aminatou (45, Hausa) complained that she had lost weight and was "malnourished like a child" because she depended on others to bring her food. Although she had previously sold millet used to make *fura* (a sour milk and millet-based porridge), she had stopped, fearing that no one would buy from her because she was ill: "To be a woman with value (*darijar*), you must make yourself useful. But with this sickness, I cannot work. So now I am poor and totally without use."

The women often said that to have value as a woman, one had to be useful. So, they reasoned, if fistula made a woman useless, it stripped her of her symbolic and economic value. In the stigma survey, 72 women expressed that they had at one point or another felt useless because of their fistulas, and almost half (48 women) felt this way most of the time.

Broken Vaginas, Shattered Identities

Fistula transformed many women's sense of self. Although Fatouma (32, Tuareg) had successfully concealed her fistula for several years from all of her social contacts, including her husband, her incontinence had profoundly affected her identity. She explained, "I accompany the women, but I am not a woman myself anymore." In a highly gender-segregated society with only two options, she was certainly not a man, but considered herself an impostor of a woman. Fatouma's belief that she was performing femininity but had become a simulacrum of the woman she used to be was shared by many women with fistula for whom womanhood felt like a masquerade. Although many were able to hide the "truth" from their husbands, families, friends, and communities through fastidious self-management and innovative strategies (as I discuss further in chapter 7), they believed that their "broken" vaginas disqualified them from membership to the sex.

Seventy women expressed that they had at one point or another felt as though they were no longer women because of their fistulas. Forty-eight women felt this way most of the time. For example, Kadi (20, Fulani) whose fistula had healed, laughed when I asked her if the injury had altered her gendered self-perception. "I didn't think about being a woman," she responded, "I didn't even feel human!" Binta (30, Hausa), who had recently developed a fistula, explained, "I don't even know if I can be healed of this sickness, so the question of being a woman, of beauty, it just isn't relevant." Talata (24, Hausa) explained, "If your vagina isn't right, you can't be a woman." To clarify the specific requirements of womanhood, I probed, "And if you have a problem with your breasts, can you be a woman?" Talata replied, "Yes, you can be." And if you are not with your husband? If you are divorced? If you cannot have children? Yes, yes, and yes, she replied. Similarly, Sa'adé (23, Fulani) explained that "a vagina makes a woman" (gindi, shi ne mace). She continued, "If there is no vagina, there is no value . . . Because you can't give birth or have sex without a vagina, if yours is broken, you have no value as a woman. Even if a man accepts to stay with you with this sickness, it will be you who still feels uncomfortable because the sickness touches your vagina." There was something particular about an illness that affected the vagina and thus disrupted reproduction that constrained the embodiment of womanhood.

These views were not uncontested, however. Saouda (30, Zarma) laughed when I asked her if she felt like she was no longer a woman because of her fistula. She had just returned to the center for a three-month postoperative checkup. After living with fistula for two years, she had finally attained continence. "I was always a woman," Saouda asserted, "even with the sickness. Sick or well, I will always be a woman. It is only men who think that if a woman is sick, she isn't a woman." Mairi (27, Kanuri), from the Niger-Chad border, explained that because of fistula she did not feel like a woman anymore, but that she would become one again if she were healed and remarried. The self-conception of womanhood was thus fluid rather than static, with women potentially entering and exiting multiple times throughout their lifetimes.

Impurity and Impiety

Although her husband had migrated to the coast for work, Hassia (20, Hausa) stayed with his parents during the year following the development of her fistula. Hassia had known her mother-in-law, who was her maternal aunt, all her life. Still, she was cruel to Hassia: "Every day she said that she wished that her son was there so that he could divorce me and remarry . . . She told me that I was dirty. She'd say I smelled bad, smelled like a camel!" Hassia was considered impure, unclean, and thus unworthy. The common slur "camel"—the debased, spitting dromedary associated with the often-denigrated nomadic Tuaregs—invoked impurity, slovenliness, and distain.

For many women, these verbal assaults on their bodily purity were particularly painful, because in Niger bodily purity is closely tied to spiritual purity, piety, personal identity, and social status. Purity is considered an integral component of Islam, the religion practiced by the vast majority of Nigériens (and all of the women with fistula whom I met). Its importance is reflected in several prophetic hadiths: "Religion is based on cleanliness"; "The key for prayer is purity"; and "Purity is one half of the belief" (Rispler-Chaim 2006, 19).[18] In order to pray or handle the Qur'an, adherents must perform ablution (*alwala*) to achieve a state of purity (*tsarki*); accordingly, before prayer Muslims wash their hands, forearms, face, mouth, nostrils, head, feet, and ankles with water, or in its absence with sand. Muslim prayer (*salla*) is performed five times daily and demands that the body be highly engaged; disciples stand, bend, kneel, and prostrate while reciting verses from the Qur'an. The act of ritual purification is negated by even a drop of urine, or small leaks of feces or flatulence (Hamid et al. 2015; Rispler-Chaim 2006). Not only are women with fistula unable to control their constant transgressive flows, but the movements necessary for prayer can precipitate or intensify leaks. As a result, some women felt that they were unable to correctly perform their religious duties.

Although female urinary incontinence is quite common globally, some scholars believe that Muslim women are more negatively affected by it than their non-Muslim counterparts because of the spiritual disruption caused by bodily impurities (Sange et al. 2008; Treister-Goltzman and Peleg 2018). The women I came to know frequently rushed through their prayers, hoping to finish before they were rendered impure. Others skipped prayers entirely, feeling that their incontinence invalidated their supplications and may have even been insulting to Allah. This left them alienated from their religious communities (*umma*) and religious identities, and placed a perceived barrier between women and Allah, a sentiment common among Muslim women with urinary incontinence (Sange et al. 2008). Some felt that this estrangement was a punishment.

When I asked Nana (56, Hausa) if fistula had changed her religious practice, she nodded: "Yes, it has changed, because I pray but I don't do it with all of my heart. You see, I pray, but I see urine, so I don't know if Allah listens to me. I don't know if I am insulting Allah." When I challenged Nana on the prohibition against prayer when impure, she shook her head. "I don't know if it is allowed. I never asked the *marabout* to see if Allah can accept the prayers of women with fistula. But I pray, and the women here pray, so that no one says, 'She doesn't pray.' We don't want people to think that we are bad women, bad Muslims, even if our prayers are rejected." Similarly, Maou (35, Hausa) continued to pray, but she noticed a shift in substance: "My religious practice hasn't changed because of [fistula], but when I pray and urine is running, I am very ashamed. I believe that Allah still accepts my prayer, but I feel dirty, impure, and ashamed." For these women, the continuation of religious practice was often performative and did not preclude a significant shift in internal identity toward shame, fear of exclusion, and self-disgust.

However, Islamic law has well-stipulated exemptions to its rigid mandates of purity for those suffering from persistent incontinence (*salas al-bawl*, Arabic). Many interpret these exemptions as requiring that those so burdened should "pray as it is" (*yusalli kadhalika,* Arabic), performing the *alwala* and praying normally regardless of any leakage in the process (Risper-Chaim 2006). Others prefer to repeat the ablution after each prayer, and religious sources advise women to close off their vaginas to prevent the escape of urine (Al-Juwayni 1994). The Shi'i Ayatollah al-Ha'iri advised *maslus* (individuals with urinary incontinence) and *mabtun* (those with fecal incontinence) to use external technologies to control leaks when praying—such as plastic pouches, waterproof materials, wads of cotton, or *tashfir* (an Arabic diaper) (Al-Ha'irir 1972, v.1–3, 82). The tactics may vary, but the general point remains: incontinence as a chronic condition does not preclude one from performing religious duties.

Although these guidelines enable substantial flexibility for individuals with chronic illness or impairments (mental or physical), they are not always well known, particularly by women who have had no Qur'anic schooling such as Nana and Maou. Other women were well versed in Islamic law and aware of their right to remain pious members of the *umma*, and they experienced very little religiously linked internalized stigma. When I asked Zina (37, Hausa) if women with fistula were authorized to pray in a state of bodily impurity, she responded, "They are not just authorized to pray, they are obligated to, because [the urine] is not going to stop in a few days like the blood from one's menses. Allah commands prayer, so despite our conditions, we must . . . Me, I pray every day. I always put on a new cloth before praying and a new pad, too." Most women at the centers prayed, and almost all explained the exception to precepts of purity in simple terms: the sickness—the leaking—was God-given. As Aminatou (45, Hausa) described her practice, "I always pray five times a day. If the urine runs while I pray, I just continue, because it comes from Allah."

Incontinence did not significantly alter many women's religious habitus; indeed, for some, fistula (indirectly) and treatment-seeking (more directly) even strengthened their religious practice, understanding, and devotion. Rachida (37, Songhai) explained, "Fistula has reinforced my faith. Some say that you can't pray with fistula, but I disagree. Fistula is a challenge to one's faith. Allah gives you fistula to see if you can prove the resolve of your faith. You must be patient and accept the condition because it is a challenge sent directly from Allah." It was at the fistula center that some women first learned to read Arabic text of the Qur'an or to recite additional Qur'anic suras. The women learned from one another, benefiting from the presence of those who were daughters or wives of *malamai* (religious scholars and teachers). Sometimes, a woman from a local mosque or the wife of a visiting Turkish or Saudi diplomat would offer religious classes to the women at the center or instruct them on proper pronunciation or form during prayer.

Importantly, the center gave women a religious community. According to the Qur'an, group prayer is more meritorious than individual prayer. Summoned by the call to prayer, Nigérien men in rural and urban neighborhoods alike gather together five times a day to worship in community. Women seldom have the opportunity to pray with others, burdened as they are with domestic chores and childcare, and experiencing limited mobility. As Barbara Cooper said, "There is undeniably a difference in the experience of *salla* [prayer] for women and men; for women, it is less associated with collective times and spaces, it is often performed alone, and it is imbued with the distractions of daily life" (2006, 380). The religious practice of women with fistula who live outside of centers is even more firmly bound to worldly concerns, as tireless self-management and worries about being seen leaking increases isolation. At the centers, though, groups of women will regularly come together at the five daily designated times to pray. After ablutions, the women place their mats in a row, and together they worship. For many women, this *umma* offers a heightened sense of religious engagement and spiritual confidence as well as a deeply comforting personal relationship with God.

Cost of Concealment

In their research on the lived experience of women with obstetric fistula in Tanzania, Mselle and colleagues (2011) focused on the heavy emotional burden that fistula causes women. They specifically identified four types of loss: body control, dignity and self-worth, the social roles of woman and wife, and integration in social life. My findings parallel theirs, with the local correlates in Niger being the experiences of shame (body control), ruined identity (dignity and self-worth), and uselessness (the roles of woman and wife). The final loss in Mselle's framework—the loss of integration in social life—was often produced by Nigérien women's attempts to mitigate, manage, or reduce the intersecting losses experienced by shame, ruined identity, and uselessness. Rather than being ousted from their social circles because of their fistulas, most women I met had withdrawn of their own accord. Through ingenuity and dedication, many women were able to disguise their incontinence for months, years, or even decades. They also significantly altered the way they spent time with other people. Most stayed close to home, ensuring their access to extra pads, changes of clothes, and showers. Generally, they reduced the time they spent with others who might witness leakage or smell urine, and their fistulas were largely invisible to the outside world. Perhaps one of the reasons that women experienced so little external fistula stigma was that so few people knew that they leaked. But the women themselves knew, and often they shouldered the emotional burden alone.

Worried that they would leak in public, women would stop attending weddings, funerals, or baptisms. They would visit friends less often. Using their money on extra fabric and perfume meant they had nothing left for gift exchanges. The women who were most successful in concealing their conditions were often seen by their kin and communities to have rejected vital tenets of relational reciprocity. Balkissa (27, Hausa) explained that because of her fistula she had become reluctant to leave her home for any extended period of time, fearing that her pad would become saturated and that she would begin to leak or smell. She began to neglect relationship obligations such as attending ceremonies or visiting friends. As a result, these connections attenuated over time: "With this sickness, I don't go out much. If I do go to a friend's house, I won't stay long. I will just greet her. My friends, they say that, '[Balkissa], she doesn't like to visit anymore.' They gossip about me because of it. But only I know why . . . Because of it [my friends] don't come very often anymore to see me. If you stop visiting someone, that person will visit you less too." Few knew the reason behind Balkissa's apparent neglect, so it was not excused. People began to think of her as a bad friend, a bad cousin, and a bad community member. With a shrug, she repeated a common Hausa proverb, *zumunta a kafa ta ke,* "good relationships depend on one's feet."

In media and humanitarian narratives, fistula is said to be the direct cause of myriad relational, emotional, and financial repercussions for women—friends reject them, husbands abandon them, and kinsfolk ridicule them. But the attenuation of women's social ties, the loss of social status within their communities, the increased poverty and decreased emotional health, the dissolution of their marriages and other social consequences may, at least in part, be the result of fistula's invisibility. For women in Niger, the illusion of normalcy comes at a cost.

AFTER THE STITCHES

After the traumatic labor that caused her fistula, Hasana (who survived her obstructed labor while her twin sister did not) was sent directly to a fistula center. She was among the lucky few who regained continence after her first surgery. Her rapid referral and operation, and its success, meant that not one person in

Hasana's community ever saw or smelled evidence of her incontinence. When she returned home after surgery, there was no physical evidence of fistula. Yet she endured more external fistula stigma than 94 percent of women I interviewed (and more internal stigma than 91 percent). Her vagina was no longer "broken." She didn't leak. She didn't smell. Her uterus was intact. She was not ill. She was strong and still capable of working in the home and in the fields. And yet she languished, mistreated by both community and family. Why?

What are women's possibilities for destigmatization—the resistance against and renegotiation of fistula stigma? Do repaired bodies lead to repaired selves and repaired social relationships? Hasana's complicated return back home helps us to understand what happens after the stiches are removed and the fistula is repaired, when women are no longer defined by physical difference. I interviewed 21 women, including Hasana, who had been healed of fistula, all of whom had fully regained continence before returning home.[19] They taught me that whether, how, and to what extent women experienced destigmatization had very little to do with the transformation of their physical bodies. Some women were able to continue with their lives, socially untarnished by their period of illness. Others felt indelibly marked.

"Once a *Fistuleuse*, Always a *Fistuleuse*"

Although Hasana was dry, and had never lived with her family while incontinent, she experienced near-constant verbal abuse and social shunning from her close kin. Her mistreatment at home was not because she smelled or leaked, for she did neither. But that did not seem to matter once her family learned why she had been away: "With [my family], as soon as I get up, they look to see if my wrapper is wet . . . My family will not eat with me, even now that I am dry. I have to rely on the generosity of friends and eat with them, otherwise I would starve." Although fistula no longer marked Hasana's physical body, it continued to mark her social body, constraining her social networks and inhibiting her chances of remarrying: "Since I am healed, a few men have proposed to me. But when the time for marriage comes, people tell the man that 'she had fistula before and she could get it again.' They convince him not to marry me; they tell him to leave me. So the men don't marry me . . . This happened last year with another man. So I came here [to the fistula center]."

Hasana sought refuge at a Niamey fistula center in an attempt to distance herself from an abusive home and unabated social injury, which had less to do with her fistula than the marginal position she occupied within her family. At the center, she helped with daily maintenance and offered her personal testimony when the center needed a face of fistula for publicity. The staff called her their "Ambassador of Fistula."

Yet life at the center was not easy for her either. She did not benefit from a "sisterhood of suffering"; instead, she was often ridiculed by the other women who yearned to return home. They could not understand why someone would *choose* to be there when they so longed to leave. Insults came at Hasana from every direction: "People mock me all of the time at home . . . If it didn't hurt me so much, I wouldn't be in Niamey. But even here, women [with fistula] gossip about me. They say, 'If she is healed, why is she here?'"

Similarly, Agaïcha (27, Zarma), who had been healed of fistula for three years, had fled to the fistula center for refuge. When we met, she had already been there for two years. She believed that at home she would always be defined by fistula: "If you are sick and you are healed, your life won't be like it was before . . . They won't forget [about your fistula]. People think that if you were once a *fistuleuse* (fistula woman, French), you are always a *fistuleuse*. Even if you are healed, that changes nothing."

For the women who experienced the worst external fistula stigma, their actual corporal state seemed immaterial to their social experience. Family members and social contacts were often skeptical of their cure and continued to mistreat and shun these women. For example, Saouda, one of the seven women who had the most extreme experiences with fistula stigma, attained continence after her first surgery, but this did little to repair her social experience. She returned home, but three months later she was back at the center, looking much thinner than she had when she left. Worry was etched into her face. Her skin had a greyish pallor, and her scalp was dotted with large splotches where she had lost her hair. When she had returned home healed, the insults persisted despite her physical transformation. She told me that her family mocked her, saying, "'You there, you've sold everything that you own. Now you have nothing!'" Few people in her community believed that she was cured: "People in the village, they say that I am lying; they think that I am not healed. They still stare at my wrapper . . . Even though I am healed, people say that I lie and that I will stay forever with the sickness."

That Hasana, Agaïcha, and Saouda experienced such acute and unmitigated external stigma *after* they were healed of fistula is powerful evidence that stigma does not solely depend on the transformation of the external "mark." The women's ability to overcome fistula stigma depended on the same factors as their ability to prevent stigma in the first place: power and status within their communities, established well before their obstetric complications.

"Fistula Changes You—It Changes Your Heart"

Many women explained that, despite an outward appearance of a reestablished normalcy after healing, their internal lives remained forever changed by the experience of illness, marked by emotional wounds and hidden anger. These women recounted selected incidents of mistreatment and spoke of their inability to excuse or forgive those who had wronged them when they were unwell. The slights and subtle betrayals were not easily forgotten, as Zeinabou (30, Zarma) explained:

If someone took care of you, if they washed your wrappers and brought you food, as soon as you have something, you will give it to them. But if someone rejected you, if someone mistreated you, you can't forget that. You will keep it with you in your heart until the day you die . . . For me, there are people like this—people who mistreated me. Even my sisters. My younger sister refused to wash my wrapper. An older sister found my wrapper soaked in urine and insulted me, asking why I would wet myself, saying that my room smelled bad. Once when she went to the clinic with me, she sent a child to buy perfume to pour on me because she said I smelled . . . Even though I am healed, even if I act as though things are like how they were before, I will always remember how they acted.

"No One Runs from Them; They Are with the People"

Conversely, many women who were healed felt that their lives had returned to how they were before fistula. This was the case with Kouloua (33, Zarma), who had developed a fistula after her seventh pregnancy. She was a reserved woman who seldom smiled. She identified as an introvert: "Unless I am close to someone, it isn't my nature to spend lots of time with people." Partially because Kouloua had managed to conceal her fistula from most of her community, partly because she did not have a thriving social life before she fell ill, and partly because she commanded some respect in her community—she was married to a well-respected son of the village chief—she had experienced support rather than ridicule while ill. "In my village, no one mistreats women with fistula—no one runs from them, no one insults them, they are with the people," Kouloua claimed.

Five months after I initially interviewed Kouloua, she underwent surgery and returned home continent. I visited her there a few months later. She lived with her husband and five children in a village about 100 kilometers southeast of Niamey. Nestled in a shallow valley many miles from the dirt road, her house was small, with only two rooms. The walls were made of mud, and the floor was loose dirt. We sat on a mat in the barren room. Her children played nearby, filling the hot air with dust, rendering each breath a challenge.

Kouloua reported that now that she was healed, she had resumed some of the social activities that she had abandoned during her illness, like attending *makaranta* (religious courses). But, she continued to struggle with the bodily constraints of her recuperation, which, due to bodily fatigue and prescriptions for rest, limited her ability to labor in the fields. She also worried about the strain that would be placed on her marriage by the extended period of mandated abstinence prescribed by clinics to ensure complete recovery. Still, she felt overwhelmingly supported and encouraged by her community, husband, and kin:

One day I went to the river to wash. There were two women, and I heard one say, "Look, [Kouloua] suffered so much this year." The other said, "Yes, now she has even gained weight! She doesn't have the sickness anymore" . . . Now when I go out, people ask if I am the same woman. I've gained weight. I've changed. People talk so much about it, I am afraid that it will attract the evil eye.[20] Before [with fistula], I didn't even want people to talk to me—I was annoyed and bothered by the company of others. I didn't want to be with people. Now I chat with people freely. I don't even want people to leave when they come to visit!

Driving home from the center as the evening call to prayer slowed Niamey's heavy traffic, my research assistant Rahmatou and I reflected on the day's interviews, discussing how fistula affected the lives of women and their social relationships. Rahmatou reflected with insight, "I agree that the main consequence of fistula is shame, but still, it is also used against women. If someone doesn't like you already and then you get fistula, they use it as a weapon." Rahmatou validated my own suspicions about fistula stigma: that fistula is just one more tool for reinforcing existing relationship dynamics. Social problems are not an inevitable consequence of fistula; rather, it heightens existing tensions in already fractured social networks. For women like Hasana, Saouda, and Fana, fistula stigma grew from—but did not create—structural disempowerment.

Fistula may engender stigma, but this stigma must be understood within a context of power. As critics of early conceptualizations of stigma have pointed out, fistula stigma cannot be seen as a trait existing within an individual, but rather as a negotiated process between individuals in the context of power differentials. Thus, processes of destigmatization are moored—dependent upon dynamic relationships and preexisting circumstances. As their narratives illustrate, some women experienced swift and unproblematic destigmatization after their bodies were repaired, but other women did not—their relationships were resistant to change. Just as fistula-related stigma is deeply entrenched in existing social fabrics and power differentials, so is the possibility of destigmatization.

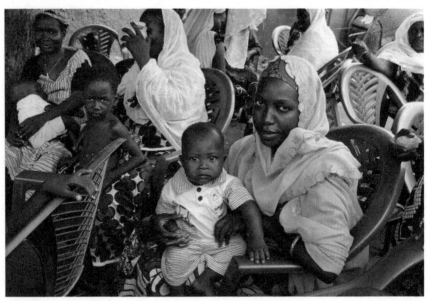
Nigérien women celebrating the baptism of a neighbor's child

3 · LIMINAL WIVES

At 15 years old, Baraka, a 37-year-old Hausa woman from the far east of Niger, was married to Ibrahim, her paternal first cousin. At 18, she became pregnant. But her labor did not solidify her role as a woman, mother, and wife: after many days in the local health center, Baraka had only delivered the head of her child. She recalled a puff of hair and placid eyes, half-birthed but no longer living. His bluish face was burned into her memory.

Baraka's husband never visited her while she stayed in the hospital, during the weeks when she regained consciousness but not continence. Rumors were circulating around her village; no one expected her to live. People stayed away out of fear, she reasoned. And when she returned to her mother's home, she did not know what to expect from her marriage. Her vagina was "broken," and her hopes of becoming a mother were shattered. What value could she have to a husband? she asked herself.

Ibrahim visited her only once at her mother's home, giving her just 2,000 Franc CFA (US$3.30). "That's all, then and after," she remembered bitterly. "I'll never forget such a small amount." With it, and the money she and her mother had scraped together, she traveled across the country to look for treatment. When she returned two years later in better health though still leaking, she found her household unrecognizable: Ibrahim had married two other women in her absence. But Baraka's story is not one of rejection and marital abandonment in the wake of illness and reproductive complications; it would be misleading to say that fistula resulted in her divorce, which took place 18 years after her return. Nor is it a story of marital strength and the redoubling of commitment in the face of injury. Baraka's marital history, like that of most women with fistula, defies simple categorization and familiar narrative frameworks. The story of her marriage moves fluidly between periods of affection and alienation, reception and rejection, and it is complicated by the dynamics of conflict and competition between co-wives.

Upon her return, Baraka's husband welcomed her home, but her two new co-wives did not. "One of his wives was so angry at him because [of me]—she protested that he would bring a sick woman to the household. She told him to divorce me." To Baraka's surprise, Ibrahim protected her: "He said he would not divorce me and chased her away instead." Ibrahim told Baraka that he loved her and he did not mind that she leaked. So she stayed with him and her remaining co-wife for almost two decades, despite her inability to birth a living child.

Everything changed after her fourth labor. This time, Baraka's baby, unlike the three before her, survived. With a child, Baraka became a renewed threat to her co-wife, rupturing the relative equanimity with which they had lived for years. Her co-wife became jealous, and their relationship soured. "She saw that even though I was sick, [Ibrahim] loved me more than he loved her. So she went to get medicine from the local healer (*boka*). My husband then spent six days without coming to my room, not during the day or the night." When Baraka had proved herself "a real woman," she (and her offspring) became competition for scarce household resources and their husband's affection. In a strategic power play, her co-wife commissioned a type of love potion to make their husband leave Baraka. The potion appeared effective, but Baraka had a plan. She gathered her few things, strapped her child to her back, and returned to her mother's house, knowing that if Ibrahim still loved her, he would come and bring her home.

Baraka spent three years at her mother's house waiting for him in vain. It was only years later, long after she had given up hope, that Ibrahim asked her to return. Angry, prideful, rejected, and still leaking, Baraka refused. She decided to sever their relationship, asking for a divorce and resuming her long-abandoned search for treatment. But Ibrahim had invested too much money and too many years in Baraka to just let her go. He denied her request to end their marriage, requiring her to seek recourse with their families, local authorities, and the local religious court, in what became a two-year battle.[1]

Twenty years after the development of her fistula, and nine failed surgeries later, Baraka sat with her then 11-year-old daughter at the fistula center, where she had recently been labeled as "incurable" and where she now lived full time. With a shrug, she explained, "Now, I am divorced. Now, this is my home."

In many ways, Baraka's story is typical of the marital experiences of women with fistula across Niger: fluidity over time, strategic deployment of separation, and the influence of co-wives on marital stability. Yet the tumult, tension, and liminality that many women have experienced in their marriages were not directly related to their incontinence. More accurately, marital disruptions were due to the interaction between injury and infertility within a context of the cultural accessibility and ease of divorce, polygyny and the constrained agency of women, and protracted absences for treatment-seeking.

MARITAL OUTCOMES IN THE WAKE OF FISTULA

Throughout West Africa, marriage is essential to female identity, social status, and the ability to transition from a girl into a woman (Izugbara and Ezeh 2010). This holds true in Niger where 88 percent of women between the ages of 15 and 49 are currently married—the highest rate in West Africa, compared with the low of 42 percent in Ghana (DHS Program 2018).[2] Due to the profound local significance of marriage, Nigérien women tend to enter unions relatively young, at an average age of 15.7—the youngest brides in the world (INS and ICF International 2013). First marriages are typically arranged by families, ideally between cross or parallel paternal (or, to a lesser extent, maternal) cousins (DHS Program 2018).[3] These unions are commonly political and considered marriages of duty and alliances, whereas second marriages are seen as unions of love. To paraphrase Inge Wittrup (1990, 123–124), the first marriage satisfies the family, the second satisfies oneself.

Although women in Niger tend to enter marriage early, they exit their marriages easily and often. Ronald Cohen (1971) found that Kanuri women may marry and divorce as many as 12 times throughout their lives.[4] Getting divorced is quite culturally accepted—but remaining divorced is not. Islam permits remarriage three months after a divorce has taken place, and most women do remarry shortly after to avoid the label of "prostitute" that is inevitably placed on premenopausal single women. These divorced women are more likely than first-time brides to enter into subsequent marriages with one or more co-wives.

Polygyny is more common in West Africa than elsewhere on the continent.[5] In Niger, just over 36 percent of women are in polygynous marriages—slightly higher than the West African average of 33 percent, which ranges from a low of 14 percent in Liberia to a high of 48 percent in Guinea (DHS Program 2018). Most Nigérien women are likely to live with a co-wife at some point in their lives because the rates of polygyny climb as women age and face illness or reproductive complications. When women develop fistula, their marriages may become fragile, magnifying a typical base level of instability born from the ever-present risk of divorce and exacerbated by the introduction of and tension between co-wives. Yet the expectation is that socially respectable women live within the safety and sanctity of marriage, so marital strain does not always (or even often) translate into divorce. Instead, it frequently leads to the rather more nebulous category of marital separation.

Among the 100 women I came to know, only 24 were divorced. The largest portion, 38 women, remained married, and almost as many, 35, were in a liminal state of marital separation.[6] Fistula had affected the women's marriages in a multitude of ways. For some, it solidified their marital bonds and exposed deep affective networks. For others, the injury led to prolonged liminal states from the protracted periods of separation. And for the minority, fistula had resulted in immediate, unilateral divorce: their repudiation and rejection.

Marriage in Name Only

Periods of separation, when a woman typically returns to her natal home, punctuate many Nigérien marriages. Women may return to their parents' home because of childbirth, illness, parental caretaking, or marital discord. Although these absences regularly span months (or sometimes years), they do not in and of themselves indicate marital disharmony. Some separations—such as for a pregnancy and birth—are considered healthy and customary; others—particularly when wives leave their husband to express dissatisfaction—may portend marital dissolution.

Periods of marital separation are not typically tracked in demographic or fistula surveys, but they serve a vital role in the marriages of women with fistula. Over a third of the women I interviewed identified as separated, meaning that they were technically still married but living apart from their husbands and experiencing uncertainty about their marital futures. In some cases, the separations appeared temporary, with the woman and her husband both actively negotiating the next step in their marriage—either a return to cohabitation, or an official divorce. But for many other couples, the separations were prolonged periods of waiting, of unknowing, that extended years or decades with no or little communication or exchange between the couple.

When Nigérien women feel as though their husbands have not lived up to their marital obligations—often due to emotional mistreatment, lack of love, neglect of financial responsibilities, or sexual inattention—they often flee to their parents' home. This visible relocation is strategic: it allows a woman to indict her husband without breaching the gendered expectations of decorum and female submission. A woman's refusal to remain makes public her distress; her husband is then forced to attend to their marriage, or to openly refuse to do so. During these periods, it is often the families who negotiate the tumult. Just as they presided over the marriage, each family represents its side to find acceptable terms of either reconciliation or dissolution.

Another kind of separation is more common among women with fistula—one that is less public and less indicting of husbands. Most women in Niger return to their parents' home around their seventh month of pregnancy. There, rather than at their marital home, women will deliver their babies and recuperate for 40 days after the birth, a custom widely practiced by younger women and known in Hausa as *shan kunu* (drink porridge) (Cooper 2006). A woman's departure from her matrimonial home for her delivery and postpartum recovery does not mark marital friction but rather allows her respite from her onerous domestic and sexual duties during the late stages of her pregnancy.

Women with birthing injuries who are reluctant to return to their marital homes and their attendant domestic responsibilities until they have convalesced frequently remain with their parents. Extended postpartum absences lasting up to several months are not unusual. But when a woman's incontinence does not eventually subside and her body does not return to "normal," she must then confront the implications of a prolonged absence from her husband and her larger social network—including co-wives, in-laws, her own family members, and curious neighbors—who may have something to gain or lose in her absence.

Asma'u (25, Zarma) had lived with fistula for three years and had undergone six previous surgeries when I met her. She described to me her uncertainty about her marital status:

> I don't know if we are still married. It has been three years since I have been at his house. He comes to visit me at my parent's, but he does not give me money. When he comes to visit, he asks me about my health; he asks if I am better. He says that if the sickness is finished, I should go back to his home, but if not, he says I should stay with my parents . . . My mother-in-law told him that he should remarry, because when she saw the state I was in, she knew that I would never be the same. She said that there would always be urine. Now, if I said that I did not want him anymore, it would not be a problem for him because he has already remarried. He has a young son . . . If I am healed and he continues to visit me, I will go back to him. But if he stops visiting, then I won't go back.

As Asma'u's situation illuminates, both husband and wife are forced to reexamine their marital configuration after the development of a fistula. They are constantly recalculating the costs versus benefits of possible futures after separation. Husbands like Asma'u's and Baraka's—and sometimes co-wives, as we will see—behave strategically during this period of uncertainty.

Only infrequently do husbands immediately divorce their wives when they develop a birthing injury; men who have already invested a great deal in their marriages tend to adopt a wait-and-see approach. The husbands may decline any further investment in the relationship during these periods of separation, no longer providing for their wives financially or emotionally. Husbands may also diversify their domestic investments, remarrying and beginning new families in case their wives do not heal. In this period of ambiguous separation—when there is a "marriage cord" (*igiyar arme*) but little substance to the relationship—a woman is prohibited from marrying elsewhere. But the husband is allowed to eschew his financial responsibilities to these women and take other wives in the meantime, thus minimizing the consequences on his household of waiting for wives' bodies to mend. Until the relatively minimal costs of waiting outweigh the potential future benefits of a possibly healed and fecund wife, few men are incentivized to pursue divorce.[7]

The gendered inequity in this arrangement is clear. Men whose wives develop fistula in polygynous Niger can marry up to three additional women, enjoy fulfilling domestic and sexual lives, and continue to father more children. Meanwhile, the lives of their wives are placed on hold. Separated women often receive little or no financial or emotional support from their partners. They cannot engage in socially recognized sexual relationships or conceive more children with other men. Additionally, prolonged periods of marital estrangement can damage their social status and perceptions of self.

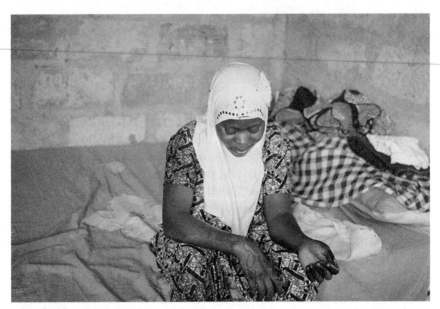

FIGURE 8. Former fistula patient during her first week in her new husband's house

Yet there are benefits of separation to women as well. Although some women with fistula do push for official divorce so that they may remarry or freely pursue treatment, many prefer to live within the boundaries of a marriage, even if that union is without financial, emotional, sexual, or social substance. These hollowed out marriages, suspended in states of separation, allow women to live within the socially normative role of a married adult (rather than slipping into the socially problematic role of an unmarried woman). Within their natal homes women live with relative independence and away from the judgment, insults, gossip, or mockery, of their co-wives. There they have the time to dedicate to the daily work of fistula self-care or to pursue medical treatment outside their communities, and they can retain hope for a future return to their marital homes (or a new husband's home) once healed (figure 8).

Cutting the Marriage Cord

Sometimes women experience an immediate marital rupture after the development of a fistula, but more often a separation followed by a divorce is a quiet, extended process. A woman may stay at her parents' home after labor, as she might have otherwise, but her husband does not give her money, visit her, or ask her to return home. The divorce is often divorce by omission—an omission of money, care, intimacy, or sex, for example. Months or years after the labor that caused the fistula, a representative of the husband's family may show up with civil divorce papers or bring the news that the husband has performed a religious divorce.[8] The news simply confirms an unspoken social fact. For example, Lahiya (22, Hausa), who had been living with fistula for two years, had not seen nor spoken to her husband since late in her pregnancy:

> When I was in the fifth month of my second pregnancy, my husband went to find work in [a town on the border with Nigeria]. He left and he didn't come back even when I gave birth. Now it has been three years, and I haven't seen him. A friend of his told him that I got fistula, so he never came back . . . I hear that now he is married and has a child . . . This year he sent me divorce papers. It is because of my fistula that he never came back. He never once called me. He never even gave me 5 Franc CFA [US$0.01].

For many husbands, the scales finally tip—perhaps the costs of waiting were too high, or (more often) the perceived benefits faded. Lahiya's husband may have wanted to wed a fifth wife (and thus needed to free up a spot through divorce). Or perhaps he was urged to divorce her by his mother, other wives, or friends, who might have argued that a leaking, sick woman would never become well enough to provide him children and only bring him (and them) financial ruin and ridicule.

Divorce is not exceptional in Niger. Contrary to assumptions about patrilineal societies with high bride-wealth (for example, see Goody 1976), Nigérien women tend to marry as early as possible, but many of these marriages do not last. Clark and Brauner-Otto (2015) estimated that within the first 20 years of marriage, 25 percent of first unions in Niger have dissolved (21 percent due to divorce, and 4 percent due to the death of a spouse). Other researchers have reported even more striking numbers in the region. Manvell (2006) found that more than one-third of married Hausa women between the ages of 31 and 40 in two rural towns had been previously divorced, and Callaway (1984) estimated that 50 percent of Nigerian Hausa women experience at least one divorce in their lifetimes. Niger's high rates of divorce and its virilocal marriage customs make Nigérien women into what Barbara Cooper (1997) calls "perennial migrants."[9]

Although divorce may seem routine in Niger, the impact of an unwanted divorce on a woman's life can be substantial. Many of the women I spoke with who had been rejected and divorced were furious at their ex-husbands. They frequently invoked religious condemnation of these men, who they considered cowardly, godless, and unethical. According to Yaha (33, Hausa), "because women are broken (*lalace*), most husbands leave, but it isn't just. It takes two to create this problem [fistula]. Keeping their promises, men do not." Souweiba (30, Hausa) explained that "it isn't right for a husband to leave. It is at his home that she got it. Men who have fear of Allah don't leave."

Yet many women decide to leave their husband's home of their own volition. They blame him for their injuries, are angry at his lack of care, or were unhappy with the marriage from the beginning. Many Nigérien marriages are involuntary, unwanted by the women (and sometimes by the men as well), and experienced as a constraint from which women are relieved to be liberated (Antoine 2002). In these cases, fistula offers an excuse. The injury can serve as a socially sanctioned point of rupture for husbands and wives, allowing either party to gracefully (and sometimes passively) retreat from a troubled union. I found that the couples who had divorced immediately after the woman developed a fistula were often unhappy to begin with.

Nevertheless, as seen in Baraka's story, a divorce is less easily attained by a woman than by a man. The man can, without justification or ceremony, simply verbally pronounce himself divorced to religiously sever his marital bond.[10] By contrast, a woman must present evidence to both her family and to a Muslim religious leader of her husband's failure in his marital responsibilities, such as demonstrating that he has severely physically beaten her (Wittrup 1990). Despite these inequities in access, women in the region are well-known to instigate a large share of the divorces, likely because they have more to lose by staying in a bad marriage.[11]

Rabi (32, Zarma) had developed a fistula just a few months before I met her. Nerve damage had left her legs atrophied and thin, and she struggled to walk with a cane. She had not spoken with her husband since her labor six months before.

> I am at my parents' house, but I am not divorced. My husband hasn't come to visit; he hasn't sent money. He didn't come to visit me when he learned that the child was stillborn. He didn't even come to give his condolences . . . He was angry with me because I had told him that I didn't want to stay with him even before the birth. When I married him, he already had a wife, but he chased away his first wife and soon after he married another woman. But his first wife came back, so then there were three of us. No; it was just too many women! I told him I wanted a divorce, even if he didn't give me my papers . . . People gossip about me. Because I refused to stay, because I left him, that's why. I've been with him for six years, and I leave him often. Before, I had always gone back. This time though, I don't think he will make me go back to him. I think now it is done.

Even before her fistula, Rabi's relationship with her husband had been strained. Although it is not clear what was best for Rabi or what she actually desired, the development of her fistula may have helped to remove her from a marriage that she "often" tried to leave.

Similarly, Zara (27, Tuareg-Zarma), who was married against her will at 11 years old, explained to me how fistula allowed her to escape a marriage that, despite her best efforts, had been inescapable in her youth: "When I returned from the hospital, my husband came to visit me. He told my uncle that if I ever healed, I could find another husband. He said that he didn't want me anymore. Even my mother-in-law came to tell me." I asked how she had felt about the divorce. She chuckled, "So happy I even laughed! This is what I had already wanted. I was joyous."

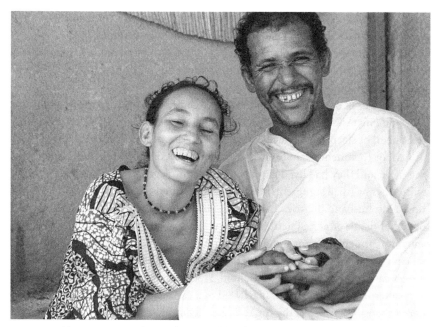

FIGURE 9. Tuareg woman joking at home with her husband

Enduring Marital Bonds

Despite the ease and accessibility of separation and divorce in Niger, some men faithfully stay with their wives, seeing them through the period of illness or awaiting their return home from the hospital (figure 9). Sa'adé (23, Fulani), from a far eastern region on the border of Lake Chad, married a Tuareg man from a neighboring town when she was 17. He had come to her village looking for work, and they fell in love; they married a year later. Sa'adé's four pregnancies resulted in two second-trimester miscarriages and two births; both babies died within an hour of delivery. After the fourth labor, Sa'adé was left with a fistula. Although she had not returned to her husband's house since then, he continued to support her, sending money, providing comfort, and visiting often: "He visits me every day at my parents' home. He brings me money and cloth and food. He sits with me in the afternoon, and we chat." I asked her if she thought he would eventually leave her if she were not healed. She responded, "No. I don't think he will leave me. He has been with me all of this time, since the beginning of this sickness. For some men, if he has the intention of leaving his wife when she gets sick, he will leave her at the very beginning, saying, 'This woman has no use. She is broken, and that's that.'" Sa'adé, who had been looking for treatment at three centers in the preceding two years, was concerned for her husband. He had no other wife—no one to look after him, cook him meals, or maintain his home. Rising above the jealousy that characterizes most women's feelings toward co-wives, Sa'adé voiced the desire for her husband to remarry: "I would like him to take a second wife because I have this sickness of urine and now I cannot be there to take care of him."

Sa'adé's story of mutual affection and selflessness, caretaking, and investment was similar to other stories I heard from women: husbands washing the urine off their bodies, laundering their clothes, consoling them, protecting them from the hurtful words of others in the community, fetching water and firewood (traditionally women's tasks), seeking out local medicines, selling off livestock to pay for treatment, or sleeping for weeks or months on the periphery of hospitals as they waited for treatment. Naio (29, Zarma) had married a neighbor she loved at the age of 14, and they had lived happily together for 15 years: "In a household there will always be small arguments, small problems, but there will also always be solutions. My husband, he tries his best . . . He is a good man." When Naio developed her fistula after her sixth pregnancy, her husband supported her while she sought treatment, accompanying her to multiple hospitals and sleeping in hospital courtyards for months. After a failed surgery, she was weak, ill, and could no longer care for herself or her household. Her mother came to stay with her, but soon after her mother was incapacitated in a car accident, leaving Naio's care to her husband. "Because of the car accident, my mother could not take care of me anymore, so my husband took care of me every day. Every day, he would bring me food, wash my body, wash my clothing. He even washed the rags I used for the urine," she explained. While Naio's or Sa'adé's stories of intimacy and caretaking were not the norm, they were also not exceptional.

Unlike Sa'adé and Naio, whose relationship had only borne the weight of fistula for a relatively short period, Ladi and Adamou had dealt with Ladi's chronic incontinence for two decades. Ladi (35, Hausa) was deemed incurable by the fistula surgeons after 11 failed surgeries. After several miscarriages and years of trying in vain to conceive, she was also deemed infertile. Because Ladi had spent so many years seeking care at a maternity hospital in Niamey, she was offered a job there as a *fille de salle,* a cleaning woman. Largely due to her relationships at the maternity hospital and her consequent increased access to health care, she was eventually able to conceive, and she gave birth via an early prophylactic cesarean section to a healthy baby girl. Nine months after our first meeting, I accompanied Ladi home to meet her husband and co-wife.

Her husband, Adamou, a paternal cross cousin, was a loving and animated man who worked at a Niamey market. He spoke to me about how Ladi's health problems had affected her, him, their family, and their relationship throughout the past two decades: "We have been together 20 years this year. It is a long time. We will stay longer . . . It is only this year that Allah gave us a chance to have a baby. [My wife] had three pregnancies, and she miscarried three times. Three times she had a miscarriage, and then we figured out that Allah is the only one who can give a child. [Our daughter] is a star, a star who, not only here in Niger, but in the world, is very important."

I asked Adamou if he and Ladi were happy together, and he explained that they were bonded through deep and unbreakable familial ties, despite the troubles they had faced.

> She and I are like a person and their shadow. You can't be separate from it, even in a dark place. It's how we are. I trust in Allah; I know [fistula] is something that came from Allah. So if you are living, you are not dead, you cannot despair . . . Ladi is my daughter, and she is my wife . . . My people and her people are the same; she is like my daughter. How can you abandon your blood? You cannot. It's like that. No one can bring any problem in this house between us. Me, her, and her co-wife, we are living in peace in this house. No problems. Everything that happened to her can happen to someone else.

Adamou stayed with Ladi throughout her struggle with infertility and her ongoing incontinence, motivated by his deep religious faith, loyalty to his family, his ethical convictions, and love for his wife. By situating Ladi both as his "daughter" and his wife, of his "own blood," Adamou positioned family marriage as a protective mechanism that ensured ongoing commitment in face of hardship.

Although these marriages were particularly loving and supportive, they were not uniquely so. These examples of caregiving and faithfulness provide a counterpoint to the prevailing grammar of masculine domination, domestic violence, and marriages devoid of intimacy that is so prevalent in the discourse about romantic relationships in sub-Saharan Africa. Despite the dominant donor and media narrative of fistula-induced marital dissolution, many women continued to live with loving and supportive partners who neither rejected nor ridiculed them because of their illness. Some women even explained that they continued to enjoy satisfying sexual lives after the development of their fistulas.[12]

MEDIATING FACTORS IN MARITAL OUTCOMES

Why do some marriages dissolve with fistula, while others adapt? I found that women's marital outcomes were determined by several factors: the context in which their marriages were entered, the influence of their co-wives, their reproductive histories, their continued sexual engagement with their husbands, and their treatment-seeking experiences.

Entering the Marriage

When a woman fell ill, the resilience of her marriage partially depended on who in her community was working for or against its continued success. The degree of familial support was particularly dependent on the conditions under which the marriage was entered—including whether it was within a family, for love, or out of obligation (see figure 10). As demonstrated by Ladi and Adamou, family

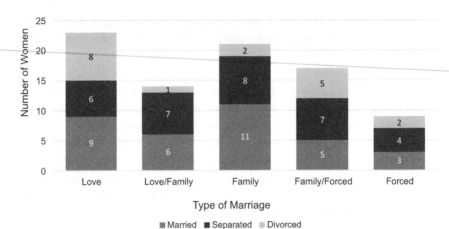

FIGURE 10. Current marital status, categorized by type of marriage, for 84 women with fistula, including 37 women with love marriages (14 of which were co-categorized as family marriages), 52 women with family marriages, and 26 women with "forced" marriages, or marriages of obligation (17 of which were co-categorized as family marriages).

marriages—fundamentally conceived as uniting two families rather than two individuals—ensured increased marital stability during times of stress. In contrast, "love" marriages—arranged by the man and woman themselves (with consent from their families)—proved less stable because neither family felt responsible for the success of the union and did not strongly intercede. Even more precarious were marriages arranged against the will of the bride (and, in some cases, the groom). Few in an unhappy union are invested in working through difficult times. Illness, injury, or infertility often offer the resentful woman or man an opportunity to be free from an undesired marriage of obligation.

The majority of women (52, 64 percent of the 84 women who responded) were in family marriages when they developed fistula.[13] Family (or consanguineous) marriages keep down bride-price, preserve property within families, and reinforce the stability of extended family bonds. Also, due to patrilineal customs and patrilocal residence patterns, when women marry paternal kin, they tend to move nearby. Family marriages are thus thought to provide young brides an additional layer of protection: proximity to their family and friends. Unsurprisingly, there is a strong preference for paternal cousin marriages (and to a lesser extent, other family marriages) among many Nigériens—particularly for first-time unions.

At first glance, families—and family marriages—appear to be an important line of defense for women against fistula's negative marital and general social consequences. But family marriages can cut both ways. When a Nigérien woman is married to her first cousin, the powerful connection between niece and aunt is transformed into a fraught relationship between bride and mother-in-law. Sides may become blurred and allegiances messy when a woman develops a fistula. As just an aunt, a woman likely would have taken her niece's side, cared for her, stood in as her second mother, kept her secret, advocated for her in periods of marital separation, and protected her from mistreatment. But as a mother-in-law, the same woman's primary concern shifts to her son and his interests, so she may gossip about her niece-cum-daughter-in-law, belittle her, and pressure her son to remarry a woman who is more likely to bear children.[14]

Furthermore, this mother-in-law may have both the incentive to harm her niece-cum-daughter-in-law and the means to do so. In the case of illness, she is still privy to the information and access restricted to closest kin. Such dynamics can make family feel a little less safe for women with fistula. For example, Jeka (28, Hausa) was married to her maternal parallel cousin, and swiftly returned to his house after her problematic labor. Back home, Jeka concealed her condition— only her husband and mother knew. But when Jeka eventually sought treatment, Jeka's aunt-cum-mother-in-law probed her younger sister (Jeka's mother). "What is wrong with this girl? You must tell me," she pushed. Jeka's mother could not lie to her own sister. When Jeka's mother-in-law learned of the cause of Jeka's departure, she forcefully pressured her son to disinvest from his marriage and begin looking for a new wife. Jeka explained: "They asked him, 'Why would you bring her home, a woman like that, a woman who has this sickness?' He said, 'No. I brought this woman to my house when she was in good health, so I cannot send her away now.' They said, 'Do not bring that woman back!' They did everything to change his mind. Because of them, his demeanor (*fuska*) changed, and he sent me away." While cousin marriages can be protective, consolidating alliances, Jeka's experience shows us how family marriages can also introduce novel complexities and conflicting interests.

The relative merits of a family marriage are not usually weighed by young women when considering future husbands, however. Nigérien women often feel powerless in their choice of spouse, fearing social, psychological, and physical consequences if they resist the wishes of their families. Twenty-six women (31 percent) categorized their current marriage (or, for divorced women, their previous marriage) as one of obligation (*auren dole* in Hausa). The majority (17 or 65 percent) of these "forced" marriages were also family marriages. For example, Zara (27, Zarma) had opposed the marriage with an older cousin, which her father had arranged when she was 11 years old:[15]

I didn't want the marriage. I didn't love him, and my family didn't give me the time or choice to pick someone I wanted. I resisted and left my father's village to stay in the village of my grandmother. But my father had conducted the religious ceremony without my consent. I was so angry. My maternal uncle gave me taxi money to run away to Ouallam, and there I met someone I loved. But it wasn't possible to marry him because according to Islamic law, I was already married. My father was angry that I ran from my husband, but he let me stay away for a few years to mature. When he thought I was ready to live with my husband, he forced me to come back . . . My husband was angry that I had resisted so long. He was hard with me. Every time I made a mistake, he hit me. My co-wife didn't like me, and she didn't like that I didn't like our husband, so she would often provoke me and my husband would hit me when she and I fought.

Love marriages were nearly as common as forced or arranged marriages, and 37 women identified their unions as love marriages they had organized themselves (with the consent of the families). Of these women, 14 said that their unions were also family marriages. Sometimes the couple had been in love for some time already when they married. "He was my boyfriend, so when he had saved enough money, he brought my parents the bride-wealth," said Karima (26, Tuareg). Other times, women described love at first sight. "He was passing through my village for a baptism, and he saw me in the market. He loved me when he saw me, so he came to ask my parents to marry me. I liked him too, so I accepted," said Amina (40, Zarma). These marriages, which have clear benefits for the couple (allowing both parties to enter into desired unions), also have drawbacks. Family marriages are securely bound in webs of reciprocity and obligation, but marriages arranged by the couple themselves have no external support; if difficulties such as health problems, infidelity, or financial strain arise, the couple's families are often less invested in keeping the relationship together.

In the face of birthing injuries such as fistula, women in love marriages that were not also family marriages experienced high rates of divorce (34 percent, compared with the average of 24 percent). Love marriages appeared just as unstable as forced marriages when confronted with fistula; rates of divorce following fistula for all love and all forced marriages were comparable (24 and 27 percent, respectively). Women in family marriages, however, had significantly lower rates of divorce: 15 percent for all family marriages, and 10 percent for family marriages not also categorized as love or forced. Family marriages also had the highest rates of continued marriage following fistula, at 42 percent (52 percent if co-categorized marriages are excluded).[16]

The Other Woman

The experience of marriage in Niger (and the likelihood of divorce) cannot be understood outside the context of polygyny. Influenced by Islamic law, if a Nigérien man can financially, and equitably, support his wives, he is permitted to marry up to four women at any given time. But the economic costs of supporting multiple women and their children are prohibitively high for many poor Nigérien men. A man can often only afford to marry a second wife once he has accrued some wealth; nevertheless, he is likely to cobble together the resources to do so if his first wife falls ill or experiences reproductive difficulties. While only 36 percent of Nigérien women are in polygynous unions nationally, of the 73 women

I interviewed who were married, separated, or widowed, 43 women—59 percent—were in polygynous marriages (INS and ICF International 2013).[17] Fistula dramatically increased the chances that a husband would seek additional wives.[18]

When a man marries multiple women, co-wives are obliged to share space, household resources, a sexual partner, and genetic entanglements (as their children are half-siblings). Nigérien women typically have no say in the other woman with whom they will share their lives. Such involuntary intimacy can lead women to feel the full emotional spectrum for their co-wives: spanning from love to hate and everything in between, including a protective indifference or a sense of resignation.

Living with a co-wife can have real benefits for overburdened Nigérien women, reducing the onerous demands of household labor, childcare, and conjugal responsibilities (Anderson 2000; Dorjahn 1988; Madhavan 2002; Ware 1979). During times of pregnancy, birth, and illness (and including periods of mandated abstinence, such as during menstruation and post-partum), the material and structural support provided by co-wives is one of the primary advantages of polygynous unions for women (Jankowiak, Sudakov, and Wilreker 2005; Tabi et al. 2010). This support can also facilitate a woman's travel outside of the home to visit family, to engage in market activities, or, vital for women with fistula, to seek medical care. And when, due to religious proscriptions, a woman's mobility is limited and her daily life does not extend far beyond the walls of her home, a co-wife can provide an important source of companionship.[19]

Despite the potential benefits and cultural normativity of polygyny, the vast majority of women admit that even when one is in good health, living with a co-wife is difficult and requires patience, humility, and control over one's jealousy. Inge Wittrup has argued that much scholarship on polygyny, which justifies the practice in terms of the practical benefits a woman may enjoy, reflect "male wishful thinking" (1990, 129). Notions of "sister solidarity" are a "male myth"; instead, she asserts, polygynous relationships are "battlefields for rivalry and conflicts" (Wittrup 1990, 131, 129). Certainly, co-wives can feel profound jealousy of and deep contempt for one another, leading to systematic undermining, merciless verbal aggression, and even physical violence. Such strategic and underhanded assaults are often waged in order to marginalize a co-wife and stake out a greater share of emotional intimacy, sexual access, and material resources from a husband.

As a result, a co-wife can negatively impact a woman's well-being and self-esteem, reproductive success, physical and mental health, and the health of her children (Al-Krenawi 1999; Jankowiak, Sudakov, and Wilreker 2005; Shepard 2013). When compared to their monogamous counterparts, women in polygynous unions are found to experience higher levels of various psychological symptoms, decreased life and marital satisfaction, and problematic family functioning (Shepard 2013). Yet, not all women are affected equally. Women's vulnerability to conflict or openness to potential cooperation differs dramatically depending on their age, their economic independence and engagement in the marketplace, their position, and the number and age of their children.[20]

Living with a co-wife provides ample opportunities for antipathy, conflict, and rejection as well as intimacy, support, and cooperation. In the face of fistula, these dynamics become increasingly complicated. A co-wife may provide an important source of care. For example, Maou (35, Hausa) explained to me how during her illness, her co-wife of many years "showed that there was love between us." "Since I fell ill," she explained, "my co-wife has taken care of me, our husband, and my children. She braids my children's hair, pounds my millet. Really, she does everything for me. She has never used my fistula against me." Maou suspected that her co-wife had even inadvertently protected her own marriage, mitigating the pressure she felt to engage in regular sexual intercourse and to produce children for her husband. This was true for many women. Co-wives enabled some women with fistula to avoid unwanted divorces by buying them time to care for their bodies and strategize about their futures while their husbands invested in second families.

Still, a study in the neighboring country of Mali found that only 21 percent of polygynous women relied on their co-wives for support during illness (Bove, Vala-Haynes, and Valeggia 2012). In fact, when a woman falls ill within a polygynous household, her co-wives may actually exacerbate her ill health. "The mere contrast between one's illness and a co-wife's good health might induce anxiety and distress in a polygynous woman who is sick. Co-wives may also affect the care that women receive . . . by interfering with the patient's relationship with her husband" (Bove and Valeggia 2009, 26).

Some women, like Maou, enjoyed continued support from their co-wives in the face of illness, but most did not. In the absence of good health, the delicate balance between co-wives' collaboration and competition is often upset. Co-wives frequently used a woman's fistula against her in order to push her out, or at least marginalize her, and thus gain power within the household. Although some women benefitted from the sharing of labor in polygynous unions, feeling unburdened from onerous household duties, others experienced this reallocation of work as a usurpation of power, and a loss of status and security within their households. Maou and her co-wife's mutually supportive relationship may be the exception rather than the rule, perhaps because Maou had lived peacefully with her co-wife long before she developed fistula. In contrast, the relationship between co-wives tends to be particularly acrimonious when women do not share a history pre-fistula, either because a man only marries a second wife after his first wife has developed fistula, or because a divorced woman with fistula enters a new household.

When a woman with fistula can no longer manage domestic (or sexual) responsibilities, either due to illness or absence, her husband often finds it necessary to take another wife to maintain a well-functioning household and ensure the continuation of his family line. Welcoming a junior wife into the household can be traumatic, even for a healthy and reproductively successful first wife; this is acknowledged in a ritual called the *maracanda* (Bornand 2005, 2012), which consists of a song between newly joined Zarma-Songhai co-wives in Niger—a socially sanctioned means to express grief, conflict, and aggression.[21] Despite the rancor, the *maracanda* is thought to help senior wives to move through the steps of mourning: anger, sadness, resignation, and eventually acceptance, with the ultimate goal of household harmony. But women with fistula often have no opportunity to air anger, sadness, and disappointment at the remarriage of their husbands. Away seeking treatment, still recovering at hospitals, or regaining strength at their parents' home, many women cannot enact the ritual transition into the role of senior co-wife and garner the accompanying respect. Instead, they become interlopers of sorts in their husband's new marriage, resented by young brides to whom they are an economic drain, unwelcome competition, and a social mark.

Mariama (50, Hausa) had lived with fistula for 30 years. Despite the close relationship that she had cultivated with her second husband, her conjugal life was full of strife because of her co-wives. Mariama was the first and only wife when she developed fistula. When her husband remarried during her prolonged recuperation, her co-wife resented her and worked to undermine her marriage.

> My husband told his wife that she couldn't [mock me] and sent her away. The next co-wife was also bad. She mocked me. She said that I sold everything I owned to find health and still hadn't. She said I just wasted all my money . . . She is a really mean person. She was jealous because our husband loved me more, despite my sickness of urine. People in the village told him to leave me, but he refused. It didn't bother him. He continued to spend the night with me. We slept on the same bed. I had seven pregnancies after the fistula. If it wasn't for him, I would have been chased away. But he is patient and kind.
>
> My co-wife was not [kind]. She would say to me, "You have an open vagina, that's why the urine pours out." She said I was dirty. She covered her nose when she walked by me. She wouldn't eat with me. She wouldn't eat the food I prepared. She would come and sit very close to me just so that she could say that I smelled bad . . . She was jealous . . . She hated to see me clean. I kept myself so clean, if it wasn't for her, no one would have known! It was because of her that the whole village learned of my sickness. She told everyone! So, because of her, I couldn't go to ceremonies. I was afraid that people would look at me and mock me. I stayed at home and never left the house! . . . When our husband found out that she had told everyone in the village about my fistula, he sent her away. But after some time, she returned. She's a bit better now because she understood that she had been punished by our husband.

Mariama's husband continued to invest in their marriage and dutifully kept Mariama's incontinence a secret from their community. Yet, her co-wife strategically circulated information about Mariama's "sickness of urine" in an attempt to discredit Mariama and gain social power within and outside of their household. Mariama's experience illustrates that while women may have supportive to semis-upportive husbands, co-wives can undermine networks of care and complicate women's coping strategies. Taken together, Maou and Mariama's experiences illustrate how a co-wife has the power both to protect and to weaken the relationship between a woman with fistula and her husband. In the most extreme cases, husbands who struggle to maintain peace at home (a difficult task even in the absence of illness) even resort to divorce, abuse, neglect, or mistreatment of their ailing wives just to appease the other women in their households. Undoubtedly, a woman's relationship to her co-wives is complex, fluid, fraught with anxiety, and often predictive of marital outcomes.

Fertility, Stability

Some studies have suggested that the typically contentious relationships between co-wives may actually improve when one woman is infertile (Jankowiak, Sudakov, and Wilreker 2005); such was the case with Baraka from the opening of this chapter. Intense reproductive competition between co-wives can be partially explained by patterns of resource allocation in households. Nigérien husbands often apportion spending money, food, and other goods between their wives based on the number of their children. In the event of their husband's death, women who bear many children are further rewarded due to Islamic inheritance systems that parcel a father's land equally between his sons (and half of what is given to sons is given to daughters). Infertility, and thus the absence of this kind of reproductive competition in a household, might promote a more cooperative and even harmonious domestic life. Fertile women receive more spending money and resources for their children and anticipate more inheritance while also benefiting from their co-wife's labor and childcare. While the deal is not as sweet for their infertile co-wives, women who struggle with their reproductive health may see a co-wife as a buffer against divorce.

Women with fistula who had no co-wives did appear more receptive to accepting a co-wife than they may have been before their reproductive complications. These women struggled with the dual burdens of illness and infertility or subfertility, and they may have felt less entitled to make demands for spousal exclusivity. For example, Sadata (45, Fulani), who had lived with fistula for 10 years, was the sole wife until she developed fistula: "My husband married two women after me. He married the first after my labor when I couldn't walk, and the second when I started coming to hospitals to find treatment." I asked Sadata if she was angry about her husband's marriages, and she said she was not. "He informed me that he wanted to remarry, and I agreed. If he had guests, who would serve them? Who would take care of him?" Although her tumultuous relationships with her co-wives (but not her husband) prevented her from returning to her marital home, Sadata recognized the importance of his remarriage to maintain his—and thus her—social status within the community.

Although women with fistula and fertility complications may have been more likely to accept an expanded household, generally the same could not be said of their husbands' new wives. Perhaps because infertility is so socially problematic in Niger, new wives tended not to view a co-wife's infertility as particularly beneficial. Instead, women seemed to feel a degree of disdain for a co-wife with fistula and perhaps a fear of the condition's moral and physical contagion. Infertility or low fertility appear to more negatively affect women in polygynous relationships than women in monogamous marriages, with polygyny associated with higher rates of infertility-related stress and anxiety (Aghanwa, Dare, and Ogunniyi 1999; Donkor and Sandall 2007; Hollos et al. 2009).

Although fistula does not cause infertility, many women struggled to birth living children. Women with fistula had fewer living children than pregnancies (figure 11). The percentage of child loss was disturbingly high among the 100 women I came to know, with on average fewer than one of every four pregnancies resulting in a living child. Child loss was highest for women who had experienced only one pregnancy, at 91 percent (meaning that only one child out of every 10 first pregnancies survived), and lowest for women who had seven pregnancies (52 percent). Women with fistula were particularly prone to late-term miscarriage and infant death during the birthing process. Physicians I spoke with offered two explanations for this. The first is that these women may be particularly vulnerable to uterine and urinary tract infections during pregnancy. The

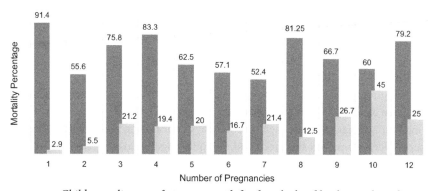

FIGURE 11. Child mortality rate of 98 women with fistula, calculated by the number of living children divided by the number of full-term pregnancies (not including first and second term spontaneous abortions). In dark grey are mortality percentages including stillbirths, and in light grey are mortality percentages not including stillbirths. The average total mortality rate is 76 percent, and the average mortality rate when stillbirths are excluded is 13 percent.

second is that whatever had caused the obstetric complications that initially led to the fistula (cephalopelvic disproportion, for example) continued to cause problems during subsequent labors.

Among the women I interviewed, most child deaths occurred during a complicated labor. Some 66 percent of pregnancies among the 100 women with fistula ended in a stillbirth, significantly higher than the national rate of stillbirth and perinatal deaths in Niger—estimated at only 3.3 percent (INS and ICF International 2013).When stillbirths were removed from the calculations, the average child mortality rates among the 100 women I interviewed dropped from 76 percent to 13 percent—a rate similar to Niger's national average for rural populations, which is 16 percent (INS and ICF International 2013).[22]

Although many of the women with fistula had been pregnant multiple times (3.7 pregnancies, range: 0–12), the women averaged only one living child each (range: 0–6 living children), and divorced women had the fewest children of all—only 0.6 on average. The low fertility experienced by women with fistula does seem to affect the status of the marital relationship. The women who developed fistula before they gave birth to living children were more likely to be divorced, and women who were competing with a co-wife averaged fewer children (1.0) than the women with no co-wives (1.3).

The causal relationship is not clear. Women without co-wives may be more sexually active, and thus more likely to eventually bear living children. Or, women without or with fewer living children may be more likely to accept a co-wife into their marriages. Either way, many women with fistula who struggle with fertility are moved into the position of the *bora,* or least favored wife, because they are unable to secure their positions within their households and their husbands' lineages through the birth of children.[23] Thus, for women who struggle with infertility or subfertility, returning home to new co-wives can be especially threatening and often demeaning.

Sexual Lives Transformed

Although rarely discussed, women's sex lives were also transformed by fistula, which in turn affected the stability of their marriages. Deterred by shame over their "broken" vaginas, many women spurned physical intimacy, preferring prolonged separations from their husbands and relinquishing the sexual work of marriage to new co-wives. Yet other women used sex to privately refute accusations of being "almost a man." For sexually active women with fistula, providing their husbands with both sexual satisfaction and with children allowed them to retain their social position and their sense of personal value.

I found a wide range of opinions regarding sex—how often, what kinds of acts, and how much pleasure was typically involved. Younger women and women from villages with greater proximity to urban centers (and thus a larger exposure to media, especially pornography) tended to be more sexually engaged in their relationships. Only in conversations with these women did the topic of female pleasure arise. Many young and peri-urban women had integrated "Western" sexual practices such as kissing, caressing of breasts, manual stimulation of both partners, and even oral sex into their prefistula sexual relationships with their husbands. For others, especially older rural women or women who were married to men they disliked, sex was seen as instrumentally valuable—a means to reproductive success—and an obligation to be hurried through. A woman's preinjury approach to sex most often predicted her postfistula sexual life. In turn, her postfistula sexual life often influenced her postfistula marital stability.

Pleasure, pain, excitement, expectation, desire, or disappointment—among Nigérien women, sex is rarely discussed, and when it is, it is almost always through euphemisms. Still, as an ethnographer who all too often traversed the boundaries of propriety, I found women willing to divulge their intimate secrets. At fistula centers, away from their husbands, homes, co-wives, and families, women had the space to bend their own boundaries.

During an afternoon lounging in a dormitory at a Niamey fistula clinic, I broached the subject of sex among a group of young women. When I asked about orgasms, there was some confusion about the concept. Only Abou (23, Zarma), who had lived with fistula for four years, seemed to understand. She explained to the other women that it was like the moment when you put a piece of candy in your mouth: "you taste the sweetness." She tensed her body dramatically and grinned. Some women knowingly laughed, many covered their faces in embarrassment. Abou openly talked about her sexual desires and the ways in which exposure to Western and Nigerian films, media, and pornography had transformed her sex life.

Most women in the room had seen pornography. According to Abou, "it is on both sides that [pornography] has changed us. Women too, they have changed by watching. Now, women understand everything." Kadigya agreed, "Yes, now we understand that there can be caressing before sex." Although women agreed that many husbands now manually stimulated their wives before sex, there was wide disbelief about cunnilingus, something many had seen in pornographic films. Abou was the only dissenting voice, suggesting with half a smile that "maybe people do this and others don't know . . ."

Women over 40 years old from rural areas seemed less affected by these shifting sexual mores. When I later spoke with another group of women, Sadata (45, Fulani) explained, "If a woman wants to kiss her husband, he will think that she is mocking him. If she wants to touch [his penis], the man will think that it is ridiculous." But this opinion was not restricted to the older generation. For example, Adama (29, Hausa) said, "At the time of sex, there isn't any kissing. It is forceful. [Men] just come like savages to satisfy themselves." I asked about how women perceive this "forceful" sex. Halima (21, Hausa) told me that "if you are already tired, if you've worked all day, yes, you want that too, so that you can rest." Many women viewed sex as a marital obligation. "In the village women work all day—they are tired. So at night, they just want to rest and eat. But she is obligated. She must accept" (Adama, 29, Hausa).

When women's bodies and self-conceptions were transformed by fistula, for many women, their sexual desires receded, shriveled by shame. But the desires remained strong for the young women who had engaged in mutually satisfying sexual lives before their injuries, even if treatment-seeking now posed barriers to their ability to remain sexually active. "I want to lay with my husband," Kadigya complained, after seven months away from him at a Niamey clinic. "I want to be close to him. Many of us do! We are just so far from our husbands. But we will desire them until we are tired."

I asked a group of women beading bracelets one afternoon, "Can women with fistula continue to have sex?" A chorus of women responded in the negative. "No. Our bodies are broken; we must be patient." "Now with fistula, we can't do what we want." But others disagreed. "Even with fistula, you *can* do what you want." "Yes! Without a problem! Your sex life can continue to be normal." "My husband wasn't disgusted. I was with him. It was good." Abou, the always outspoken advocate of mutually pleasurable sexual experimentation, explained, "There will always be urine running, so it will be a little different . . . But for [my husband] it isn't a problem. If I can have children, our lives will be like they were before. It is only me who cannot feel at ease with this sickness."

To save their marriages, reduce their own shame, and enhance their pleasure, many women found inventive ways to mask the effects of fistula during sex. Women spoke of tree barks and "Chinese market medicine" that dried up the vagina, counterbalancing the increased moisture from the urine. Others described elaborate fasting schedules that ran parallel with their schedules of sexual activity, ensuring that there would be little liquid to leak during nights with their husbands. Women even cooked up schemes ranging from preparing their husbands extra heavy food to encouraging notably energetic sex—to tire their husbands out to ensure they wouldn't notice the women sneaking out to wash and dry their bodies, cloths, and pads.

Although not all women discussed their sex lives with me, many had continued to be sexually active after developing fistulas, evidenced by and resulting in multiple postfistula pregnancies. Although 55 women developed a fistula during their first pregnancies, only 34 women had experienced only one pregnancy.[24] For women like Abou, sex was not only about personal gratification or marital obligation, it was strategic. With a coy smile, she explained, "I give [my husband] too much pleasure to push me away. I think he will want me whether I leak or not." And if a child came from it, all the better.

Waiting for Treatment

Waiting, the subject of chapter 5, defines women's experiences with fistula treatment. Ironically, the act of seeking treatment can inaugurate a marital rift. When I first interviewed Agaïcha (29, Hausa), she had been at a Niamey center for nine months without having yet received an operation. Agaïcha believed that her second husband divorced her because of her decision to seek treatment. "He knew my problem [fistula] when he married me. He accepted it. But I told him I would go to Niamey to look for health. He said to me, 'If you go to the hospital in Niamey, consider yourself no longer my wife.' He said, 'If you go, you won't be leaving as my wife.'" Although Agaïcha's husband had accepted her incontinence—he married her after she had developed fistula—he refused to accept her prolonged absence from his household. Her decision to seek care came at the cost of her marriage.

Dr. Youssoufou, a Nigérien fistula surgeon who claimed to have operated on 1,300 women with fistula since 1997, noted that often fistula itself did not cause divorce—it was the long separations due to treatment-seeking. "You have seen that there are women who've left their homes two or three years ago—most husbands won't wait that long. There are some women who have been looking for treatment for 15 years. So it is clear that it will cause a separation, and the husband of course will take another wife . . . Often, it isn't the fistula itself; it is the absence that can cause divorce."

For many women in Niger, the long absences weakened their social networks; they became increasingly peripheral to social life back in their marital villages.[25] Women were often consumed with anxiety at the centers, unsure about when or if they would receive treatment, or whether the treatment would be successful; they were anxious about what was happening at home in their absence. The women worried about their children, wondering whether they had enough to eat or were being well taken of. They were concerned about their marital stability, knowing that each day that passed might bring them closer to divorce, or that their co-wives' exhortations might eventually prevail. As one 34-year-old Zarma woman explained, "One day, even if your husband loves you, if you are not there, one day he won't be comfortable with you. He will listen to what your co-wife, his family, or your neighbors say." To secure their position in the household, some women preferred to delay treatment until they birthed and weaned additional living children, carefully managing information about their condition while they waited at home.

Fistula did not always cause an inevitable and definitive rupture in marital status. Sometimes, it actually solidified marriage bonds and buttressed structures of support between women and their husbands and co-wives, kin and community. Other times, fistula treatment-seeking—a woman's quest for bodily and social normalcy—resulted in separations and periods of conjugal uncertainty, offering either partner an opportunity to be liberated from unhappy or undesired unions. After the development of a fistula, often both husbands and wives acted strategically as they determined what the injury's impact on their marriage would be. Fistula could offer a socially sanctioned point of marital rupture, freeing a woman from the obligations and responsibilities of marriage, or stripping her of the marriage's benefits and social protections.

While the women were seeking health care and navigating new reproductive, corporeal, and sexual realities, their husbands typically did not immediately divorce them. The husbands tended to adopt a wait-and-see approach, often diversifying their assets by investing in additional wives and children. Frequently, the principal marital threat came not directly from a woman's husband but from his other wives. Smoothly functioning polygynous households require both a prudent husband who is just and equitable with his wives and has sufficient household resources to diminish the potential resentment and silent warfare over resource allocation between wives. However, such equitable distributions of time, money, sexual interest, and emotional closeness are rare, particularly in the face of fistula—a condition that may result in substantial economic loss, long periods of absence, and sexual abstinence due to a woman's incontinence.

Fistula often increases household tension between the co-wives and between the woman with fistula and her husband. Although co-wives can materially and emotionally support women with fistula during times of illness, jealousy and intense competition over resources can mean that fistula damages the delicate household calculus of conflict versus cooperation between co-wives. Fistula may be leveraged to gain power within the household, damage a co-wife's status within the community, and alter or dissolve a co-wife's relationship with a shared husband. Many women's co-wives protect the integrity of their households, caring for the husband and children while the woman with fistula is too ill to do so or away seeking treatment, but this protection comes at a cost. Often co-wives actively attempt to push out their leaking competition.

Writing about the social consequences of fistula, journalists, humanitarians, and scholars frequently describe women as having been "abandoned" by their husbands (see, for example, Alio et al. 2010; Brugière 2012; Kristof 2003; Michaelson 2018; Miller et al. 2005). However, these reductionist typologies transmit very little of the texture of women's conjugal experiences, and they obfuscate the multifaceted transformations in marriages affected by fistulas. The category of "abandonment" forces diverse marital configurations and their meanings to be understood through a singular lens of victimization. But only rarely did fistula result in victimization—in experiences of asymmetrical, uncontested expressions of power or domination. As so many of these women's narratives demonstrate, the onset of fistula did not cause an inevitable and definitive rupture in marital status; instead, fistula affected Nigérien women's marriages in unexpected ways, often characterized by overlapping experiences of love and disappointment.

PART 2 CLINICAL ENCOUNTERS

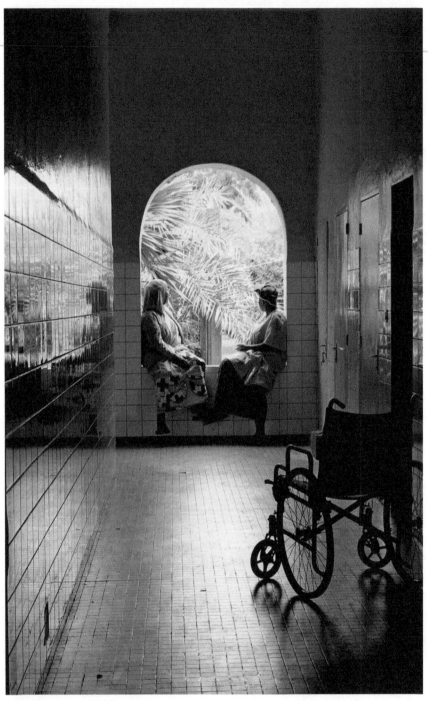

Midwives taking a break at the Maternité Issaka Gazoby in Niamey

SIX BEDS, SIXTY MINUTES

Just like traffic patterns, the hospital had its own rush hours. "Monday mornings are the worst," the nurse told me as we plodded through crowds of women at the Maternité Issaka Gazoby. "Women wait at home all weekend, then come to the hospital after things have become urgent. You haven't finished with one patient before three or four more urgent cases need your attention." As we walked, the nurse dressed me in an oversized white coat, the sartorial symbol that opened all doors. She left me in the emergency triage and treatment room, where women from all over Niger were referred for eclampsia, obstructed labors, advanced gynecological cancers, and other gynecological and obstetric problems.

I had first come to Niger in 2010 as a doctoral student in anthropology to study maternal health. In the summer of 2013, I found myself at Maternité Issaka Gazoby, the top public hospital for women's gynecological and obstetrical care in Niger. So many of the women with obstetric fistula in Niger, women I had come to know over the years, had eventually found themselves at this center, the last link in a broken referral chain. I was looking for answers to the question, "What went so wrong?"

The emergency and triage room was small, filled with six narrow examination tables, leaving vacant only a single, person-sized aisle. With space for little else, the room was spartan: one standing yellowed light, a box of blue latex gloves, a bookshelf buckling under the weight of thousands of pink intake folders, and a few weathered chairs pushed along the perimeter. Within these walls, within a single set of patients, within the rotation of a clock's big hand marking one single hour, are the quotidian realities of maternal health and reproductive injury in the African Sahel—both the challenges practitioners face and the battles women fight. Here are six stories from a single hour in this room.

BED 1: SUFFERING IN SILENCE

At 9:00 A.M., a woman arrived with a half-delivered baby boy. She was torn, and he was stuck. After some expert navigation by the midwife, the baby was delivered; despite his difficult delivery and a few noticeable anomalies, miraculously he was alive. His mother, however, was the worse for wear. As the midwife stitched up her gaping flesh, the woman grimaced, and she clenched her teeth. Silently, feverishly, she massaged her abdomen each time the needle plunged back into her skin. The midwife had not given her anything to dull the pain. "If she needs it, we will give her Tylenol after," the midwife assured me. "I hear in your country, women fear pain. I hear that women take medicine so that they feel nothing. They can't really consider themselves mothers." The midwife shook her head as the needle sank again into the new mother's torn flesh. Blood trickled down her legs and pooled beneath her. Still, she did not make a sound.

BED 2: TRANSGRESSION AND TRICKERY

At 9:10 A.M., a woman with wide facial features and a haggard red and black wig shuffled in. She made pained expressions. She groaned. She screeched. "She's not Nigérien," a midwife told me with visible disapproval. "That's why she's crying, that's why she's making a scene. It's shameful. Nigérien women aren't like that. They are courageous." The woman and I chatted, and I learned that Grace was from Togo. She had moved to Niger to marry, but it had not gone well. Her husband was inattentive, and they were struggling financially. When she discovered that she was pregnant with an unwanted fourth child, Grace felt out of options. With cautious whispers and darting eyes, she confided that she had taken medicines from a local healer to abort the pregnancy. I wondered if Grace's grimaces and moans were born from pain—the physical consequences of an unsafe abortion in a place with no legal means for a woman to choose—or if they were instead performative, a theatrical attempt to conceal her transgression of the law.

Grace asked me in a hoarse whisper, "They will take it out, won't they?" She looked at me with pleading eyes. "I have three kids already, and there's no money now for another. There is just no money. I need work. They must take it out." The emergency room filled up—two dozen people squeezed inside a space no bigger than a bedroom. The smells of sweat and blood and vomit and amniotic liquids mixed in the air, a vile potpourri. Grace quieted down, reanimating with displays of pain only when a nurse caught her eye.

BED 3: THE INVISIBLE CRISIS

In the early morning, the third bed had been occupied by a woman with a transverse fetus, then later by an older woman with a large vaginal tumor. Both women had waited silently, until they disappeared behind a tattered screen. Around 9:15 A.M., the room was no longer so tranquil. A young Fulani woman was wheeled in, just referred from a rural health clinic. It was not clear if she was conscious. Her neck was limp, and her head dangled off the back of the wheelchair. Suddenly, her head shot up as she vomited repeatedly down her front, soiling the silver *hijabi* pulled down around her neck. She jerked and began to fall toward the tile below.

My hand braced her shoulder as I struggled to keep her upright. "Let her fall," the midwife instructed. The young woman tumbled to the floor, arms and legs akimbo as eclamptic seizures gripped her body. Workers, patients, and clinician stepped over her in their own race to heal or be healed.

BED 4: WHO YOU KNOW

At 9:30 A.M., a woman in an embroidered white dress with a plump face and round belly drew the attention of all the nurses and passing doctors. Other women were losing blood, losing consciousness, losing continence, and losing babies, but I could not tell what this woman might risk losing. Her urgency was not visible. She would get up every twenty minutes or so and walk to one place or another, undergoing blood tests, ultrasounds, and consultations with specialists. In her absence, women would slip onto her bed, hoping to be seen by the nurses in the interim. When the young Fulani woman from bed three sprawled on the floor and began to seize, I stepped backward and bumped into an immaculately dressed *Hajiya* (an affluent woman who has made the pilgrimage to Mecca). After apologies and introductions, I learned that the *Hajiya* was the hospital's former director. The inexplicably well-cared-for woman in bed four? Her daughter.[1]

BED 5: THE MALADY THAT MUST NOT BE NAMED

At 9:45 A.M., an older woman contorted her face in pain as she slowly, with careful attention, removed her blouse. Her left breast hung low—a flat and flaccid marker of her fruitful reproductive years—but her other breast was hard and high like an oversized artificial breast, but blooming with red and white sores, pus, and exposed tissue. The sores had consumed her nipple, which was no longer visible, and blossomed underneath her arm at her lymph nodes. This is breast cancer in the Global South, where the disease is often a taboo and undocumented illness (see Livingston 2012; Van Hollen 2018).

"It is a neuro," the doctor told the elderly woman. She did not know that a neuroblastoma is a malignant cancerous tumor in nerve tissues, but that was the point. "Sometimes," the doctor told me, "I tell them it is a tumor, but we never use the word cancer here." Cancer is thought of as a death sentence, and patients lose hope, he explained; instead he endorsed an unspoken policy of paternalistic beneficence. Just from a quick glance, the doctor knew that the woman's cancer had metastasized. He could see it in her lymph nodes. He could see its movement across her body. With few words, and even fewer answers, he left the elderly woman alone on the plastic table, struggling to dress herself, clutching a prescription for acetaminophen (Tylenol).

BED 6: THE LIVES THAT COUNT

At 10:00 A.M., a thin woman curled up on a mattress on the floor, and next to her was a shadow of a baby—a skeletal thing that had come into the world too soon. The mother was severely anemic and could not produce any milk. For four days, this three-pound infant had not had a drop to drink or eat. He was quiet. There was no elasticity to his skin. Through his nearly transparent skin, every rib was visible. His rapid heartbeat sent vibrations across his chest. His mother rocked him, but the movement seemed dangerous, as though it risked shattering this child who resembled a sculpture made of blown glass.

"Can't we do anything for this baby?" I asked the nurse. "Is there no artificial formula for babies like this?" "Why?" the nurse asked me in response. "The mother isn't well. What happens if the child lives and the mother dies? And even if the mother lives, so you feed the baby today. Look at that woman; she can't afford formula. What happens when you are gone? Who will feed the baby then?"

In Niger, where rural child mortality is over 16 percent (down from 35 percent in 1992), few mothers expect all their children to make it past the age of five; nearly half these children die in infancy (DHS Program 2018). Parents wait a week to give a baby a name, and when a baby dies, parents mumble prayers of renunciation and acceptance: Allah did not intend for this baby to continue on earth. It was not its time. It was not Allah's destiny. As this mother held the fragile being, shaking him a little too fast, holding him a little too hard, I wondered if she had already resigned this life to "destiny."

THE THRESHOLD BETWEEN LIFE AND DEATH

I had come to Maternité Issaka Gazoby in an attempt to retrace the steps of women with obstetric fistula. Many of the women I knew had at one point found themselves at this hospital, or a regional hospital like it elsewhere in the country. In Niger, the maternity hospital is the terminus of a catastrophic delivery gone awry. As the fees at Issaka Gazoby are often 10 times as high as those at lower-level centers, few women go there who do not have to. Often women woke in an unfamiliar room with blood seeping through bandages on their abdomens— the stinging from their emergency cesarean delivery the only clue as to what had happened to them. Some had been unconscious when they came through Issaka Gazoby's doors, sometimes after days of referral after referral, up through a long chain of mid- and low-level health centers. Many of these women could count themselves as near misses—women who barely made it off the delivery table with their lives. Many who survived were permanently marred from a long battle with their own body, their own child.

Although my research took place mainly in four fistula centers across Niger, I had come to the Maternité to observe how emergency obstetric care was administered. What kind of patients found themselves in the hospital's crowded wards? Who left surrounded by their family, with an infant nestled in their arms? Who hobbled out, arms empty, leaking urine? And which women were covered unceremoniously in cloth and carted from the hospital without breath? I had come looking to understand the context, to get a fuller picture of maternal health in Niger.

Walking the grounds of the maternity hospital, I watched as women sat on woven plastic mats in the sandy outdoor passages, cradling sick children in their arms. Older women sat patiently with their own adult daughters, whose *hijabai* tumbled over their pregnant bellies but failed to hide the worry and pain that flickered across their faces. I walked through the halls of the hospital rooms, where laborers threw buckets of soapy water to chase the blood out over the low thresholds into the sand.

In a hospital like Maternité Issaka Gazoby, I am always reminded how different the experience of pregnancy and birth is in much of sub-Saharan Africa, where each labor is a risk—where women go to great lengths to hide their pregnancies until they are safely home with their baby. *Ta cin wake,* ("she ate beans"), one says of a pregnant woman among the Nigérien Hausa, afraid of attracting the attention of evil spirits, superstitious that just saying the words out loud might somehow jinx her or her child. The concern with the fragility of mother and child during pregnancy is understandable. In Niger, over 5 percent of infants die before they reach one year of age—10 times higher than the infant mortality rate in the United States in 2018. The disparity is even more striking for women. In Niger, 550 out of 100,000 women die from preventable causes related to pregnancy and childbirth (World Bank 2018). In the United States, the maternal mortality rate is 14 out of 100,000; in Greece, it is 3 out of 100,000. The probability of death from a maternal cause for Nigérien women is at least 165 times higher than for women in the United States.[2] In Niger, each pregnancy is a gamble, and the risk compounds over a lifetime. This is the context within which fistula occurs.

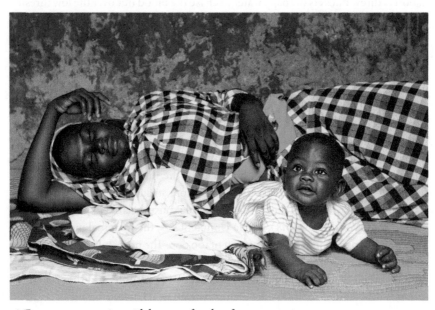

A Zarma woman resting with her son after the afternoon prayer

4 · THE "WORST PLACE TO BE A MOTHER"

Raha's story was difficult to follow. Her narrative bounced across decades, husbands, and biomedical and supernatural understandings of the world. Frequently she would stop midsentence, critically eyeing my research assistant, Rahmatou, or pinching my biceps or belly. "You two are too thin. Are you sick? Aren't you hungry? You should eat something," she would exhort, reminding me more than a little of my own grandmother. Raha spoke quickly. She was 60, or maybe 40, but possibly 70, she told me. "We villagers don't have a good sense of time."

Raha, married at the age of 20, had carried 12 pregnancies, had endured 12 deliveries or miscarriages, and had mourned the loss of all 12 babies. She had struggled with infertility throughout her life, and claimed to have carried a single pregnancy for 10 years, evoking the Islamic concept of a "sleeping fetus."[1] Her first husband was a maternal cousin, and after 17 years, with only 12 small bodies buried in her yard to show for the time gone by, she left him. "People would gossip about me. Once people saw that I was pregnant, they would begin to say that I would miscarry or deliver a dead baby," Raha lamented as she strung together bracelets of iridescent plastic beads under the uneven shade of an acacia tree. "Women the same age as me no longer wash [menstruate], many have more than 10 children. My sister-in-law was married the same time as me and now she has 14 children. But I have none. One of my sisters says that I am not even a woman because I don't have a single child." Raha paused her beading, then added, "I believe that she was right."

In Niger, as in many places across the globe, children are conceptualized as a source of wealth and personal value (Izugbara and Ezeh 2010; Hörbst 2015; Wall 1988). Nigérien women are defined largely by their reproductive capacity and are not considered fully adult until they have children (Janssen 2007). Because adulthood and individual worth is so strongly linked to reproductive success, being childless in Niger incurs high emotional, social, and financial costs for women. The inability to bear living children can cause extreme anxiety about the future, social vulnerability and marginalization, personal devaluation, and familial shame (also see chapter 3).

Some women told me that their incontinence posed fewer social problems than did their lack of living children. Raha, who developed a fistula during the protracted delivery of her twelfth pregnancy, claimed to manage her incontinence quite effectively (although uncomfortably) with a catheter and black plastic bag tied to her thigh. But there was no parallel way to manage her infertility, no way to hide what she and her community believed to be a malediction. Her "broken vagina" resulted in excoriated thighs, money spent, and delicate social maneuvering. But Raha believed that her "cursed uterus" rendered her socially irredeemable. Childless, not a mother and so not quite a woman, she was a "waste of life."

The intense social expectations surrounding fertility often drive women and their partners into an unrelenting "quest for conception" (Inhorn 2003). For Nigérien women, infertility's social and emotional consequences are often amplified because, in high-birth rate Niger, infertility is a kind of "barrenness amid plenty" (Van Balen and Gerrits 2001). Such reproductive realities constitute what Marcia Inhorn calls the fertility-infertility dialectic: very high rates of infertility often occur where fertility is highest (2007). Both primary and secondary infertility are particularly prevalent in West Africa generally, and in Niger specifically, in part because of untreated reproductive tract infections, unsafe abortions, harmful obstetric practices, and poor access to quality care.

According to most recent estimates, in 2010 just over 2 percent of child-seeking women in Niger were unable to attain a live birth, and 10 percent were unable to have a second child (Mascarenhas et al. 2012). These figures represent a decline in rates of infertility in sub-Saharan Africa since 1990, probably associated with general improvements in maternal health in the Global South, where maternal mortality ratios have fallen by as much as 44 percent worldwide, and by 37 percent in Niger (Mascarenhas et al. 2012; World Bank 2018).

These are the numbers—wholly abstract and perhaps of questionable accuracy (Oni-Orisan 2016). But numbers do not tell us much about the real experience of infertility or birth in Niger. As Claire Wendland reminds us, "Indicators have power in part because they make statistically—and politically—malleable stories in ways that individuals' lives do not" (2016, 77). These deeply-flawed statistical artifacts reveal nothing about the experience of reproduction in a country regarded dubiously, by the global media and humanitarian community, as "the worst place in the world to be a mother" (BBC 2012; Save the Children 2012).[2]

In a place where motherhood is at the center of a woman's identity and social value, what are the social and emotional costs of childlessness and infertility when one's body "fails" or is failed by the health system? What is the experience of birthing in such hostile terrain? What risks are women willing to take to achieve motherhood? These questions are particularly salient given the poor, often hostile care that women regularly receive in Niger's rural health clinics. Through ethnographic engagement with women's painful recollections of their labor stories, we can better understand how women fall through the cracks of Niger's health care system.

It is surprising that so many women dutifully continued to give birth in decaying health centers that are crippled by structural inadequacies, practitioner corruption, and patient mistreatment and mistrust. "Despite widespread discontent with unsatisfactory and often blatantly discriminatory practices, everyone lined up to visit the doctor," Adeline Masquelier noted of a Hausa health clinic (2001a, 287). Perhaps, Masquelier suggested, the fantasy just out of reach, the "illusion" of progress, prosperity, cleanliness, and care, was better than no care at all. I found that women were also compelled, both emotionally—shamed by public health interventions focused on moving birth out of homes and into clinics—and financially, facing fines for laboring at home. In rural Niger, parturient women enter into what Masquelier calls the state's "hollowed out" health system. The encounters within the health care system between patients and practitioners, whose interests continuously collide, is rife with obstacles and moments of friction.

FAILED WOMANHOOD

In Hausa, the word *wabi* denotes a woman whose children all die. As women with fistula tend to experience higher than average percentages of child mortality (see the previous chapter), this pejorative term was a familiar one around fistula clinics. For example, Tamoutan (age 40, Tuareg), who had had eight pregnancies and no living children, explained that although no one treated her poorly because of fistula, she was mistreated because of her failed fertility. "Some people would say, 'You there, *wabi!* You don't even have children. You just give birth to dead kids. Get out of here!'"

Women frequently claimed that children protected them against the harmful social consequences of fistula—particularly divorce. Many women who were divorced after fistula attributed their marital dissolution not to the condition itself but to fistula's implications for their future fertility. Zuera (26, Hausa), with three previous pregnancies and no living children, explained that childless women are ridiculed, rendering them especially vulnerable to divorce or marital mistreatment, as husbands are affected by community members' gossip. "People will say, 'She only eats and shits; what's her use?'" Ashamed, and perhaps afraid that people will suspect that it is he who is impotent or otherwise to blame for the infertility, a husband's feelings toward his wife may harden.

Children are extremely important in Niger. Rural Nigérien women birth an average of 8.1 living children, slightly higher than the national total fertility rate (the world's highest) of 7.6 living children per woman (INS and ICF International 2013). Of women aged 45 to 49 who have completed their families, 37 percent have birthed 10 or more living children (INS and ICF International 2013). Many Nigériens consider numerous children both an economic asset and a religious mandate, an opportunity to provide Muhammad with more disciples on Judgment Day. In an economy firmly rooted in agriculture and pastoralism, a large family translates into laboring bodies. Children also allow women to concretize familial alliances, enter into perpetual cycles of gift and debt within extended relations, secure their place within their households, and ensure support in their old age. Despite their utility, children in Niger are not conceptualized as a means to wealth but as wealth itself—a notion known in Hausa as *arzikin mutane* (wealth in people). Their value transcends the practical.

Lacking the social and emotional ties created by children, the childless women I met perceived a social invisibility, vulnerability, and discredit that left them unmoored in social space, jeopardizing their place within their social networks, households, and communities. Infertility also struck women at the core of their identities, redefining who they were as women and as adults. Hadjo (18, Zarma), who had no living children, explained that "you can't be a woman when you aren't married, and you can't stay married without having children. It is only young girls that aren't married and have no children—not adult women." Hajo's claim that fertility is crucial to successful marriage is supported by research. When Nigérien women were asked in a national survey how many children they would have if they could plan their ideal family, women reported an ideal fertility size of 9.2 living children, increasing to 9.5 among married women (INS and ICF International 2013). Nigérien men, in the same survey, reported an ideal family size of 11.5 children, increasing to 13.0 children among married men. For women like Raha, Tamoutan, Zuera, and Hadjo, who will never be able to give a partner the dozen children they desire, constrained fertility severely restricts marital prospects, and is socially aberrant and personally distressing.

The social and emotional pain of childlessness and thus failed motherhood— seen as failed womanhood, and to some extent, failed personhood—was particularly acute for women like Raha, who had suffered a high number of stillbirths. These women dealt with the parallel challenges of incontinence and illness management and the repeated traumas of infant death, social alienation, increased vulnerability to divorce, and internalized identity loss that infertility brings. In Niger, where the common Hausa proverb *haifuwa maganin mutuwa* (only birth cures death) prevails, remaining childless was not a socially viable option. So despite the high costs to them—potential repeated pregnancy loss, dangerous complications, and physical injury—women who had previously faced obstetric disaster continued to try for children.

THE IDEALIZED BIRTH

For Nigérien women able to conceive and maintain a pregnancy to term, the act of labor is imbued with cultural meaning, providing women with the opportunity

to demonstrate their courage and patience through the mastery of pain and suffering. Women are expected to birth silently and alone. Although women recognize that the "ideal" birth cannot always be achieved, the enduring preference to
birth alone is tied to a desire to accrue social status and avoid spiritual risk.[3]
Through silent and unassisted births, Nigérien women hope to avoid evil spirits
during a dangerous and vulnerable time of transition; to demonstrate courage,
strength, stoicism, and patience in an effort to achieve an idealized womanhood;
and to prevent the social repercussions of a poorly performed labor.

Regardless of age or ethnicity, the women I spoke to agreed that showing too
much distress during labor, including verbal and physical signs of pain such as crying or flailing, brings shame on a woman and to some extent on her family
(through an unspoken transitive property). Shame is particularly prominent in
the lives of women in Niger (see chapter 2), mediating most interactions and
impacting women's sexuality and reproductive health. Shame, or modesty, dictates
that a young woman avoid broaching inappropriate topics, calling her husband
or first child by name, or making direct eye contact or speaking familiarly with
those to whom she has a relationship of respect. It also dictates various reproductive health decisions (Pierce 2007). Among the Hausa (of Niger and Nigeria),
kunya or shame (also translated as deference, modesty, or respectful avoidance)
plays an important role in daily life. Similarly, Zarma women's relationship to *haawi*
(shame) dictates the boundaries and exigencies of relationships and social
constraints on personal conduct. Fulani have an analogous relationship to shame
or *semteende,* an integral component of *pulaaku* or "Fulaniness." For women in
Niger, shame (*kunya, hawi,* or *semteende*) is a way of life.

Aminatou (45, Hausa) explained, "If you cry, or let the pain get to you [*jin
zahi,* literally, feel heat], you will feel nothing but shame after." To avoid shame,
insults, or community gossip, laboring women must avoid complaining, being
alarmist, talking too much, excessive movement, screaming, kicking, flailing, or
any visual or audible cues of suffering or struggling. Because mastery of one's
body in the face of extreme pain is difficult, many women prefer to birth alone.
Freed from the gaze of onlookers, a woman's grunt or whimper, tear or flail is
unobserved and so, has no social consequences.[4]

Nigérien women from all ethnic backgrounds share the ethos of the idealized
lone birth. Although birthing norms are rapidly shifting due to increased national
and international efforts to move birthing into clinics, more than 70 percent of
births in Niger still take place at home, and approximately 20 percent of births
are completely unattended.[5] In comparison, the rates of unattended birth among
rural populations in Niger's neighboring countries range from 1 to 6 percent.[6]

Because an unassisted birth holds so much cultural and personal value, local
Nigérien midwives support women in the prenatal and postnatal periods but do
not typically assist in deliveries.[7] Among the Hausa, *ungozoma* (local midwives)
serve as ritual officiates of pregnancy and childbirth, administering ritual baths

after delivery, caring for and inspecting the new child, and properly attending to the powerful placenta.[8] Although some women recounted stories of *ungozoma* or elder female kin or neighbors gently guiding the fetus during delivery, either through light abdominal massages to "wake up" the baby and encourage its descent or by attaching fabric around a woman's torso to stop the baby from ascending (also see Smith 1954; Wall 1998), most women were adamant that *ungozoma* "don't do anything" until the labor has finished. During labor, the *ungozoma's* value lies elsewhere—she is trained in the Qur'an and capable of reciting prayers of protection. Nearly all laboring women drew on these prayers, amulets, and (to a lesser extent) herbal tisanes to encourage the healthy progression of labor.[9] Yet, when birth complications arise at home, in the absence of a skilled local birthing expert there are relatively few practical interventions upon which rural Nigériens can rely.

Women and their families spend large sums of money on religious and herbal remedies during halted or otherwise problematic home labors, but these strategies also cost women precious time. As families rush to find an *ungozoma or a malami* or *marabout* (Muslim religious specialist, teacher, or scholar) able to write, or at least recite, prayers, or a *boka* (local healer) capable of finding or mixing remedies of barks or herbs, the obstetric complications worsen. With little infrastructure in place to facilitate the quick movement of people or procedures, a rural Nigérien woman facing an obstetric complication at home awaits a host of delays.

UNDERSTANDING MATERNAL MORBIDITIES

An estimated 15 percent of pregnant women globally develop complications during pregnancy or delivery (Essien et al. 1997). When these complications are not treated expeditiously by trained practitioners, women are at risk of morbidities ranging from damage to pelvic structures to infertility to so-called near-miss events, in which women nearly die but survive. Time is of the essence during obstetric complications. With hemorrhage, death can occur within two hours of the onset of bleeding. Eclampsia can kill a laboring woman within 10 hours, and obstructed labor within 72 hours (Bates et al. 2008). Just as quickly, a woman can sustain serious, life-altering disabilities.

Given the importance of rapid treatment for obstetric complications, Sereen Thaddeus and Deborah Maine developed the three phases of delay model in 1994 to identify the types of barriers to timely treatment of obstetric complications and the resultant poor outcomes. The first phase is the delay in deciding to seek care after the onset of complications. Second is the delay in reaching a health facility once the decision to seek care has been made. Third is the delay in receiving medical care once the facility has been reached. First-phase delays (prolonged laboring at home) often result from a complex interaction between objective factors surrounding available health care (such as distance, cost, and quality) and one's subjective experience (perception and expectation of care), synthesized within a broader context of gender, household decision-making processes, and socioeconomic and educational status (for example, the expectation in Niger that women give birth silently and alone). Second-phase delays (prolonged laboring on the road) are physical barriers to reaching health care facilities, including transportation, cost, and facility distribution. Finally, third-phase delays (prolonged laboring at health care facilities) reflect inadequate health care systems lacking in skilled staff, supplies, medications, and organizational efficiency, or practitioner bias based on their perception of patients' wealth, ethnicity, or social status.

Many of the women experienced all three phases of delay during the labors that ultimately resulted in their fistulas. The experience of Habsu (20, Kanuri) illustrates this. Habsu resisted her marriage to a maternal cousin, and once married, they fought mercilessly and she often fled from him. They were both young and intractable, and they did not care much for each other. When the contractions of Habsu's first labor began, her husband punished her out of spite by hiding her cell phone and forbade her calling her grandmother. "He said that I didn't need help; he said I could be strong and courageous and birth alone." Alone in her room, Habsu labored for three days. "During these three days, I knew that there was a problem. For three days I couldn't walk around, I couldn't urinate. I knew that I was broken." On the night of her third day of labor, Habsu felt panic. "Will I die here?" she asked herself. Driven by fear and excruciating pain, she furtively slipped from her house while her husband slept and called her grandmother for help. "She said that my husband wanted me to die, that's why he didn't bring me to the hospital."

Here, Habsu experienced a first-phase delay—prolonged labor at home.

By the time her grandmother made the long journey across the Niger-Nigeria border to Habsu, the child's head had been delivered, but the rest of his blue body was still stuck inside her. The nurse at the local health center took one look at Habsu and shook his head—there was nothing he could do. Habsu's grandmother hired a mule cart to take them to the nearest hospital. The roads were poor and the distance long, and with Boko Haram active in the area, they were forced to take an even more circuitous path. The trip took them nearly 18 hours.

Now, Habsu experienced a second-phase delay—prolonged labor on the road.

When they arrived at a Nigérien health center, Habsu's grandmother heard rumors from other family members waiting there that the hospital's doctor exploited women in need. Habsu elaborated, "There was a man who operated on women there, when he performed surgeries, he would also profit by taking out organs from the women to sell. The women told us that if he operated on me, I would die. They said that just that day, there were two women who died because of him. So my grandmother refused to let him operate on me."

Habsu believed that the hospital staff were angry with her for refusing care (and thus, she reasoned, denying them an economic opportunity), and that they punished her for it: Habsu was left for a full day and night without any intervention. Eventually, the long-dead child was removed with forceps.

Finally, in the practitioner's denial of expedient care, Habsu experienced a third-phase delay—prolonged labor at the health care facility.

The next day, Habsu asked her grandmother, "Women that give birth, does their urine run like this?" She lifted her wrapper to show her grandmother the urine that had pooled between her legs. "The nurses said that they didn't know what I had. They sent me home, and it wasn't until the next year that we heard of this sickness of urine."[10]

The Nigérien Health System

In the context of an obstetric complication, rapid entry into a system of quality care is essential. Unfortunately for women like Habsu, the shortcomings of the underfunded and understaffed Nigérien health system can result in increased danger, not its resolution. The public Nigérien health system is organized into a pyramid with three levels. At the bottom of the pyramid, community health centers (*cases de santé*) throughout the country offer preventive care and the most basic health services. These health centers often serve as birthing women's entrées into the health system. Low-level health centers are intended to rapidly identify birthing complications and refer women to higher levels of care. In the middle of the pyramid are integrated health centers (*centres de santé intégrés*, each headed by a nurse), district hospitals, and regional hospitals. Yet the efficiency of the pyramidal structure frequently breaks down: referrals are delayed and they often move horizontally rather than vertically. Additionally, the quality of care at these midrange canters is often poor; fewer than half of Nigériens have access to the minimum package of health services at integrated health centers (République du Niger 2017). The top of Niger's health pyramid consists of national hospitals (of which the Hôpital National de Lamordé is one) and a single national maternity hospital (Maternité Issaka Gazoby).

Paralleling this public health system is a private health system of missionary and nonprofit medical centers and for-profit health centers, including hospitals, specialists, and laboratories. Many private for-profit health centers are staffed by physicians who also work in public hospitals; for a premium price, these clinicians offer patients evening and weekend access to their services.

Niger is divided into eight regions and 36 districts; six of these districts do not have any health facilities at all and 11—nearly one-third—have no hospitals or maternities (Blanford 2012). In six of the eight regions in Niger, there are approximately two doctors for every 100,000 people. In all of Niger, there are only three doctors for every 100,000 people; for comparison, in the United States there are 255 doctors for every 100,000 people, and Cuba has 750 doctors for every 100,000 people (République du Niger 2017; World Bank 2018). Approximately 650 doctors, 5,500 nurses, and 1,000 midwives care for the entire population of more than

20 million Nigériens (République du Niger 2017). In addition, the Nigérien system's caregivers are concentrated in urban areas, leaving rural areas with little medical coverage. Although fewer than 6 percent of Niger's population lives in its capital city, over half of all doctors, 22 percent of all nurses, and 45 percent of all midwives are concentrated in Niamey (République du Niger 2017).

Given that Niger's fertility rate is the highest in the world, women are repeatedly exposed to the risk of obstetric complications throughout their lifetimes. The understaffed and unevenly distributed health care workforce means that women are unlikely to receive high-quality maternal health care. The dynamics of the health care system partially explain why birthing injuries such as obstetric fistula are so prevalent in Niger.

First-Phase Delays: Prolonged Laboring at Home

Habsu experienced dangerous delays throughout her birthing process—on the road and at the health center—but the first delay she faced was at home when she wasn't allowed to leave. Although most women's first-phase delays were structural and logistical, some were due to locally held meanings, values, prohibitions, and practices.[11] In Habsu's case, she lost precious time because of gendered inequalities—a woman's lack of decision-making power or autonomy. Similarly, Laraba (26, Kanuri), who had fled from her husband, was in labor for two days before heading to a health center. When I asked her why she waited so long at home, she explained, "I couldn't go by myself—I couldn't decide by myself to go. I had to be brought. It was up to the family to decide when it was time to go. I had been chased away from everywhere, so I had to listen to my aunt. I didn't have options."

Other women were delayed by the reliance on and belief in the efficacy of local treatments (such as herbs, prayer, or light touch), the suspicion of and mistrust in biomedical health facilities, and the shame incurred by the inability to birth alone and unassisted that is implicit in birthing at a hospital. Young primiparous women in Niger lack autonomy and the perceived experience to decide when to seek biomedical care for birthing complications. They must rely on more senior members of their household. But because residence patterns are patrilocal, young brides may feel extra shame (*kunya*) in voicing concerns to their husband's mother, father, stepmothers, or aunts. Recall the cultural taboos around sex and birth (discussed in chapter 2), and the centrality to Nigérien and Islamic culture of the sense of shame (which also encompasses a kind of deference or respect). Because of the shame that surrounds sex and birth in Niger, and the heightened humiliation that women feel when they are unable to achieve the idealized Nigérien silent, solitary, stoic birth and must access biomedical intervention, women of all ages are often triply reluctant to voice concerns about their births and their bodies when they suspect problems.

Most fistula prevention and eradication efforts focus on reducing prolonged laboring at home (first-phase delays). The reasons behind these delays are presumed to be primarily "cultural." The assumption is that because of familial negligence, "traditions," or "ignorance," women wait too long at home before seeking emergency obstetric care. Habsu and Laraba are exemplars. For example, in a study on fistula in Niamey, Idi Nafiou and colleagues concluded that a woman with fistula is "a victim of traditions dictating early marriage and delay in the search for obstetric care, even when such care is urgently needed" (2007, 573). The president of the nongovernmental organization (NGO) Dimol explained, "Fistula is a problem that mostly affects women in rural areas where the women have no access to health services, where ignorance and tradition prevails over common sense" (IRIN Staff 2007a). In these formulations, women like Habsu, restrained by their kin and husbands, refrain from seeking health services until the physiological damage has already been done. As a result, fistula prevention efforts often discourage home births, encourage prenatal care (to familiarize women with health care systems and thus increase the chances that they will use health services during delivery), and focus on persuading husbands, parents, and in-laws of the importance of rapidly seeking care for parturient women.

But Habsu's story was not the norm. For most women I met, protracted labors at home were not due to familial negligence, overt gender violence, or "tradition," nor could they be attributed to ignorance. Rather, the delays in evacuating women with complicated labors from homes to health centers were most often due to the confluence of multiple political, economic, and logistic factors.

For some women, political instability rendered travel to health centers unsafe. The Islamist militant group Boko Haram has terrorized northern (and particularly northeastern) Nigerians with brutal and indiscriminate violence since 2009.[12] Rahila (25, Hausa-Tuareg) had been living in a village outside of the northeastern Nigerian city of Maiduguri, the epicenter of Boko Haram's violence. She labored at home for four days before seeking care at a health clinic. When I asked Rahila why she waited so long at home, she explained at first, "It is the Tuareg tradition to stay at home and labor," but then added, "It was a period with a lot of political activity—campaigning and propaganda—so the roads were very busy and not very safe." Rahila's husband had been abducted and hanged just two months before her due date by men affiliated with Boko Haram. Paralyzed by fear, she tried not to leave the house during the remainder of her pregnancy. Despite her complicated delivery, Rahila considered traveling during labor to be less safe than remaining at home and attempting to manage the complications herself.

The prohibitively high cost of hospital or clinic births was enough to keep other women home. Women worried about the aggregate costs of birthing outside of their homes, including the costs of transportation, clinic fees, medicine, and opportunity costs, both their own and to those who would accompany them (who, as a result, could then not sell goods in markets, work in fields, or tend to responsibilities at home). Tshara (40, Hausa) was in labor for four days at home before

deciding to seek care at a clinic. She explained that "to give birth in a hospital fin-
ishes all of your money" (*haifuwa asibiti, kashin kudi ne*). People in her village,
particularly the old women who often attended births, advised Tshara's family to
wait, knowing that a hospital delivery was expensive and potentially avoidable.
So, she said, "We waited to see if I could do it on my own." When it became clear
that she could wait no longer, Tshara's mother took her to a hospital. But they did
not go to the closest clinic, which was missionary-run and charged for deliveries
and for the hospital bed. Instead, they traveled over 100 additional miles to Sokoto,
Nigeria, where they knew that a hospital delivery was free.

Many women expressed a need for time to prepare for their long journey to a
health facility. For example, although Yaha (30, Hausa) intended to birth at
the health center, she labored a full day at home first because she and her family
had to "prepare ourselves and find the money to go." Women were often delayed
by waiting for family members or their husbands to return from fields or markets
to accompany them on their journeys to hospitals.

Women also explained that it was not clear at what point a normal, unproblematic birth became complicated and in need of specialist intervention. In
fact, it was not always clear to the women when their labors had begun. Naio
(29, Zarma), who had given birth five times previously without complications, was
told by a nurse during prenatal screenings that she had a high-risk pregnancy
and needed to give birth in a clinic. She was not told what was wrong or what to
look for, but she and her husband agreed to a clinic-based birth. Still, Naio spent
over three days at home before going. She explained, "For each time before, when
the labor began, it always started with a stomach ache—then the child would
move. But [this time] it started with the liquid running, and I wasn't used to seeing
this, so I didn't really know what it was or what to do." When Naio decided to go to
the health center on the second morning of her labor, no one else was at home, and
she had no means of contacting anyone. Unwilling to travel alone a long distance
while in such pain, she waited until her mother and husband returned from the
market and distant fields. Many women who labored too long at home explained
delays as a function of uncertainty about when labor had begun and whether it was
progressing normally, compounded by delays in preparing for the journey and
waiting for accompaniment.

Second-Phase Delays: Prolonged Laboring on the Road
Second-phase delays refer to the obstacles women experience in reaching a health
care facility once the decision to seek care has been made. The anticipation of
second-phase delays may also prolong first-phase delays: lack of transportation,
poor roads, unsafe passages, distant facilities, and prohibitively expensive evacu-
ation affect families' calculations regarding care seeking, encouraging women to
wait until a concern has become a crisis. Second-phase delays are thought to be

such an important factor in the development of fistula that the Hamlin Fistula Hospitals in Ethiopia concluded that "fistula is the result of obstructed labor and obstructed transport" (Hamlin 2004).

In Niger, public transportation is limited and personal car ownership is extremely rare; as a result, transportation is predominantly by foot or animals such as mules, camels, or horses. For 25 percent of the population in Niger, the nearest health center is a 4 to 24-hour walk (Blanford et al. 2012). Journeys take even longer during the wet season when many of Niger's roads (90 percent of which are unpaved) become impassable. After the rains, more than 75 percent of the population must travel more than an hour by foot to reach health care (Blanford et al. 2012). For some women in the Agadez and Zinder regions of Niger who must pass through the Ténéré Desert, the journey to the nearest health center can take between two to four days (Blanford et al. 2012).

Although among the women I talked to second-phase delays were not as significant as the first- or third-phase delays, Nigérien women did express concerns regarding the cost of, access to, and safety of transportation and the distance to health centers. Saouda (30, Zarma), who was in labor for three days, explained that only on market days (held once a week) were there ever any cars in her village. When she experienced complications in her delivery, her husband hired a mule cart to take her on the several-hour journey to the nearest health center. Gripped by disorienting pain, Saouda fell out of the cart twice during the bumpy ride. When she could no longer continue in the mule cart, she and her husband waited several hours on the road until a car passed and took them to a health center.

Sakina (20, Fulani) labored at home for two days before her family decided to send her to a health center. However, because no regular transport was available, her family had to raise over 100,000 Franc CFA (approximately US$161) to rent an entire taxi for her (the cost is typically shared among many passengers). "My family had to sell a cow to get the money. It took some time for them to find a buyer. We waited a very long time for my father to get the money. By the time we reached Zinder [hospital] I was already unconscious," Sakina recalled. Mariama (50, Hausa) never even attempted to travel to a health center. She spent her entire labor at home. She explained, "In my village, there were no cars, no motorcycles, no mule carts. Nothing! If someone was sick, a group would carry her above their heads on a stretcher. Like that it would have taken days to get to the health center."

Third-Phase Delays: Prolonged Laboring at the Health Center

Fistula prevention campaigns and the logics that surround them situate fistula predominantly as the result of first-phase delays (prolonged labor at home), but women like Habsu underscored the harmful effects of delays in receiving appropriate care at the health care facilities as well. The quality and timeliness of biomedical care received by rural Nigérien women may be the most critical factor in mediating morbidity risk. Of the 97 women whom I worked with who developed fistula due to childbirth (three women did not), only 16 did not at any point during their labors seek biomedical attention.[13] The remaining 81 women sought biomedical care, 38 either immediately or within 12 hours of the onset of labor. These women were not "late to care"—they were failed by care.

Recalling the births that caused their fistulas, women struggled to count the hours or days when they labored in vain. The 97 women who developed fistula due to childbirth labored for an average of 3.1 days in total, with labors ranging from 4 hours to 11 days. Women spent nearly as much time laboring at health centers as they did at home.[14] Although there may be several confounding variables, the tragic outcomes of women's prolonged labors indicate that the quality of care they received at health centers was poor.[15]

Access to care is not the same as access to quality care. Fistula can be caused by a poorly trained clinician keeping a woman at a center for far too long, refusing to refer her to a higher level of care, or performing forceful and inappropriate interventions in the face of an obstetric complication. This decenters the popular public health prevention approach targeting only first-phase delays, which assumes that "changing the culture of birthing" and "raising awareness" about the importance of birthing at a health center will lower the incidence of fistula.

Gomma's narrative of the protracted delivery of her twins captures the frustration, physical pain, neglect, and referral disarray experienced by many rural Nigérien women. In a largely futile attempt to access care, Gomma (25, Hausa) spent over a week moving between four health centers and two hospitals.

> I started my delivery at home, and I spent two days in labor before I went to [Health Center 1] to seek care. There, they told me to go home. I was in too much pain, so I spent two days at that health center, but they didn't even touch me. I finally went back home and spent another day in labor. The baby wouldn't come, so my parents put me in a mule cart and took me to [Health Center 2]. I had gone there for a prenatal consultation, and it was the day of [prenatal] consultations when I arrived. So I had a consultation but did not tell them I was in labor. The midwife saw that I was in labor, but she sent me home anyway. I spent another day at home before returning to [Health Center 2], but the doctor wasn't there, and he refused to come. After a day, he came and gave me a shot—my pain was very strong then. The doctor went back home, and I spent the night alone there. The pain was too strong, so [my husband and parents] decided we would leave to go to [Health Center 3]. But at [Health Center 3] they said they could not do anything for me and sent me to [Health Center 4]. There, I finally gave birth. I spent one week there before I lost consciousness.
>
> Finally, the nurse called an ambulance to send me to [Regional Hospital 1] because there was still another baby inside me. I wasn't conscious and don't know

what happened there, but I was told that the nurses used their hands to get the rest out. When I woke up, they didn't tell me anything, but saw there was a leak and they sent me to [Regional Hospital 2] because they didn't have medicine for my sickness. I went to [Regional Hospital 2] and waited for seven months there before receiving surgery [for fistula]. I was still very sick and couldn't even stand up.

Of Gomma's seven days in labor with her first child (and seven more laboring with her second), only two days were spent at home. While actively laboring, Gomma was refused care by three practitioners and was referred horizontally (to health centers with similar capacities) rather than vertically (to higher levels of care) once. Ultimately, she visited four health centers and one hospital before being referred to a sixth health center where she was treated (unsuccessfully) for the devastating trauma incurred by her poorly managed obstetric complication.

Nigérien obstetrician and accomplished fistula surgeon Dr. Youssoufou explained to me that referral delays might not be caused by practitioners' malice, but by their inability to recognize when a delivery has stopped progressing.

It isn't that the person [nurse or midwife] refuses because they want to refuse. Maybe it is because the person isn't competent enough to see that there is danger . . . The question is does the midwife have the competence to know when the situation surpasses her skills? Once I received a case of uterine rupture. When the woman couldn't walk anymore, she went to a [mid-level health center]. The nurse there didn't understand what was happening, he didn't see how serious her symptoms were, and he didn't do anything. The family saw she wasn't getting care and asked to be referred. I assume they asked many times, because [the nurse] eventually wrote that he was referring her against his own wishes. He wrote "referred by repeated demands of parents" to excuse himself for what he thought was an unnecessary referral. But the referral saved her life.

As Dr. Youssoufou's reflected, the system of referrals in health centers is political. Referral delays expose practitioners' attempts to negotiate between their professional responsibilities and their personal reputations. Practitioners feel shame and embarrassment when referrals are considered by their peers to be unnecessary, but this anxiety about their standing must be perpetually weighed against their accountability for health outcomes and the acknowledgment of their own limitations. To reduce practitioners' anxieties, state-issued guidelines have unambiguously outlined for nurses and midwives which patients should be referred and when. Still, according to Paul Bossyns and Wim Van Lerberghe, "the referral system in Niger exists on paper but hardly in practice" (2004, 2). Most nurses practicing in rural areas disregarded state referral guidelines, and some "never" followed them. One of Bossyns and Van Lerberghe's interlocutors believed that if nurses referred as the guidelines stipulated, "We would become a mere entry point for hospital treatment." Another nurse rationalized referral delay by explaining, "We'd lose all credibility in the eyes of the patients" (2004, 3). Nurses are reluctant to refer because there are no clear benefits from referring, and in doing so the practitioners risk "losing face" with their patient base.[16]

Disinclined to refer, low-level practitioners frequently use referral letters (as noted by Dr. Youssoufou) to exculpate themselves. This was the case with Binta (30, Hausa), who was blamed by the health center in the death of her own child. Binta knew that her fifth labor was not normal. She felt a pain unlike that she had experienced in her previous labors. Although she went quickly to the health center, she spent three days moving through a series of three horizontal referrals. When she arrived at the final center, her referral letter framed her as a "bad patient." "On my referral paper, it was written that I didn't come on time to the center, that it was my fault. But I had spent the previous three days in the health center! The nurses scolded my mother and asked her why she left her daughter to suffer until the baby's head had already come out. The nurses were very angry at us. They blamed the death of the baby on my family's neglect!"

Most of the women I interviewed were referred to two or more health centers before finally delivering. Women regularly experienced referral delays and horizontal referrals to health centers of similar levels of care rather than vertical referrals to better-equipped health care centers with better-trained clinicians. Still, many women were blamed for their disastrous obstetric outcomes.

Clinical Negligence

Lahiya (26, Hausa) was refused care due to confusion surrounding a large fibroid that obstructed her labor for three days. The government-trained midwife in her local health center mistook the visible fibroid for the head of the child and assumed that Lahiya's inability to deliver was due to a "lack of courage." Lahiya's referral to a higher level of care was delayed for two days, and the midwife did not acquiesce until her family offered a large bribe. Even after Lahiya was referred to a higher level of care, the midwife called the regional hospital to state her opposition to the referral, suggesting that Lahiya should not receive a cesarean delivery but be forced to "show courage" and deliver vaginally. The hospital's practitioners heeded the midwife's counsel, leaving Lahiya for two days before performing the cesarean surgery. "They left me alone, in total pain. I felt my body breaking." Unattended in a corner bed, Lahiya lost consciousness and eventually—like so many women—continence. Her story demonstrates the politics of referrals, the inadequacy of practitioner training at lower levels of care, and the ways in which the idealized birth that prioritizes stoicism and the mastery of pain affects the provision of emergency obstetric interventions in rural Niger.

Similarly, Zeinabou's (30, Zarma) labor story also reflects the clinical negligence, or at least its perception, that is common in Niger's centers of care.

My fistula, it was the fault of the nurse in my town. I went to the health center as soon as my labor began. When the complications began, I asked that he send me to another center, but he looked at me and refused. He said that he didn't see any complications. He pushed on my stomach with too much force. Some people have hard hearts.

"Abdominal expression," where a strong force is placed on a woman's abdomen (specifically, the fundus of the uterus) to encourage the expulsion of the fetus, risks uterine rupture, tearing, cognitive disabilities in newborns, and breaches the standard of care.[17] Abdominal expression has been documented throughout West Africa and is still common in many low-level health centers across Niger (Jaffré and Olivier de Sardan 2002; Phillips, Ononokpono, and Udofia 2016; Tebu et al. 2009). The practice is not limited to West Africa; although now prohibited, an estimated one in five women in France reportedly underwent abdominal expression during their labors, for four in five women, their consent was not sought (Kammerer 2017).

Zeinabou, after being subjected to "abdominal expression" for an entire day, requested a referral letter, but the nurse refused. Zeinabou's experience at the health center caused anger within her community. "Many say it is because the nurse didn't refer me early enough that I got this sickness. They think it is his fault. Other women have had bad experiences there too. A neighbor lost her two children because of what the nurse did, because he pushed on her stomach. Now, women will not wait there anymore." Women in Zeinabou's village preferred home birthing, fearing the center and its perceived outcomes, but they no longer had the right to stay home. "In my village, now if a woman stays at home, she is fined 5,000 Franc CFA [approximately US$8], but at the center she only pays 1,000 Franc CFA plus soap . . . Women who have money don't go to the center. They would rather pay 5,000 Franc CFA than go there and be mistreated. Or if a woman's family is from another village, she can go back home and not have to go to the center. But for the rest of the women . . . well, the rule isn't just, but I can't do anything about it."

Criminalizing Homebirths

As in Zeinabou's village, many women reported that their village chiefs, working closely with local health agents, had banned home births. This move may have been in an effort to decrease maternal mortality and morbidity rates thought to be caused by prolonged first-phase delays, and perhaps also to increase the profitability of local health centers and the power of their practitioners. Women who refused to birth in the local *case de santé*, or health center, were subject to a fine, the amount of which varied from village to village. Many health centers were little more than an empty concrete building with few, if any, supplies and often staffed by a nurse with insufficient training. Adeline Masquelier has called these local dispensaries in Niger "places of emptiness," which, despite their decay, "effectively rule over patients through the management of inequalities and the routine impo-sition of discursive techniques that produce control, if not health" (2001a, 270). These centers become loci of corruption, discrimination, and control, reflecting a state whose authority derives from its power to deny and confine.

Hadjo (18, Zarma), who developed fistula after her first delivery, was in labor for seven days, all at health centers. In her village, there was also a steep fine, 20,000 Franc CFA (approximately US\$32), for home birthing. As soon as Hadjo's labor began, she went to her local health center. But these "safe motherhood" initiatives only work when the care women receive in clinics is safer than no care at all, and Hadjo did not believe that this was the case. "The nurses there do not care for women well. If women go to consultations, the nurses and midwives insult them for no reason. Sometimes they call the women 'bastards,' other times they won't even consult them and send them away."

Hadjo paid the nurse 10,000 Franc CFA (approximately US\$16) plus the cost of all medicines and supplies, which was quite expensive compared with other health centers that typically charge between 1,000 and 5,000 Franc CFA for an uncomplicated vaginal birth. "They didn't give me any medicine, and they wouldn't let anyone enter the room—not even my mom to give me food . . . They hit my mom when she tried to come in to see me and give me something to eat. I spent three days without eating," Hadjo recalled. Hadjo also underwent abdominal expression. "There were three women working at the center. Two women would hold down a [laboring] woman, and the other would push on her belly or sit on her . . . The nurse pushed on my stomach, and a fat midwife sat on my stomach." When Hadjo was in the delivery room, four other women were also in labor. None was allowed visitors. One woman died "because they used so much force trying to get out the baby." "After they finished with that woman, they came to me. I was scared. When the nurses left the room, I snuck out and ran away. I found my mom and explained what happened." With the other women who had also run from the center, Hadjo and her mother rented a taxi to go to another health center in the nearest large town.

At the next health center, Hadjo waited three days before anyone would con-sult her, and again, the workers tried to push on her stomach. She explained that they even used a piece of wood to hit her stomach. "They didn't do a cut [cesar-ean] because there was a power outage. One woman was being operated on when the power went out, and she died. So my parents refused to allow them to do this procedure on me." Knowing the dynamics between clinicians and patients in rural centers (and the disdain many practitioners have for noncompliant patients), I asked Hadjo if the staff had punished her for refusing the recommended cesar-ean. She responded that they did. "They ignored me for another three days before even looking at me again."

On the seventh day of her labor, Hadjo had lost consciousness and was sent to Niamey. Within an hour of her arrival, Hadjo was operated on. She did not regain consciousness until a week after her surgery, finally waking to the news of a stillborn child, a fistula, and an emergency hysterectomy. Rendered incontinent "like a child," Hadjo learned at 17 years old that she would never have children.

Whether they went of their own initiative or were incentivized by steep fines, women reported heading to health centers as soon their labors began, only to birth alone in unmanned buildings. They were referred horizontally; were monitored by untrained village health assistants; were left unassisted when nurses' or midwives' working hours ended; were forced to bribe nurses, midwives, or health assistants for referrals; were punished for noncompliance or failure to consent to procedures; or were subject to ineffective and dangerous interventions such as abdominal expression.

Nigérien fistula surgeon Dr. Youssoufou explained that many obstetric morbidities in Niger are due to a lack of competence in health centers practitioners.

What could save mothers and children, what could avoid fistula, is to give birth with a *qualified* attendant—to give birth in front of a *qualified* person. This is different than giving birth in a center. If the person [nurse or midwife] at the center isn't competent, if he can't follow a partogram, he will not have a good attitude toward women.[18] He may mistreat them. One can't just build a center and assume that maternal health will improve. Who will work there? What is the competence of the attendants? ... The quality of the training of midwives and nurses isn't good here. There is a recruitment problem. Anyone can get in [to nursing programs]. There is also a lot of corruption—you pay tuition and you are in. Many people who get a [nursing] diploma don't have competence ... There are midwives who go through three years of training, three years of school, and still don't know how to follow a delivery! How can she get a diploma? She pays for it! A midwife or a nurse who works with delivering women—if that person can't say if the birth is going well, there is no reason to let a woman go there. In the bush, if these people see the head of the child, they think that if they use force and push [on the woman's abdomen] it will come out. And sometimes it does. But other times, it doesn't. And when a woman is tired, they will try everything.

Across sub-Saharan Africa and the Global South generally, scholars have noted that the arrival at a health center does not always mark women's entry into a safe system of health care.[19] Neglect, negligence, carelessness, inexperience, and incompetence are the more insidious counterparts to abuse and torture—all are forms of obstetric violence, regularly experienced by birthing women in rural Niger. Previous studies in Niger show the ubiquity of non-patient-centered medicine, with practitioners regularly demanding extra fees and "gifts," threatening women with physical violence or unwanted interventions, administering unnecessary treatments like the uterine stimulant Syntocinon during labor to charge women and pocket the money, and holding patients (or important documents such as birth certificates) hostage until they pay these unforeseen charges (see Jaffré and Olivier de Sardan 2002; Masquelier 2001a; Olivier de Sardan 2001). The worst infringements of patients' rights in Niger are in delivery and emergency rooms, where the practitioners frequently show incivility and contempt toward patients, extort extra money, and exhibit systematic bias against poorer patients (Jaffré and Olivier de Sardan 2002; Jaffré and Prual 1994; Körling 2011). It is of little surprise that in a 2001 study Jean-Pierre Olivier de Sardan found that midwives matched custom officers as the most feared civil servants, seen as attacking the destitute and making arrangements with the powerful with impunity (Olivier de Sardan 2001; Østergaard 2015).

Women in underresourced health care settings across the globe have associated poor quality of care with both passive neglect and active abuse, but many practitioners see desensitization to patient suffering as an essential survival strategy, the only way to continue working day after day in dysfunctional structures mediated by dire local economic and social realities (Abramowitz and Panter-Brick 2015; Redfield 2013). Nigérien nurses and midwives shifted the blame for "imperfect" care to health system constraints such as the lack of materials and the shortage of clinicians, which impeded them from effectively performing their jobs. The providers felt that being understaffed, underpaid, undersupervised, and overworked forced potentially dangerous triaging decisions and sometimes compromised care.

Forced to reconcile their highly academic, theoretical training with the rather bleak realities on the ground, clinicians must "improvise" or adopt "coping strategies" (Livingston 2012; Olivier de Sardan 2001, 2002; Street 2015). Inexperienced clinicians are expected to provide care beyond their capacities and without supervision. According to Olivier de Sardan (2002), with a mix of "initiation and disenchantment," clinicians just out of training come to internalize and reproduce the local norms of the professional health culture. Postcolonial African medicine suffers from not only a "bureaucratic indifference" generally, but a "medical indifference" specifically, integrated into the professional culture of practitioners, modeled and reproduced in everyday care (Olivier de Sardan 2002). Like all other civil servants, health care providers in bureaucratized contemporary West African states experience a conflict of interest. On the one hand, they are pressured to profit maximally from their position and its privilege (and to spread those benefits throughout their close network); on the other, they encounter a work environment that is "profoundly frustrating"—unstimulating, nongratifying, nondirected, and nonproductive. So "many of them give up, or simply protect themselves (from the situation, from the powerlessness, from the outside pressure, also from the suffering and death of others), by establishing psychological or behavioral barriers between patients and themselves" (Olivier de Sardan 2002, 179). Corruption is certainly present in Niger's health care sector (see chapter 5), particularly for laboring women, and Olivier de Sardan has demonstrated its flagrance and its cruelty, as well as its logic.

PERCEIVED CLINICAL HARM

Many women in Niger have a deeply engrained mistrust of biomedical care. As Zara (27, Zarma-Tuareg) explained, "women are afraid to give birth in centers—it is the fear of dying. If women go to centers, they will suffer much more than at home . . . Most women who die, they die at the health center. Most babies too." Women consider their bodies as completely capable of unassisted and non-medicalized birth, and often, even in the face of an obstetric complication, they blame fistula not on a birth gone awry, or on lack of access to care, but on medical intervention itself.

Iatrogenic fistula, a fistula provoked inadvertently by a practitioner during medical treatment (often a cesarean delivery or emergency hysterectomy), is thought to account for approximately 10 to 15 percent of fistulas worldwide. However, these numbers may be rising, perhaps due to efforts to increase access to cesarean deliveries—a government supported initiative pushed heavily by the WHO. In one study, one-fifth of Uganda's fistulas were found to be the result of "human error" during health interventions, typically from cesarean deliveries. The study's author positioned this as "a dark irony, given that cesarean sections are also needed to help prevent fistulas" (Kardas-Nelson 2013). In Ethiopia, the numbers of new cases of fistula are falling, but the number of iatrogenic fistulas are increasing, and now represent 25 percent of fistula cases (Wright, Ayenachew, and Ballard 2016). Thus, although cesarean deliveries are widely understood to be key to the prevention of fistula, they are also a risk factor of its development (figure 12).

A Sudanese fistula surgeon who visited Niamey as the head of a surgical mission believed that the prevalence of human error was due to the lack of legal or political accountability for practitioners in Niger.

> The problem here is that they don't talk to the patients. Sometimes if I take out a uterus, I explain that it was to save your life. Here I think that they don't have respect for the patients. It is just a personal feeling . . . It is totally different in Sudan—we have a medical council there that will follow you if you make mistakes. A doctor has rights, but so do patients. There are consent forms, and women must sign them before surgeries. The situation is totally different here . . . There is no accountability for practitioners if they make mistakes. Here they have a policy of training doctors to do a lot of cesarean sections to reduce fistulas, but they are actually causing them. I am trying to find an excuse for these doctors, like the working situation . . . . The lights flicker—sometimes they don't stay on for a minute. And in a bad situation, saving a woman's life might be more important. But this can also be an excuse for bad work.

Medical malpractice is certainly an issue in Niger. Still, given the context of biomedical mistrust, more women may *perceive* that their fistulas were caused by

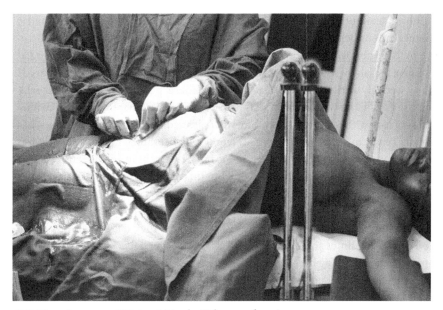

FIGURE 12. A woman at Maternité Issaka Gabozy undergoing an emergency cesarean delivery

medical intervention than actually were. Approximately 20 percent of fistulas in sub-Saharan African countries are suspected to be iatrogenic, but a larger proportion of women may blame biomedical practitioners for their fistulas. When the topic arose among the 100 women I interviewed, 29 expressed a belief that their fistulas had been caused by a biomedical health care provider. For example, Aminatou (45, Hausa) explained, "It comes from Allah—still, *all* of the women here have it because of hospitals, because of midwives."

As has already been made clear, many women receive atrocious care from midwives and other local health care practitioners, which affects how they interpret obstetric morbidities. This dynamic is not limited to Niger; among 86 women with fistula in Nigeria, Beth Phillips and her colleagues (2016) found that 73 percent believed that medical negligence factored into the development of their fistulas, especially the 30 percent of woman who specified a traumatic bodily experience during hospital labors, 20 percent of whom described wailing in agony as practitioners forcefully sat on their abdomens. Similarly, in a study in Uganda, Maggie Bangser and her colleagues (2011) reported that 84 percent of women believed that their fistulas had been caused by practitioners accidentally puncturing their bladders or using force or dangerous instruments (such as forceps) during delivery. In a retrospective analysis of hospital records in the Democratic Republic of Congo, Mathias Onsrud, Solbjord Sjoveian, and Denis Mukwege (2011) reported even more dramatic findings. They found that that 55 out of 229 women (24 percent) who delivered via cesarean had an iatrogenic fistula, but *all* women who underwent vacuum extraction, cesarean, hysterectomy, or other obstetric interventions believed that their fistulas were caused by those procedures.

A Nigérien woman who undergoes a cesarean delivery after a prolonged obstructed labor (when the damage to her pelvic tissue may have already occurred) may wrongly attribute her fistula to the procedure, perhaps because of her relative unfamiliarity with and fear of the procedure, and perhaps due to the coarseness of care with which the procedure was delivered. Because the government has made cesarean deliveries free for all women, the cesarean rate has slightly but steadily increased from 0.9 percent in 1992 to 1.4 percent in 2012 (DHS Program 2018; INS and ICF International 2013), but this rate remains comparatively very low (in the United States, 32 percent of all deliveries are via cesarean). Maou (35, Hausa) explained, "For me, I think that it is the operation. I had never had a [cesarean] before. All I know is that when they operated they cut something. I gave birth so many times and didn't have fistula, but I never had a [cesarean]." Maou's probabilistic thinking here reflects the fact that for many women the delivery that caused fistula was their first encounter with biomedicalized birth.

Many women are suspicious of biomedical intervention's efficacy and safety. This is understandable considering the sample sizes for unassisted and biomedicalized births. Most women in rural Nigérien villages have seen large numbers of home births, and they may have had personal experiences with uncomplicated and safe prior home births of their own. Although Nigérien maternal and mortality rates are high in relation to more developed nations, they are still low enough that a woman in a small village may know of very few women who have had severe negative outcomes from birthing at home. Their sample sizes for biomedical births are small, and they have inherent bias—health centers are typically used only for emergencies, when the outcomes are likely to be poor. Women may therefore perceive an exaggerated risk in biomedicalized births. The prevalence of poor health care (particularly poorly trained practitioners) and the lack of confidence in these systems reinforce the underutilization of the health care system, which likely increases the first-phase delays.

Since the early 2000s, the Nigérien state has made laudable efforts to increase access to maternal and child health care. Many district health centers have invested in ambulance services and have experimented with mobile technology to help bridge the gap between local communities and health care providers. In 2006, the government decreased financial barriers by eliminating user fees for prenatal care, cesarean sections, gynecological cancers, contraception, and all health care for children under five years of age (thus increasing mothers' familiarity and comfort with health centers; Ousseni 2011). As a result, the use of these health services has markedly increased. Between 1992 and 2006, the percentage of rural women in Niger who delivered in a health center remained between 5 and 8 percent, but in the six years between 2006 and 2012 the percentage almost tripled, with home births dropping from 91 percent in 2006 to 77 percent in 2012 (see DHS Program 2018; INS and ICF International 2013).

Many maternal health interventions in Niger, including fistula prevention campaigns, position the reductions of first-phase delays (or prolonged labor at home) as a cornerstone of the strategies to reduce maternal mortalities and morbidities. But fistula is often the result of all three phases of delay: women waiting too long at home, then taking too long to get to a clinic, and then, when they do arrive, waiting too long to receive appropriate care—which may never come at all. The three phases reinforce one another.

Global health campaigns overemphasize cultural and individual access barriers, overlooking the principal factors that contribute to the development of fistula: the structural problems with health systems in Niger that produce second- and third-phase delays. For example, an article entitled "Niger: Why Are So Many Mothers Dying?" suggested that the high rates of maternal mortality and morbidity in Niger are due to individual poverty (preventing women from paying for adequate care), low levels of education, reliance on "religious officials and traditional healers," and "a lack of awareness of women's rights" (IRIN Staff 2007b). The article concludes by quoting a UNFPA officer: "We could have the best health care facilities in the world here, but if people don't understand why it matters, they won't go" (IRIN Staff 2007b). Birthing at clinics is uncritically framed as the key component to fistula prevention. Fistula eradication campaigns assume that the fewer women who birth at home, and the less time they spend there, the fewer fistulas they will get; therefore, they focus on discouraging home births rather than investigating why women opt out of clinical deliveries in the first place.

But most of the women I met *did* access biomedical care—and the quality of the care they received was often exceptionally poor. The clinics are burdened by chronic shortages of trained personnel, drugs, equipment, ambulances, electricity, and running water. Women frequently experienced broken referral chains, the refusal of care, poor-quality care, and inappropriate interventions. For the rural residents of the Sahel, health care does not always or often mean quality care. Unfortunately, women's encounters with the health care system did not improve much once they found themselves with fistula.

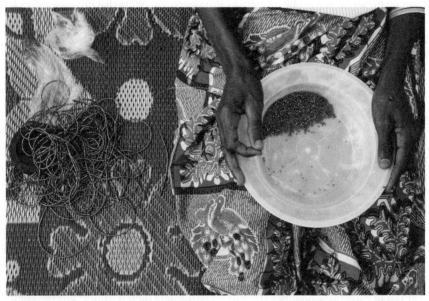

A woman with fistula passing the time at a Niamey fistula center by beading bracelets to sell

5 · THE INDETERMINABLE WAIT

The three of us sat silently under the late afternoon sun. I could hear the sound of a pestle banging spices against a mortar from a few houses down. If I strained my ears, I could make out a voice on the radio wrapped in static praising *Ikon Allah,* the power of God. An occasional rooster let us know that it was still daytime. We sat languidly, waiting. Just sitting. Just waiting.

I had been invited to a friend's house for dinner. I watched Ouma's cousin Saratou prepare *tuwo,* a thick corn-based paste, something she had been at for a while. It was the original "slow food," without Alice Waters' romanticism and a lot more boring. Pots simmered and Ouma and Saratou waited, half listening to the radio's crackle. Quiet and statuesque, seemingly uninterested in chatting, the women sat. Waiting is something that most Nigériens have mastered. Is boredom even a concept that exists among Nigériens? I asked myself. Or the concept of maximizing one's time? After no more than 90 seconds of sitting, I felt the need to look for something productive, or at least distracting, to do. A book? Interview notes? Hausa flashcards? Except for a few Maggi bouillon cubes and a package of paracetamol, my bag was empty. I was woefully unprepared. Watching me wriggle restlessly, my toes boring holes into the yard's orange sand, Ouma reproached me as she might a child, as she had many times before: *Sai hankuri, Aliassu!* "Be patient, Ali!"

Here, patience is a way of life. Don't have enough to eat? *Sai hankuri.* Stomach pain? *Sai hankuri.* Death of a loved one? *Sai hankuri.* When I ask about birthing practices, women tell me that if a woman cries, complains, or moves around too much during delivery, it brings her shame. Why, I ask? *Rishin hankuri,* I'm told, and few things are worse here than demonstrating a lack of patience. *Sai hankuri,* women with fistula tell me when I ask about their experiences with the condition. "Allah gave me this condition; I only need the patience to understand why."

If I had to point to one cultural division between me and my interlocutors (or between the United States and Niger more broadly), it would be that of *hankuri.* I am impatient and obstinate in equal measure; to me, the idea of letting things sort themselves out with time was foreign and unpalatable. And yet each day in Niger was a lesson in patience—one that I could not seem to learn.

Every day I spoke with Nigérien women who had endured hardships beyond what I could imagine, women who seemed forgotten and deprioritized. I spoke with women who had waited months hoping to be scheduled for an operation. I interviewed women who had traveled through a dozen clinics across Niger, Nigeria, and Burkina Faso before arriving to the fistula center in Niamey, only to wait months or years for an operation that never seemed to materialize. Many had left behind parents, siblings, spouses, and children, departing alone on their quest for health. Rahila (age 25, Tuareg) explained, "To me, Niamey was as far away from my home as I could imagine. After Niamey, there was only the great unknown. I cried for three days before leaving my village. But I was assured that here they would fix me. Here I'd regain my life."

Full of anticipation and anxiety, these women make their way to the big city. For months, they wait patiently. Some learn to make small crafts like beaded bracelets or knitted hats, others learn to recite suras—verses of the Qur'an—in Arabic. Mostly, though, they just wait. After months of waiting without having even been seen by a doctor, some conspiratorially whisper among themselves, losing confidence, quietly questioning. Still, few ask directly. No one pushes. It would be unthinkable to demand. Rahila had been waiting at a clinic for over a year and still had not even been consulted by a doctor. She lamented, "Since I've been here, my life has gone by. My sisters and my cousins have given birth. Some have married. But I wasn't there. I missed it all because I was here waiting."

Nafissa, a Zarma woman with high cheekbones and radiant skin, was somewhere between 35 and 42 years old—meaning that she had lived with fistula for between 20 and 27 years. A quarter of a century before, Nafissa had been referred to three low-level health centers when her birth went awry. She labored for seven days. Due to both the length of her labor and bad luck, Nafissa's injury was particularly severe. She had been waiting at the fistula center for four months for her third repair surgery, an operation that she hoped would restore her continence. Yet as the months passed and visiting foreign surgical missions came and went, Nafissa never saw the inside of the operating room. After quick examinations, the surgeons left notes in her chart like "huge fistula," "very difficult," "no cervix," "no urethra/small gap for urine," and "total destruction of uterus." Instead, they operated on simpler cases with better chances of success.

In *Pascalian Meditations*, Pierre Bourdieu wrote, "waiting implies submission," and so it is with many women like Nafissa, whose marginality dictates their temporalities (2000, 228). Nafissa was told little about her body and injury, about the center's timeline, or about her chances for a cure. Powerless, she was told to wait; she was told to pray. So she waited, and she prayed. "I really don't know why I'm waiting," Nafissa told me. "[The doctors and staff] always tell me that they are going to do the operation . . . They say to be patient."

A year after I completed my fieldwork, when I returned to visit the center, Nafissa was still there—sitting on the same prayer mat at the same fistula center, still waiting for treatment. After swapping stories and sharing a meal, I asked Nafissa how long she had been waiting. "Four months," she guessed—the same estimation she'd given me more than a year prior, as though time in the center had ceased to advance. When I probed, Nafissa agreed, "It's a lot. It's more than 12 months . . . We must have patience," she said, turning her head to hide a tear. "I'm just waiting until Allah makes it better." It is difficult to estimate how many years of the two decades that Nafissa had lived with fistula that she had spent on the campuses of fistula centers across Niger, waiting for an as-yet-illusive cure to her incontinence.

Nafissa's experience was common at the four fistula centers where I spent my time in Niger. Surgery for obstetric fistula is frequently described by donor and media narratives as a rapid, low-cost, and highly successful intervention—a panacea, a magic bullet. However, I found instead that repair surgeries were frequently difficult for women to access, and less successful when they finally take place. Women may move through half a dozen to a dozen fistula centers, traversing regional, ethnic, and sometimes national borders.[1] And still, after multiple operations and even more years gone by, so many of them are left incontinent.

Surgical repair is not a discrete event but a process, a waiting game that may take many years (sometimes decades), several surgeries, and an abundance of patience. In the postcolonial, philanthrocapitalistic terrain of Niamey, where fistula care is commoditized and frequently outsourced to visiting teams of foreign surgeons, repair surgeries were maddeningly infrequent. The theme of waiting was woven through women's illness narratives, a complex temporality that shaped their lives as they navigated their bodies, identities, and social worlds. The exigencies and consequences of waiting factored into women's calculus of care-seeking as the liminal state it induced jeopardized their piety and caused social alienation.

THE TEMPORALITY OF WAITING

Waiting is a manifestation of subordination. To dominate is to make others acquiesce to one's timeline, to bend and comply. As Pierre Bourdieu says, "The all-powerful is he who does not wait but who makes others wait" (2000, 228). While power translates into speed, efficacy, and the ability to assert temporal domination, the inverse is also true. For those who are poor, dispossessed, and vulnerable—society's marginal populations—waiting for care or essential services is distressing and disempowering. Waiting is inherent to the human experience (waiting for rain to come, traffic to move, illness to pass, kids to call), but the "raw waiting" that results from structural inequities and power imbalances—waiting that cannot be avoided and must be endured—is a categorically different experience (Sutton, Vigneswaran, and Wels 2011). This type of raw waiting is experienced as less agentive than ordinary forms of waiting or waiting by choice. It situates people in a state of prolonged uncertainty that is "endured because it is fueled by a mixture of despair and hope" (Sutton, Vigneswaran, and Wels 2011, 30).

Sustained by faith in a biomedicine, but often experienced as helplessness, fistula care in Niger was defined by striking imbalances of power. Dispossessed of power, these poor, largely rural and unschooled women inhabited an alienated time ordained by the state, surgeons, bureaucrats, and nongovernmental organization (NGO) workers—the possessors of power. Far from home, unable to feed or clothe themselves at the distant centers, and without the vocabulary or opportunity to engage in a dialogue regarding their health care, women with fistula are obliged to, as Bourdieu describes, "wait for everything to come from others" (2000, 237). The disruptively long waits at fistula centers led to induced passivity, entrapment, and confusion, what Javier Auyero calls the "indignities of waiting" that erode emotional and psychological well-being (2012, 76). And for many women, long waits were a significant barrier to care.

So why did so many women with fistula in Niger continue to wait at the centers? Was it their continued hope for cure? Their fear of challenging the centers' directives? Logistical constraints that made leaving difficult, if not impossible? Yes, it was all of that. But why did women have to wait? Was it unavoidable—dictated by perpetual shortages in the center? Or was it poor organization? Exploitation? Although waiting can be partially attributed to the structural inadequacies of the health care system, women's experiences of waiting in Niger can also be understood through a lens of everyday corruption. Waiting in Niger was a symptom of a health care system heavily influenced by half a century of neoliberalism and its policies of exploitation, which allowed fistula organizations to profit from women's subordination.[2] The women's particularly long waits at the Niamey fistula centers can be explained by three features of Niger's health care system: exploitation and everyday corruption common in postcolonial health care, the ultimately disempowering "gift" of free care, and ineffective care as revealed by the surprisingly high rates of surgical failure.

WAITING PATIENTLY ON THE THRESHOLD OF CONTINENCE

The 100 women I interviewed had waited, on average, 5.8 months by the time I first interviewed them; some had been waiting as long as six years. These times mark how long a woman had been at the center where I first interviewed her, not how long she waited for her first surgery, which may have come many months later, if at all. Many women continued to wait at the centers throughout my research period, and they continued to wait after my departure from Niger. No woman at the Danja Fistula Center had waited longer than three months, but this was not true for the three fistula centers in Niamey, where the average wait jumped to seven months (with a median of four months); but some women had spent eight or nine years of the previous decade at these fistula centers.[3] By the end of my research period, the 100 women had undergone a combined total of 278 previous operations in their lifetimes, and 44 percent of them had endured between three and 11 previous surgeries. For many women, the time at clinics did not represent physical, social, and emotional transformation but one surgical failure after the next, with long waits in between.

The fistula centers claimed to offer a variety of programming for women while they waited—the typical suite of gender-based development training promoted across sub-Saharan Africa and the Global South for the past two or more decades. These include literacy classes and education on income-generating activities, such as sewing, weaving, soap-making, and small-business management courses. Although these courses (see chapter 7) are well intentioned, they deflect attention from the institutional failure that waiting represents, reframing it as a deliberate intervention into women's health. Similarly, women were presumed to benefit from the "sisterhood of suffering," drawing strength and support from other women like them. Fistula centers thus purported to offer these socially marginalized and economically vulnerable women a respite from the hostile social landscapes they were thought to face back home. Fistula centers reframed the experience of waiting, presenting it instead as an opportunity for social, emotional, and economic transformation.

However, the daily existence of women at the three centers in Niamey typically did not contain scheduled programming. The women's days consisted mostly of sleeping, chatting with other women, praying, learning Qur'anic suras, and beading bracelets (figure 13). During my time at the Niamey centers, I witnessed only a handful of training sessions or activities organized for women. Mostly the women helped to cook or clean the center, braided one another's hair, and focused on their own personal hygiene, spending a good deal of the day washing themselves and their clothes, fastidiously avoiding the smell of urine. The women described their main activity at the center as "sitting with patience." Waiting at the centers was particularly trying for women, both because of the duration of the waiting and their physical confinement. Women rarely left the centers; most had no money to spend, nowhere to go, and no one to take them there.

Besides the monotony of everyday of life at the fistula centers, the act of waiting tests women's piety, reshapes their identities, and situates them in a perpetual state of unknowing regarding their bodies and their futures. Waiting has both a religious and moral valence in Niger. The conception of time is co-constructed by local ontologies (be they Hausa, Zarma, Tuareg, Fulani, Kanuri, or others) and by Islam, where time spans both earthly and heavenly existence. Under these various conceptions of time, patience is one of the most central Nigérien virtues. This is reflected in many common Hausa proverbs, such as "patience is the world's medicine" (ha'kuri maganin duniya) and "by bearing troubles patiently one soon sees the end of them" (kome ka yi ha'kuri da shi ka ga bayansa). Waiting is also

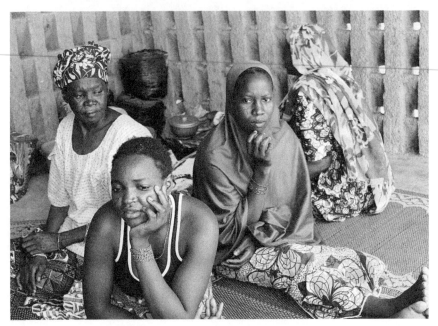

FIGURE 13. Women waiting at a Niamey hospital

given moral texture, as the virtues of patience are exalted frequently and fervently throughout the Qur'an. "And be patient. Indeed, Allah is with those who are patient." "And seek assistance through patience and prayer" (Qur'an 8:46; Qur'an 2:45).

Pati, the Latin root of patience, means to suffer, to endure. And for so many women, patience was painful. As women waited, many confronted their feelings of anger, frustration, and injustice. These feelings were often channeled toward the fistula centers and sometimes toward their families—particularly their husbands—who may have failed to support them through their protracted periods of treatment-seeking. Without work and taken away from households where they might enact the most important marker of female identity—motherhood—many women felt adrift. While some women found comfort through redoubling their religious practice, prayer offered others little respite from their isolation and uncertainty. In the face of these feelings, women struggled to maintain the religious, cultural, and gendered virtue of patience.

THE FOUR CENTERS

One reason behind the long waits is the way surgical interventions are structured in Niger. Although all four sites were considered "fistula centers," they were quite distinct and were characterized by a spectrum of services and opportunities for women. Only one of the four sites (the Danja Fistula Center in Maradi state) provided regular surgeries for women. Another (Dimol) billed itself as a "waiting and reintegration center," offering women a place to live, eat, wait, and receive various training but not medical care (although the women themselves were not aware of this). One center (the National Hospital of Lamordé) operated on only one or two women a week, and these surgeries were halted completely within months of my arrival. The fourth center (CNRFO, or Centre National de Reference des Fistules Obstétricales/National Reference Center for Obstetric Fistula) was the only purveyor of fistula surgeries in the capital for most of the time I was there. The CNRFO was capable of independently providing surgeries to women, but due to financial incentives, it depended heavily on foreign surgical missions. Some centers offered women activities and programs; others offered women little more than a shaded place to spend their days, months, or years waiting. The quality and content of "care" in fistula centers across Niger therefore varied remarkably.

Clinics might be imagined as highly technocratic, medicalized spaces, but this too varied. While Danja was staffed by a full-time surgeon, several nurses, aides, and administrators, the Niamey centers were often staffed only by a guard. At CNRFO, the fistula surgeon rarely visited, leaving all daily administrative and medical responsibilities to one very dedicated head nurse (*major*). Although social workers and a psychologist were technically employed by the state to work at CNRFO, they rarely came; when they did, they spent their short hours in their office, away from the women. The operation theater—largely unused and spatially segregated—became a representation of immobility and inactivity as women waited across the courtyard for its locked doors to open.

National Hospital of Lamordé

L'Hôpital National de Lamordé (the National Hospital of Lamordé) was Niger's only university hospital. Tucked into a corner office near the hospital parking lot, one nurse and a social worker managed the dozens of women seeking fistula surgeries. Lamordé was intended to house women in the short period immediately before and after surgery, but it became an improvised institution of longer-term housing as the women had nowhere else to go during the long waits. Of all the centers, Lamordé afforded women the least space, privacy, or dignity. Lamordé's accommodations were the most basic, consisting of a small, walled-in area located in a highly trafficked part of the hospital grounds near the hospital's main entrance. Often, all 18 plastic mattresses were occupied, and all spaces under the semiprivate, covered concrete structure were claimed by sleeping mats, leaving many women to sleep in the small, open outdoor yard bordering the hospital's main access road. Women frequently complained of vandalism, losing money and cell phones during the night, and they were embarrassed by the treatment they received from passersby.

Women could wait months on end in the small space near Lamordé's parking lot. Fistula cases competed for time with all other urogynecological surgical cases (such as women with pelvic prolapse, who unlike the women with fistula were expected to pay for their procedures), so only a couple of fistula cases were operated on a week, leading to an ever-expanding backlog. For political reasons, some months into my fieldwork the fistula operations at Lamordé were discontinued indefinitely. The women were relocated over the Niger River and across town to the Centre National de Reference des Fistules Obstétricales. Except for the occasional overnight visit for a blood test, X-ray, or ultrasound on the hospital grounds, women with fistula were no longer sent to Lamordé.

National Reference Center for Obstetric Fistula (CNRFO)

Located in a northwest, middle-class neighborhood of Niamey, near the cemetery of Yantala, the Centre National de Reference des Fistules Obstétricales (CNRFO) received both simple cases and referrals for complex fistulas from across Niger. In May 2013, a surgical suite that had been constructed many years before on the campus of CNRFO (but had never been fully operational) was officially opened. In theory, CNRFO would now be able to provide holistic care within the center's walls, and women no longer needed to leave. With six rooms, 35 beds, several administrative offices, outdoor bathroom facilities, two operating theatres, a consultation room, a sewing room, and an outdoor shade structure, the center offered women moderately comfortable longer-term housing. However, during my time there, it remained understaffed; only one nurse and a driver worked regular hours at the center, and a guard and his family lived there full-time. A social worker and psychologist were on the payroll, but their hours were unpredictable. The head of surgery, the center's director, and other affiliated clinicians spent their days at other hospitals and made only irregular visits.

Although the administration told donors (as they had initially told me) that women did not stay longer than three months, women regularly lived at the center for several months at a time and spent as long as two years waiting to be scheduled for surgical interventions. Despite having two onsite operating rooms and the necessary resources to perform surgeries, during my research period there were no regular operations at CNRFO. Instead, every three to six months foreign surgical missions came to the center, resulting in short bursts of surgical activity that benefited only a fraction of the women each time.

The surgical mission came from various countries such as the United States, Turkey, Sudan, or the People's Republic of China. They were often funded by their governments, by large multinational nonprofit organizations, by Islamic charities, or the by Saudi Arabian government as part of broader Islamic humanitarian work. There was some indication that the foreign surgical missions may have offered "bonus pay" to Nigérien staff for their participation, thus disincentivizing the local staff to conduct operations independently. However, the foreign surgical missions came for only a few days at a time, and irregularly at that. This meant long periods of inactivity at the center, and many months of women waiting.

Dimol-Niger

The building that housed CNRFO was built and established in 2004 by the NGO Dimol-Niger (a Fulani word meaning "dignity"). The organization Dimol was one of the first NGOs in Niger to become involved in fistula prevention, treatment, and reintegration work. In 2008, the government took back the land the Dimol center was built upon (effectively taking the center) under claims of mismanagement. This land then became the home of government-run CNRFO.

Believing that the state's actions were unjust and that a judicial injunction would return the center to them, Dimol staff rented a three-bedroom home across the street from the center, hoping to house the women temporarily until they could return to their original land. In 2016, eight years later, they were still located in this house and had no immediate plans to relocate. The rented house had 20 beds that filled two bedrooms and the living room, leaving the third bedroom as an office and consultation room for the on-staff midwife and social worker.

The NGO Dimol bills itself as a "reinsertion" or "reintegration" center, terms used in the fistula world to refer to the process by which a woman with fistula who was once stigmatized due to her condition is healed and returned home with new social (and economic) tools to facilitate her reentry. However, Dimol had an extremely strained relationship with Niamey's sole purveyor of fistula surgeries, CNRFO, because Dimol believed that CNRFO had stolen its land and center.[4] The staff at Dimol refused to take patients across the street to CNRFO. Thus, with no other surgical options in Niamey, Dimol was not actively involved in securing surgeries for women.[5]

How can women be reintegrated if they were not being repaired? In reality, Dimol was more of a fistula waiting house than a reintegration center, housing, feeding, and (some claim) exploiting women for indefinite periods of time as they waited for improbable surgeries.

When I interviewed Dimol staff, each made it clear that their job was to offer women support through the surgical process and to provide postoperative services, not to secure surgeries—a task that they asserted was the woman's alone. Yet all the women waiting at Dimol who I interviewed or with whom I spoke informally claimed to be unaware that they alone were responsible for locating a surgery. When I revealed what the Dimol administrators had told me, women were shocked and felt betrayed. They had been told by staff to wait; they had been told that eventually they would be scheduled for an operation. So the women waited—and they waited for years. They were deaf to Dimol's double-speak and were unaware that Dimol's administration accepted that they would not be surgically repaired. Meanwhile, Dimol continued to receive substantial funding from various national and international donors to house and train women with fistula.

The Danja Fistula Center

Compared to other health care facilities in Niger (and the three other fistula center sites in this study), the Danja Fistula Center (DFC) had the most impressive facilities, the highest standards of care, and the best implemented holistic treatment program. Twice a week, the on-staff fistula specialist, a Cuban-trained surgeon from Burkina Faso, and his nursing staff held a clinic to examine all patients in the 42-bed ward and "the village," the hostel area where women lived and waited. Once a week the DFC staff performed operations. In contrast to the centers in Niamey—even those dedicated to fistula surgery like CNRFO, where women waited for months—the DFC offered many women rapid intervention with the aim of respect and dignity. Although the DFC had been conceived as a training center for fistula repair in the region, at the time of my research the on-staff surgeon was relatively new to fistula surgery and lacked the expertise to operate on complicated cases.[6] As a result, women with particularly complicated cases had to wait months for a more experienced fistula surgeon associated with the center to pass through.

Danja's problem was not the capacity to operate; as mentioned in chapter 1, women were being channeled away from the DFC because of fistula politics— the patterned dynamics of competition over the resources that women with fistula could indirectly command. State systems of referral put in place in the capital meant that even patients from the district hospital in Maradi—only 12 kilometers away—were seldom sent to Danja. Local rumors about Christian proselytizing at the DFC fueled the problem and provided the government with justification for bypassing the center.[7] While the centers in Niamey were awash in patients anxiously awaiting surgeries that never seemed to come, the rural center in Danja had a surgeon, nurses, an anesthetist, medicines, and a full staff—but few patients.

During my fieldwork, I came to understand that the politics surrounding fistula were toxic. Fistula had caught the attention, and the wallets, of Westerners; fistula meant money, and many important people wanted to corner the market. Certainly, I saw good intentions in Niger—humanitarian interest, dedicated practitioners, and quality programming. Yet the dark side of fistula politics, in which women were used as political pawns, all too often dominated the fistula scene, particularly in Niamey.

Information is power, and it does not flow freely. In Niger, communication from funders to administrators often never makes it to center staff, and most certainly never gets to the waiting women. I spent a great deal of time in Niamey seeking information about why women were not receiving operations. I met willing staff after hours, away from the centers' structures and inquisitive eyes and ears. Often I felt more like an investigative reporter than an ethnographer, although I was woefully unprepared for the clandestine meetings and off-the-record divulgences. Still, just as physicians take an oath to do their patients no harm, anthropologists take an unspoken vow to understand and expose systems that prey upon and oppress the marginalized and vulnerable. I heard stories of political intrigue, mismanagement, and corruption. Women were waiting for longer than they should have; women were used as pawns in a political game, because in the fistula world money was at stake. Whatever the politics were, it was not the women who stood to gain from those maneuverings.

In the next sections, I discuss the politics of international aid and the provision of fistula care in Niger. These might be generalizable to other sub-Saharan African contexts, or even the Global South more broadly, but there are particularities in the politics of fistula in Niger. I thus write with this caveat: women's experiences with fistula in Niger are specific to a place and time, and many fistula centers around the world operate effectively and efficiently, which drastically changes women's experiences seeking care.

THE POLITICS OF WAITING AND THE MARKET OF EXPLOITATION

"But why?!" I asked a friend who had been waiting for nine months at Dimol, a center that was neither providing nor actively seeking surgeries for its patients. "What are you waiting for? Why don't you leave? Why don't you go to CNRFO (where surgery is being performed, however irregularly) yourself, or find another hospital?" Zouhera's response evoked the Nigérien concept of shame/respect, patronage, and the submission of those who receive gifts that they cannot reciprocate: "They give us food. We are in their place. We are guests. They told me to be patient. So I will wait until they tell me otherwise." Although she spoke of the responsibility to forbear, her expression betrayed frustration edging on anger. Zouhera could see what I could not: as a neoliberal subject with almost nothing to give, she was not entitled to care.

At independence, many African nations embraced the position that it was the duty of the state to provide universal, quality health care, along with other services, to its citizens. Despite these ambitious goals, left with a rudimentary, under-staffed, and urban-focused health structure—largely designed to ensure the health of Europeans and African civil servants, not the general public—universal free care in Niger was more an aspirational philosophy than an executable policy (Arzika 1992). With few means to provide care throughout the vast nation, the state relied heavily on unfunded and poorly trained community health volunteers (Körling 2011). Medicines were largely unavailable, and rural access was poor (Masquelier 2001a).

But even these modest efforts to actualize the state's responsibility for the health of their citizens through the provision of free health care were derailed by the economic crisis in the 1980s. Niger's growing debt resulted in intervention from the

International Monetary Fund (IMF) and the World Bank, organizations guided by neoliberal agendas that imposed conditions on loans: cuts in government spending, devaluation of the local currency, the withdrawal of the state from public services, the imposition of user fees, and the decentralization of government. The result of these structural adjustment polices on health services were catastrophic: the health system was crippled, users were disempowered (even though individuals were now actively responsible for keeping themselves healthy), and unregulated and often unsustainable NGOs eventually moved in to fill in the gaps in care left by the retreating state. The Nigérien state could not reliably pay salaries, maintain facilities, or ensure the restocking of essential medications, all of which encouraged more venal forms of corruption.

I write with reticence about corruption in Niger. Women like Zouhera are without a doubt victimized by a system within which they have little power or voice, but by structuring the argument with the explanatory logics of "corruption," I fear I am reinforcing prevailing dichotomies of corrupt Africans and Western "watchdogs." As Daniel Smith (2007) has noted, Western donors and development agents' best intentions may have the unintended consequence of reproducing and reifying harmful stereotypes about African corruption. In the process, the discourse of illicit exchange and extortion fails to identify the embedded moral and social economies at play, where manipulations of the system are required for elites and ordinary Nigériens alike who struggle to uphold their parts in relationships of patronage, reciprocity, and obligation. The familiar narrative of corruption sidesteps an in-depth examination of the structures that constrain even the best educated Nigériens from getting ahead in an economy fettered by unfair global political and economic policies.

It is too easy to tell a story of corruption that highlights the exploitation of the innocent. And in the fistula clinics of Niamey, this story takes on a new urgency. But, in the process, let us not efface the larger context: corruption in Niger is a symptom of staggering inequality. As Daniel Smith (2007) recalled from his time working with USAID in Nigeria, a local NGO employee regularly earned one-fifth of his less-qualified, expatriate junior—who was also provided free housing, a guard, and household help. Might the local development workers who divert project resources into their own pockets, Smith asked, see their actions as a kind of compensation for gross inequities? Could the same be said of the Nigérien practitioners working at fistula clinics who are vastly underpaid by the state (assuming that their salaries arrive on time or at all)? How might this influence how we come to understand their reallocation of resources?

As I have explained, for over half of a century Western countries have promoted neoliberal policies that favor market-driven solutions to both economic and social problems in the Global South. The fallout of neoliberalism across sub-Saharan Africa has been staggering, resulting in a massive restructuring of civil society, state pullback from services, and expansive decentralization. Health care has been privatized and marketized, and often NGOs are relied on to assume the responsibilities abrogated by the state. NGOs have proliferated across sub-Saharan Africa, and funding has followed. In 1990, 60 NGOs operated in Niger; today more than 2,600 do (Soumana 2017). By 2010, donor financing contributed nearly 30 percent of total expenditures in the health sector (World Bank 2013). This deep financial investment of international NGOs has, in turn, birthed countless local NGOs—counterpart organizations able to profit from the windfall.

Smith has suggested that development programs provide cover for egregious forms of corruption, within which entrepreneurs "seek advantage and advancement in circumstances of great constraint" (2007, 88). Elites have manipulated the neoliberal promises of "development," diverting resources from the intended beneficiaries—internally displaced people, AIDS orphans, girls seeking an education, women with fistula, whatever the fundable cause—to their own bank accounts and those of their closest contacts.[8] The financial incentives to profit from fistula has resulted in routinized care practices oriented more towards maximizing income generation rather than best clinical or social outcomes.

Fistula care in Niger exists within this neoliberal backdrop, where it is predominantly under the purview of NGOs and thus subject to the demands of the market and the unstable interest of global funders. Everyday acts of corruption may come to seem morally justified to those involved, who may have received no salary for months and must rely on money "on top" to feed and house their extended families. In the field of health, practitioners may charge patients more than the official rates for services, make extra money through the *ristourne* (a share of clinic revenues), administer superfluous—but chargeable—services, expect money to navigate bureaucratic barriers, or demand cash "gifts" (Jaffré and Olivier de Sardan 2002; Körling 2011). However, those working with fistula cannot expect these on-top payment from their patients, who arrive to centers nearly penniless, socially isolated, and largely without access to funds. Not only do the women have no money to give, but the funders have—and are willing to give—much more. So common acts of "everyday corruption" adapt: if women cannot be the source of money, they may be used to attract it.

As Vincanne Adams's (2012, 2013) research in New Orleans after Hurricane Katrina has demonstrated, structural forces keep disaster alive by design. Neoliberal policies have made the exploitation of humanitarian relief easier—or perhaps have even encouraged it—as "disasters are turned into market opportunities for profit" (2012, 186). Adams and Naomi Klein (2007) have examined the exploitation of the poor during large-scale tragedies such as war or natural disasters; however, the recent international attention paid to women with fistula has created a kind of disaster capitalism rooted in philanthropy, or philanthrocapitalism—it takes advantage of a market opportunity to capitalize on *individualized* suffering. In the Nigérien fistula care industry, women are continuously exploited by both private and state-affiliated actors for whom potential fistula funds from development and humanitarian agencies such as UNFPA, USAID, Oxfam, or the International Red Crescent may represent a local actor's best opportunity to not just scrape by but to get ahead. At some centers, the women become de-facto employees—their uncontracted labor is their mere presence. Filling beds at fistula centers is often more lucrative than fixing holes.

The long wait times in fistula centers, particularly in Niamey, reflect a distinctive manifestation of corruption in Niger. Some entrepreneurial Nigériens have identified women with fistula as lucrative sources of funds. As they fill beds, are exhibited to donors who pass through, and are counted on patient rosters, the women with fistula attract money to centers from both international and local funders. Some of that money can be diverted to the pocketbooks of those at the top, although this does not always happen. Women at some centers become the faces of fistula, whose wages are paid in room, board, health care, and perhaps the promise of some sum of money when they eventually depart. But they ultimately benefit little from their labor—profits rarely trickle down.

The centers that are funded for women's room, board, and various training schemes (rather than strictly for surgeries) have little financial incentive to quickly move women through surgery and back home, not when their presence can create both institutional and individual financial gain. There is reason to believe that the incidence and prevalence rates of fistula may be overestimated, leading the centers to become increasingly unlikely to move women along as the fear increases that the patient populations (and thus the funding and organizational raison d'être) are drying up.[9]

The Real Price of Free Care

The fistula care system that now seems so broken originated with the best of intentions. Early in the international movement to provide fistula care, it became clear to public health officials, donor agencies, and clinicians that due to the unique demographic of women most at risk for fistula—poor, rural, and living far from treatment centers—women were often unable to pay for care. Even nominal fees could pose insurmountable barriers to care. Hence, all fistula centers in Niger (and nearly all in the Global South) eliminated "user fees." Surgery, medicines, and room and board were provided free of charge.[10] The cost of care for women at the fistula centers has been provided primarily by donor organizations such as UNFPA, USAID, or the International Islamic Relief Organization, largely with funds from global publics.

This policy, referred to as *"gratuité des soins"* (free care), was in step with a larger movement in the country, and sub-Saharan Africa generally, to eliminate user fees for most maternal and child health care (see Booth and Cammack 2013; Burgess 2016; Diarra 2012). The covered services included comprehensive care for children under five and selective care for pregnant and laboring women, including prenatal consultations, cesarean deliveries, and treatment for gynecological and breast cancers. These reforms were implemented in Niger in 2006, but without any supporting accompanying measures they nearly resulted in the collapse of the whole health system. The state has not been able to afford the cost of the increased demand for services. After six years, the state owed the health facilities 1 billion Franc CFA, and the deficits grow annually. Delayed reimbursements from the state resulted in a hollowing out of health centers across Niger, which could no longer afford to pay staff salaries or restock essential medications.[11]

The policy of free care does not cover the costs of vaginal deliveries or emergency transport, and women are often left heavily indebted—transportation to referral centers can cost more than a cesarean delivery. In recognition of these barriers, most fistula care centers tried to provide women with transportation to and from the center (although not all centers in Niger were consistent in this), hygiene products (such as soap), and small amounts of money or other goods attached to some sort of "reintegration" or "reinsertion" program at the time of a woman's departure from the center. Often small donors attached themselves to the centers, regularly giving women gifts, including fabric, perfume, rice, cell phones, money, milk, sugar, tea, and other goods.

Despite the complete *prise en charge,* or centers' assumption of financial responsibility on behalf of women, women frequently complained of having no money and feeling infantilized. Women felt disempowered by their inability to buy food from local purveyors when they were hungry, phone credit to call home when they were lonely, or new sandals when theirs broke. As women could not farm at centers, they had very few opportunities to provide for even their most minimal needs or desires. Women complained that they had not foreseen the long periods of time that they would be expected to wait at centers, and thus had not come to centers with adequate financial resources to meet their everyday needs.

Additionally, centers—particularly those in Niamey—were often unresponsive to women's desire to leave, occasionally withholding transportation money for the trip home. Sometimes centers did not have the money to reimburse women's costs for transportation to the center; sometimes the terms of transportation reimbursement were inconsistent, leaving women with large debts back home from transportation to the center purchased on local credit. Despite the fistula centers' generous funding for the care of women, financial anxiety consumed many women during their time at the centers. And many center administrators saw women as greedy, expecting funding, refusing to pay any portion of their own care. Considering, however, how many surgeries most women were expected to undergo and how many trips to and from the center such treatments required, it was simply impractical for women to contribute financially to their care.

The tension between women and administrators arose out of a tension inherent to philanthrocapitalism—a power dynamic that characterizes the gift economy within a capitalist market more broadly. As Marcel Mauss has established in the seminal work *The Gift* (1925), giving incurs reciprocal responsibilities. Gifts are never given entirely freely but come with strings attached, binding the giver and the receiver in relationships of expectations and obligations. According to Mauss, when reciprocity fails, the gift economy exists at the nexus of honor, shame, and moral breakdown. Like waiting, receiving is a form of submission; Mauss explains that "charity wounds him who receives" because "to give is to show one's superiority . . . to accept without returning or repaying more is to face subordination, to become a client and subservient" (1935/1973, 63,72).

This power relationship has previously been observed in the context of medical philanthropy. In discussing the relationship between donors and recipients of drugs to treat parasitic infections in Tanzania, Ari Samsky explores the ways that gift giving reinforces hierarchy: "The gifts come, as they always do, with many strings attached, and rather than creating empathy and goodwill between the donor and the recipient, they act to reinforce their separate identities, to valorize the partner who gives and who withholds certain things, and to emphasize the subaltern position of the recipient" (2012, 327–328). In Niger, the gift of surgery, care, room and board, and reintegration—none of which can be reciprocated—reinforces the subordinate position the women already occupy within the health care system (due to their gender, poverty, class, lack of Western education, and general social marginalization). This "free care," in the context of the women's lack of access to money, structured the women's relationship with the centers and with the marketplace around them.

La gratuité des soins partially explains the long wait times at the centers; women are positioned as beneficiaries of "gifts" of care rather than as clients of paid services with rights to demand high-quality, rapid interventions. Indebted and bound by the benefaction of the center, women are often silenced, unable to make demands or speak on behalf of their interests or rights.[12]

SURGICAL FAILURE

If given the space to speak, what would women with fistula ask of centers? Undoubtedly, the answer is surgery. Because biomedicine has been accepted and naturalized as a hegemonic site of power in Niger, surgical procedures are uncritically forwarded by donors, practitioners, and women themselves as an absolute good. Yet, the faith in biomedicine can also cause harm; the unusual complexity of fistula cases in Niger and the frequency of surgical failures leads to consequentially long waits for women.

Citizens of contemporary Niger are ever aware of the "haunting presence of the colonial," a specter of violence and appropriation reflected in underperforming systems, poor governance, and institutionalized assumptions (Good et al. 2008, 5). These postcolonial and capitalist systems inevitably result in illness and social suffering for Niger's poor, particularly those with intersecting identities of marginality. Politics of exploitation engender disparities, exacerbate poverty, and ultimately inflict wounds upon the bodies of Nigérien women. Biomedicine is forwarded as the singular solution to address these broken bodies. But biomedicine is designed to treat only symptoms of ill health, never the systemic, structural diseases of inequity. Highly technical, noncontextualized, and vertical interventions that undergird biomedicine are framed as apolitical, concealing the genesis of ill health: structural violence and systematic inequalities, exacerbated in sites of postcolonial disorder in the Global South (Ferguson 1990; Good et al. 2008).

As is common of "African biomedicine" (Wendland 2010)—where the line between healing and harming can blur—biomedicine often fails Nigérien women. Biomedicine is held up as the gold standard of care for most practitioners and many patients, but a persistent lack of resources fundamentally transforms the practice of biomedicine throughout sub-Saharan Africa. "Evidence-based medicine" and "best practice" as developed and regulated in high-income countries do not account for the technical, social, financial, and even biological conditions mediating the standards of care in much of sub-Saharan Africa. Subject to long waits, exploitative practices, and frequent surgical failures (which then lead to longer waits), biomedicine overpromises and underdelivers for Nigérien women with fistula.

Surgery and Western biomedicine are not a magic bullet for fistula in Niger. Donor and media fistula narratives emphasize the relative ease and inexpensiveness with which women with fistula can be healed through surgical intervention—reporting that fistula surgery successfully "cures" between 75 and 95 percent of cases, with the most common figure being a 90 percent success rate (for examples, see Clinton Foundation 2014; Engender Health 2014; Fistula Foundation 2014; Menard-Freeman 2013; "Obstetric Fistula" [Wikipedia] 2014).[13] However, a handful of peer-reviewed studies have suggested that surgical outcomes vary widely depending on particular fistula characteristics. For example, Rathee and Nanda (1995) found success rates that ranged between 17 percent and 100 percent depending on particular defining attributes, or categorizations, of the fistula. Successful surgical outcomes largely depend on such factors as the fistula's size and location, the degree of scarring and tissue loss, the damage to the urethra, bladder capacity, prior surgical attempts, postoperative care, and the surgeon's expertise and experience. Indeed, not all fistulas are the same, nor do they all have the same likelihood for repair. When fistula surgery is performed under ideal conditions, on ideal patients (women with "simple fistula" who are "new cases"), surgical intervention *can* be quite effective (de Bernis 2007). But the majority of fistula cases in Niger are neither simple nor new.

Although there is no internationally agreed upon classification system, "simple" fistula is frequently defined by some combination of a lack of previous failed surgeries, lack of involvement of other continence mechanisms such as the urethra, and a measurement of less than 3 centimeters in diameter (figure 14). "Complex" fistulas are generally large in size and are associated with severe vaginal

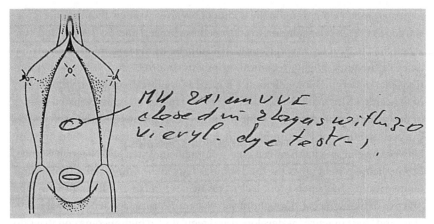

FIGURE 14. The clinical file of a woman with a simple, small fistula measuring 2 × 1 centimeters. This fistula was closed surgically and the woman was negative in her dye test, meaning that no liquid leaked from the fistula (she was continent). Simple fistula may represent the minority of fistula cases in Niger.

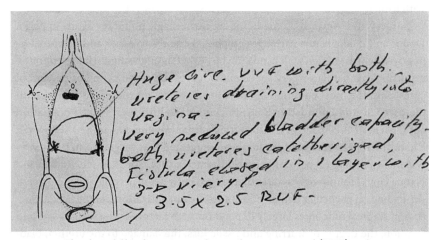

FIGURE 15. The clinical file of a woman with complex vesicovaginal (VVF) and rectovaginal (RVF) fistulas. She developed fistula after her ninth pregnancy. The picture above notes that she had a "huge circumferential VVF with both ureters draining directly into the vagina," "Very reduced bladder capacity," and a large RVF measuring 3.5 × 2.5 cm. She had undergone three previous unsuccessful surgeries.

scarring and reduced bladder volume (figure 15). There is wide agreement that simple fistulas are likely to have good surgical outcomes. But because women who have labored for days without relief often have extensive damage, between 65 and 80 percent of fistulas in Niger are complex, which alters the prognosis (Cam et al. 2010; Falandry 2000; Karateke et al. 2010).

As with simple fistula, women with no previous history of fistula repair, the "new cases," experience much higher rates of surgical success. Surgical failure increases with the number of previous surgical attempts, during which a woman accumulates scar tissue, likely changing a simple fistula to a complex fistula (see Arrowsmith, Barone, and Ruminjo 2013; Cam et al. 2010; Castille et al. 2014; Creanga and Genadry 2007; Karateke et al. 2010; Maulet, Keita, and Macq 2013). Hence, her chances for success become increasingly slim. One study found that the failure rate of surgery increased threefold for "old cases" or women who had experienced one or more previous repair attempts (Holme, Breen, and MacArthur 2007). Similarly, in an 18-month cohort study conducted with 120 fistula patients in Mali and Niger, new cases (with a mean of 1.5 surgeries) were found to have a success rate of 74 percent (23 out of 31). However, only 22 percent (17 out of 78) of old cases (with a mean of four surgeries) attained continence (Maulet, Keita, and Macq 2013). The authors concluded that new cases "stand a good chance of rapid continence gains" while old cases "cling to hope" (Maulet, Keita, and Macq 2013, 531).

And even if a woman's fistula is "successfully" closed following surgery, she may be forced to wait for yet another operation. Researchers estimate that anywhere between 26 and 55 percent of women whose fistulas have been surgically closed will suffer from residual incontinence (Arrowsmith, Hamlin, and Wall 1996; Browning 2004; Frajzyngier 2011; Wall 2016). What Lewis Wall (2016) calls the "continence gap" can be caused by many factors, including the loss of bladder capacity, compliance, sensation, and motor innervation; the loss of coordination between bladder and sphincter; the formation of bladder stones; reduced urethral length; or sphincter disruption or destruction (Arrowsmith, Barone, and Ruminjo 2013; Wall 2016; Wall and Arrowsmith 2007). These women are promised surgical solutions to their residual incontinence, and so they wait at centers even longer for specialists to pass through.

I found that when women were finally able to secure surgeries after months (or sometimes years) of waiting, their surgeries frequently failed (table 3). Of the 61 women who underwent surgery during the clinical stay at which they were interviewed (out of 100 women, 86 were actively seeking surgeries), only 22 women (36 percent) attained continence, and 39 women (64 percent) remained incontinent after surgery.[14] Of the 22 women who attained continence, 16 women (73 percent) were new cases, having previously undergone no surgeries or one surgery before the research period; only six (27 percent) of the newly continent women had undergone two or more surgeries before the research period.[15] The outcomes varied slightly by fistula center: CNRFO/Lamordé had a 31 percent continence outcome, and Danja had a 41 percent continence outcome.[16] Although many factors (including a small sample size) may account for this variation, temporary surgical platforms—such as the short-term surgical missions like those frequently relied upon at CNRFO—have been shown to result in

TABLE 3   Outcome of surgery by repair attempt for 61 women

| Surgical cases | Surgical Outcome* | | | |
| | Continence | | Incontinence | |
	N	%	N	%
New cases				
No previous surgery	11	—	10	—
1 previous surgery	5	—	8	—
0–1 previous surgeries	16	73	18	46
Old cases				
2+ previous surgeries	6	27	21	54
Total	22	36	39	64

*In total, 22 women were continent (36 percent), and 39 women were incontinent (64 percent).

worse outcomes for patients (Shrime, Sleemi, and Ravilla 2015).[17] My data are supported by a country-wide survey by Niger's Ministry of Public Health and Statistics in 2017, which reported that of all 623 women with fistula operated on in Niger in 2016, 52 percent attained continence, with significant variability by center: 35 percent at CNRFO and 43 percent at Danja (République du Niger 2017).[18]

And, of course, a significant portion of the women I came to know did not undergo surgery at all, which is another kind of surgical failure. Twenty-four of the 29 women who did not undergo surgery during the research period were excluded from the operation blocks due to long wait times, infrequent surgeries, and the surgeons' tendency to operate first on the simple cases (which had better chances of success).[19] The majority of these waiting women (15 of the 24) continued to wait at the centers after I left Niger. But a few—nine women—decided that the cost of waiting was too high. "Too discouraged," these nine women "gave up" and returned home without receiving surgeries.[20]

Although the wait times were long for all women, particularly for women at the centers in Niamey, they were also markedly unequal. Women with several previous failed surgeries or with extensive damage tended to stay at the centers months or years longer than new cases or women with simple fistula. Many women who were seeking but did not receive surgical interventions had very large, complex, and potentially "incurable" or "inoperable" fistulas. Some surgeons demonstrated a preference for women with simple cases, no previous surgeries, and thus a higher probability for success.[21] Additionally, under external pressure from funders to produce "better data," or higher rates of surgical success, the fistula centers frequently excluded from operation blocks the women who, like Nafissa, had the most extensive damage (and thus lowest probability of surgical success) (see Heller 2018). Few of these women were instructed to return home; like Nafissa, they were told to wait.

Of the 32 women who were healed at the end of the research period (including 10 women who were dry at the beginning of the research period), 16 (50 percent) were healed after their first surgery, but as the number of surgeries increased, the success rate declined.[22] Women received up to 11 surgeries, but not a single woman was healed after the seventh surgery. Yet many women underwent one failed surgery after the another, spending years at the centers.[23]

"Incomplete" yet "necessary" and "vital," biomedicine in sub-Saharan Africa operates within cycles of promise and despair (Livingston 2012). Despite frequent surgical failures, biomedicine's promise of renewal transcends the data, and the hope for a cure endures—for women, practitioners, and donors alike.

Despite the enduring hope in and promise of surgery, as women watched their friends undergo surgeries but continue to leak when their catheters were removed, they began whispering among themselves. Rather than questioning the potential of a surgical cure, they blamed the surgeon. "He doesn't have eyes. He doesn't fix anything. He only makes it worse," Sadata (45, Fulani), who had had eight previously failed surgeries, said of the fistula surgeon at a Niamey center. "Yes! He complicated everything. He ruined everything. It was worse after the operation than before," agreed Mairi (27, Kanuri), who had had four previous surgeries.

These are not the women of the donor narratives—a cohort of young women, recently crippled by the injury, with high hopes for a quick, successful surgery and easy reintegration into her home life. Instead, 44 percent of the women I came to know had, by the end of my research period, undergone between 3 and 11 previous failed surgeries, making up a cohort of chronic sufferers. As time marched on, their prospects for restored continence decreased, and the social costs of pursuing treatment increased.

CONSEQUENCES OF WAITING

Sadata (45), who had been waiting at CNRFO for her ninth surgery, explained to me how the time away had affected her social network at home. "I've now been here five months. They said they wouldn't operate during Ramadan, but it is now well after, and look—we are still waiting. They say, have patience . . . The problem is, there aren't operations here. I haven't had news of my family. Those who come from far away, it's the same for them. Some women have phones, but most do not. It is hard. And at home, they don't know what's going on here. Some even think that the woman has died when she has been gone for so long. There is no way to know."

Only a few academic studies have examined the long wait times at Nigérien fistula centers—their prevalence and their impact on women's lives. In a study of fistula care in Niamey's National Hospital (l'Hôpital National de Niamey, which stopped performing fistula surgeries in 2011), the long wait times were found to compound social problems of dependence, stigmatization, and social rejection

(Ndiaye et al. 2009). Another study of 52 women with fistula at Niamey's National Hospital also described long wait times, noting that 46 percent of women had waited between six months to one year, while 35 percent had waited more than one year (Harouna et al. 2001). An 18-month cohort study conducted in Niger and Mali investigated the prolonged and tortuous care-seeking process, and found that the median time spent in fistula centers during the study period was seven months. Nine women did not leave the center at all during the entirety of the 18-month study (Maulet, Keita, Macq 2013); of these nine, all had already undergone previously failed surgeries, eight of the nine were incontinent, and two were deemed incurable. Women in this study felt that they were "on hold" during their treatment-seeking process, and they demonstrated an "infinite patience" (Maulet et al. 2015). All these findings—the average wait times, the felt experiences of waiting, and the significantly longer stays of women who cannot achieve continence—match my own findings, bearing out Sadata's story.

The complex reasons for the waits—and the complex reasons for which some women decide *not* to wait—are not part of the dominant narrative of fistula care. This is in part because much of the fistula literature and the media and donor narratives emanate from East Africa, and particularly Ethiopia, the location of the first, the largest, and the most successful fistula centers that are dedicated to fistula repair surgeries—the Hamlin Hospital and their regional fistula hospitals. As noted in chapter 1, at a regional fistula repair center in the northwestern region of Ethiopia, the average patient stay was only 18 days (Hannig 2017). In Ethiopia's sophisticated fistula care system, which dominates the fistula narrative, the long waits experienced by women in Niamey are unheard of. And because waiting does not find its way into the dominant fistula narrative, women who choose not to wait for surgery (or choose not to seek it out at all) are often misunderstood. Women who make an informed choice to return home rather than suffer through prolonged periods of separation from their communities, are rendered invisible. The media narrative assumes that these women do not access care because of ignorance; they are framed as being "unaware" that a treatment for fistula exists or that this treatment is free. For example, the Society of Obstetricians and Gynecologists of Canada's International Women's Health Program explains that despite the affordability of fistula surgeries, many women do not access the procedure because of ignorance: "While most cases of obstetric fistula can be cured by surgical procedures costing approximately $300 to $450, in the developing world, women with fistula may live their entire life with this preventable and treatable condition. Many are unaware that there is a cure and others simply don't have the financial means or access to the procedure" (IWHP 2009).

However, understanding the difficulties women endure at the centers, particularly the long wait times, enables us to see another possibility: that some women make an educated decision to stay home, preferring to live with chronic fistula rather than endure years away from home, thus avoiding the damage such an absence may wreak on their social networks.

These long waits and protracted absences from home have serious consequences for women's social and conjugal lives, often resulting in marital friction or divorce and the attenuation of social bonds as women become increasingly disconnected from their social life back home. It is difficult to keep in touch over long distances in Niger. More than 80 percent of the population lives in rural areas with little to no electricity, limited cell phone reception, and little cash with which to buy phone credit. In these circumstances, women have restricted or no ability to remain in contact with their families once they have left home.[24] In Niger, where polygyny is common, women risk deterioration of social ties, specifically with their husbands, and particularly when co-wives remain at home, vying for position and resources (see chapter 3). This risk alone was often enough to discourage women from continuing to seek care. In deciding whether to embark on, or continue, a quest for continence, the women were far from ignorant; rather, they performed a complicated calculus, constantly weighing the hope for physical health against the risk of social harm.

Women learned upon their first visit to a center that the biomedical solution to their conditions would be neither quick nor certain, and that the process of treatment seeking would itself be costly. So women constructed strategies that balanced their care for their social well-being with their continued treatment-seeking efforts. Sometimes women punctuated prolonged stays at the center with visits home. Women with particularly complex cases for whom the center could not offer immediate surgical solutions or women whose surgeries had repeatedly failed experienced a pattern not dissimilar to seasonal migration—returning home for holidays or for the rainy season to labor in the field with their families, then returning to the center in hopes for cure or for economic reasons.

After months of waiting in vain, Sadata and Mairi sat under a tree at a Niamey fistula center and weighed the relative costs of clinging to hope versus accepting their conditions. Mairi reflected, "Some say that they have had enough with the operations and that they will be patient and live with it. I have a friend, Fati, she had seven operations and said that she had enough. She went home. She got married with [fistula]!" Sadata listened intently, but retorted, "There was one woman I know who was operated on 11 times, and it wasn't until the eleventh time that she was healed. But now she is healed. Sometimes I want to say that I will go home and live with it, but her story gives me hope. It teaches me to be patient. Still, my little brother told me to leave the operations and come home, to be patient and to live with the leaking."

When hope is destroyed or disappointment total, the power of "making people wait" is greatly diminished. Bourdieu reminds us that outside a context of absolute power, an individual can only be "held" and made to wait to the extent that she is invested in "the game"—wherein the person with power and access "delay[s] without destroying hope" and the "patient" is controlled through aspirations and expectations (2000, 228–231). Many women "opt out," accepting (or at least tolerating, then managing) their bodies as they are, and thus regaining power. These women enact a politics of refusal; they return home, still leaking, hoping to salvage what is left of their marriage, friendships, and community connections. Hope of corporeal transformation is exchanged for hope of social harmony.

Health centers and hospitals are often places of imagined transformation—corporeal, emotional, social, and sometimes economic. Yet for these 100 women in Niger, these biomedical centers were less a place of renewal than of stasis and immobility. Paradoxically, while the women's bodies were infrequently altered—only 36 percent of women who underwent repair surgeries during the research period attained continence—their social lives were often unexpectedly affected by their prolonged periods of treatment-seeking. These prolonged wait times on hospital grounds were justified by the fistula centers that assumed the women's social ties had already been dismantled due to fistula, so the long wait times, which benefited the fistula centers in material ways, were infrequently examined. So for months, years, or decades at a time, women attempted to demonstrate that most Nigérien of all virtues, patience—sometimes to their detriment.

PART 3 THE MARKETPLACE OF VICTIMHOOD

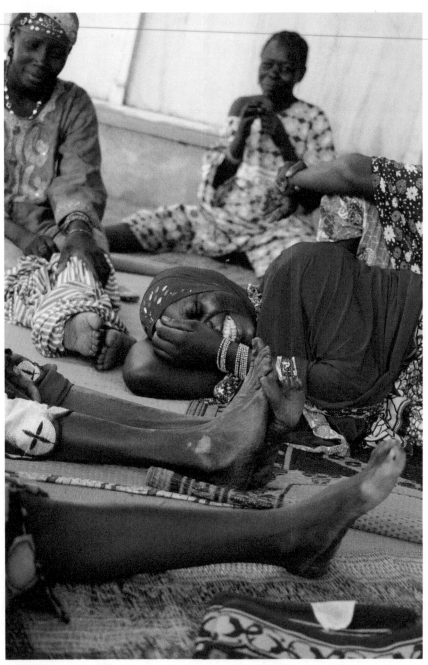

Women lounge outdoors, joking, and telling stories at a Niamey fistula center

ARANTUT'S STORY
The Other Extreme

Fistula has become a symbol of the physical consequences of harmful culture on the quintessentially innocent. Donor agencies and the global media that generate and circulate the narrative of a monolithic (often young and powerless) sufferer do so to bring resources and attention to women with fistula—aims that I share. However, my experiences in the field complicate this narrative of a single type of suffer. As I parsed together story after story of Nigérien women seeking treatment for obstetric fistula, I found neither archetypical sufferers nor archetypical experiences of suffering. The women's stories were as diverse as they were: they were young, and they were old; they were rejected, and they were embraced; they were forced by parents to marry before menarche, and they themselves chose when to join their lives with the men they loved.

Still, the discourse surrounding obstetric fistula presents an archetypical narrative: a woman—a girl, really—is abandoned first by her husband, then by her community, then by her family, until finally she is alone. She is ridiculed, poor, and hungry. She is enshrouded by the indelible odor of urine or feces. And yet, out of the 100 women I came to know, and the dozens more with whom I have informally chatted, I can count on one hand the few who fit this description. The archetypical fistula sufferer—young, abandoned, and crippled by shame—does exist, but she is at the far end of a multidimensional spectrum.

If I placed the women I met on this spectrum, the stories from the extreme ends are both revealing and real, but they are not accurate reflections of the majority of women, who find themselves somewhere in the middle. As a counterpoint to the young victims of fistula who populate donor organizations' pamphlets and reporters' columns, here is the story of a woman who deviates from the norm as much as these abject few. She is the other extreme.

I met Arantut, a Tuareg woman with olive skin and a wide smile, at a Niamey fistula center. Just two weeks prior, Arantut's catheter had been removed, and as she whispered over and over *Alhamdulillah* ("praise to Allah"), not a drop of urine fell. After a yearlong quest for continence, Arantut had arrived.

Arantut was married at 20 years old to the man of her choosing. It was mutual love, *soyayya muke,* between them, she told me. He was her first cousin, but her *auren gida,* or intrafamily marriage, did not bring her problems as it sometimes did for other women with reproductive complications. Instead, she explained to me that because her husband was family, and her mother-in-law was her aunt, they had no choice but to support her, love her, and have patience until Allah saw her through. And they had. She said that through her sickness, her husband never said a bad word toward her. He refused her nothing. He never took another wife. He waited patiently during a year of abstinence while she lived with a catheter.

Arantut developed a fistula during her fourth pregnancy. At a prenatal consultation she was told that her child had a deformation, an enlarged head that could make a natural birth difficult, if not impossible. Such an abnormality was not unheard of where she was from, deep in the Saharan desert where women were regularly exposed to dangerous levels of radiation from nearby uranium mining. So she and her husband prepared. As soon as her labor began, her husband rented a taxi (with money he had been saving since he heard the news of potential complications). By the time she arrived at a health center, she had birthed the hands and feet of her child, but as expected, she was unable to birth his head. The nurse reported that the child had already died; he was cut out of her, piece by piece.

Soon after, urine began dripping down Arantut's legs. She had never heard of any sickness that rendered a woman incontinent; so, she went home and tried to wait it out. But the wetness did not dry. Eventually, after a long and convoluted chain of misdiagnoses and referrals, Arantut found her way to a fistula center. The center had a long backlog for surgeries and was subject to the same political tensions that make fistula repair surgery unattainable for many women. So the center opted to try an older technique: inserting a catheter for a prolonged period, hoping that a respite from urine leaking on the raw tissue in the vagina would allow the hole to heal on its own.

Arantut lived with the catheter, which connected to a small bag to collect her urine, for eight months. She told me that while the catheter was physically irritating and sometimes painful, and she worried that it would not fix her fistula, she never experienced any mistreatment from anyone. No one refused to eat the food she prepared. No one called her names. No one spit when she passed. Despite the discomfort, life went on. And because she lived close to the fistula center, she spent every night during her year of treatment at home with her family.

"You will see," she said to me when I met her at the fistula center. "Come home with me, and you will see. My family will be there waiting. They will say, 'Arantut is home! Thanks be to Allah, Arantut is back!'" Curious, and wondering if perhaps she was withholding experiences of mistreatment, I took her up on the offer—one perhaps made more for rhetorical purposes than an actual invitation, but such awkward impositions are standard, arguably necessary, for anthropological fieldwork.

We passed through the mud archway of her home in a labyrinthine neighborhood inhabited principally by Tuareg migrants from the north of the country. Arantut pushed aside the woven grass mat that acted as a door, and her sister ran to us. Her twelve-year-old daughter flung her arms around Arantut's torso. They ushered us into a small room with mats on the floor—the only room of the house. Her husband, Mohamed, came in grinning, placing Arantut's four-month-old niece into her arms. Her father, who reclined in the shade, beckoned us. I spent the afternoon with her family, listening in as they joked, laughed, told stories, and shared tea.

We reclined on mats and as the sun began to set, I asked Mohamed how Arantut's fistula affected him specifically. "I didn't pay attention to my worries or suffering because it wasn't anything compared to Arantut's suffering," he replied. "Some husbands throw away their wives when they get sick. There are two reasons for this. First, they don't have a strong family connection like we do, so they don't have a strong relationship—Arantut and I grew up in the same house. I was there when she was born. Second, they didn't have strong mutual love (*soyayya*) to begin with, even before she was ill! But we have so much mutual love between us." While Mohamed spoke, Arantut poured herself some tea into a cup already half full of sugar, and laid down on the ground next to her husband. When Mohamed pronounced his love for her, Arantut laughed and playfully pumped her fists in the air in triumph.[1]

Perhaps beyond that placid afternoon, Arantut's neighbors did gossip about her condition, or her friendships did suffer, but the truth remained that Arantut's experiences of fistula were at worst mixed: equal parts of suffering and frustration and social support and compassion. If we accept only one fistula narrative—if we deny that for some, the illness does not disintegrate social networks but reinforces them—then we cannot understand what makes Arantut different from women at the other end of the spectrum. Can it all be boiled down to luck, or is there some confluence of factors (age? parity? ethnic group? severity of fistula? conjugal dynamics? length of time away from family?) that predictably determine where on this spectrum a certain woman will fall?

In 2010, after my first research trip to Niger, my first instinct when I heard versions of the global fistula narrative was to question my data. Why were the stories I heard from the women I met so different from the stories I read in newspapers and donor publications? It took time to realize that perhaps the stories were not so different after all. One woman told me how she often thought things would be better if she were not alive. Another woman recalled how, frustrated by her genitals and how they had betrayed her, she had attempted to slice off her entire vulva with a straight razor. Still, these stories were in context. They were points that punctuated a life narrative, a narrative consisting of both highs and lows. Pain and pleasure. Alienation and acceptance. The same woman who had told me about suicidal ideations also recalled stories of warmth and care from her

friends and neighbors. Her mother rubbed her back as she tearfully remembered these moments of hopelessness. The woman who had attempted to slice
away her leaking genitals also told me of the sacrifices made by her father, uncles,
and brother to find her care, the months they had spent sleeping beside her at
multiple fistula centers across Niger and Nigeria. Perhaps the stories that populate
op-ed columns and hover above red "donate" buttons on fistula organization
websites are not untrue; they simply are not contextualized within the complexity of a life experience.

There is no formula explaining why some women with fistula find themselves
rejected and mistreated while others find themselves embraced and cared for
(although I do offer a few theories); most women find themselves somewhere in
the middle. So I begin by looking at the middle of the spectrum for a more nuanced
and cohesive fistula narrative. What ties these women together? And what can
anthropologists pass on to clinicians to encourage more experiences like Arantut's and fewer from the other extreme?

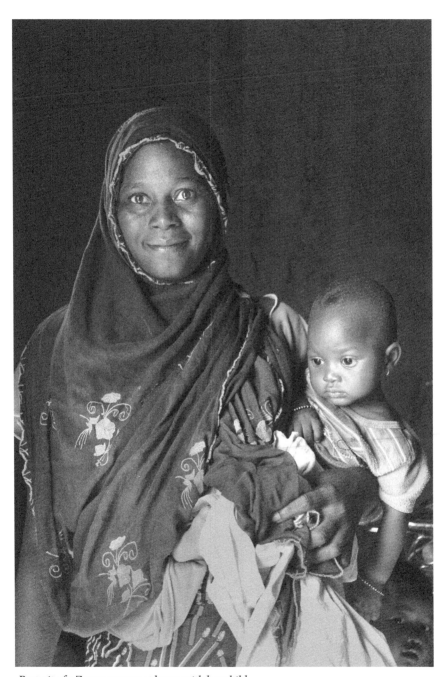

Portrait of a Zarma woman at home with her child

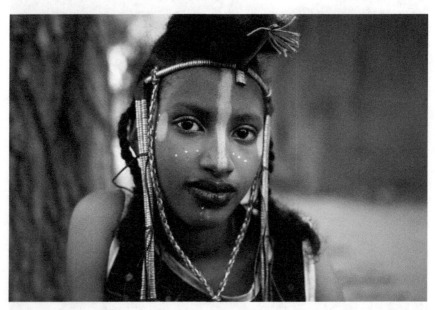

Portrait of a young Fulani woman in Niamey, Niger

6 · SUPERLATIVE SUFFERERS

In May 2013, I spoke over the phone with a reporter at CNN. She was working on a piece about obstetric fistula in Africa to be published in commemoration of the tenth anniversary of the United Nations Population Fund's Campaign to End Fistula. When we spoke, I underscored not just the suffering caused by fistula but the social support it generates. I spoke not only of humiliation but of hope—of resilience, tenacity, and diversity. So I was surprised to eventually read the article's headline: "A Fate Worse Than Death for Scores of African Women" (Winsor 2013). I had spoken with the reporter for two hours, yet only the stories of young girls, gruesome deliveries, shame, fear, and the most severe injuries made it to print.

Typical fistula narratives told in Western media nearly always share the same elements. The sufferers are girls forced into "child" marriages. Due to their youth, potential malnutrition, small stature, and lack of negotiating power within their households, they suffer through a complicated labor for up to a week without any medical intervention. After the birth, when the leaking begins, they are abandoned by their kin and exiled from their communities. Finally, they are physically—but also emotionally, socially, and sometimes religiously—transformed through biomedicine, often at the hands of Western practitioners and the organizations that financially support them.

At first glance, this narrative arc does not appear especially problematic. Simplistic and reductionist, yes, but it speaks to a humanitarian-minded Western audience, inspiring sympathy, offering hope, and setting forth a plan of action. In a world inundated by the relentless noise of catastrophe, the frequencies emitted by individual crises are often out of phase. The destructive interference from the clamor of so much need has rendered the sound waves of global suffering fuzzy, indistinct, or even silent, producing a pervasive apathy. As an ethnographer, I too work to amplify the voices of those who struggle. How will their plight be distinguished from the rest? How will they be heard? In many ways, I share the mission of donor and media organizations: to work on behalf of the disempowered, to elevate their voices, and to set out a path forward. I recognize the substantial hurdles donor organizations and the media face in attracting and sustaining public interest. To draw in the limited and fleeting attention of donors (both large and small) and consumers of media, the humanitarian organizations and the media forward this formulaic and reductionist fistula narrative in which young girls, victimized by their cultures, are ultimately redeemed through biomedicine.

We in the West absorb these narratives, and narratives powerfully shape our perceptions of the world, helping us to "order experience" and even to construct reality (Bruner 1986; Marcus 1998; Mattingly and Garo 2000). Through narrative, we give texture to morality. But when one narrative dominates, it erases the multiplicity of experiences, perceptions, and perspectives. When we retell these dominant narratives, we make a series of political choices. As feminist theorist Clare Hemmings warns of historical narratives, "which story one tells about the past is always motivated by the position one occupies or wishes to occupy in the present" (2011, 13). The same may be said of dominant narratives concerning contemporary events, crises, people, and places—they are political, and they have stakes. These narratives, reproduced and repeated, affect the ways in which we think about an imagined "Africa" and about African women—their bodies, their cultures, and their alleged victimization. Why do we tell the stories we tell about suffering in the Global South? The explanations may be manifold, situated in the logics of humanitarian engagement in a capitalist marketplace, our historically embedded schemas of the Global South and its inhabitants, and gendered patterns of engagement with race and cultural pathology.

THE FISTULA NARRATIVE

First, what is the typical fistula narrative? Like Kristof's article about Jamila (chapter 1), most popular and academic treatments of fistula follow a well-rehearsed formula that includes an array of elements working together for a particular effect. At the center of the narrative is an innocent, typically young, woman, who likely married too young and became pregnant too soon. Divorced, abandoned, and exiled, she becomes an outcast once she develops fistula. It is through biomedicine that she finds hope and renewal. In hospitals, often by Western hands, she is transformed. The names of the women and the sub-Saharan African country that is their backdrop change, but the general contours of the story do not. Individual scholars have contradicted some of the main tenets of this narrative—often one piece at a time.[1] Yet the shape of the narrative remains fairly constant across the various forms of media and organizations that champion the cause. Three primary tropes—or plot devices—constitute a recognizable fistula narrative: innocence taken, superlative suffering, and surgical redemption. Stitched together with the familiar threads of loss and salvation, these narratives reveal as much about their audience as their subjects.

First Plot Device: Innocence Taken

> Poor obstetric care was not the only reason for the fistulas. The other big
> problem was, and still is, that of child marriage … Girls may be betrothed at
> the age of eight and can be married as young as twelve … They are not
> mature enough, emotionally or physically, to cope with a sexual relationship.
> It is rape, really—condoned by their parents.
> —Catherine Hamlin, *The Hospital by the River* (2001, 130)

The first, and most basic, element of the fistula narrative is the portrait of the
woman with fistula herself. The fistula narrative brings into focus a singular
sufferer—young and innocent. She is a victim in all senses of the word. She is a
passive receiver of injurious decisions made by her male kin or husband regarding
her life and her body. She is the Madonna, representing an almost religious purity.
The power of this narrative comes in its moral clarity. In stripping her of any agentive role in the development of her fistula, she is also stripped of agency in its
remedy. She is no longer the protagonist of her own narrative. Organizations, clinicians, and, ultimately, donors are the heroes of her redemption story. Just as she is
harmed by others, she is healed by others through the "gift" of a cure.

The central figure of the fistula narrative is usually portrayed as a mere child,
referred to as a "girl" rather than a woman (for examples, see Hamlin 2001;
Kristof 2005; LaFraniere 2005). She is thereby systematically stripped of the
agency that is assumed to accompany adulthood. As the narrative goes, these
girls are vulnerable to the predation of men. They are wed to men they often do
not know and are carried off against their will at an early age, becoming "child
brides." They become pregnant as soon as they are biologically able, and this
leads to a devastating labor that culminates in the development of fistula because
the bodies of these girls are too small and "immature" to birth a fully developed
child (Wall 1998). Fistula is framed as the physical evidence of corrupted cultural
practices, invoking images of despoiled youth, tainted innocence, and predatory
male elders.

Second Plot Device: Superlative Suffering

> She was never dry, her clothes always soaked, and she dribbled all day. The
> bladder and its urine quickly became infected and foul-smelling. In no time
> her labia, her thighs, became wet and macerated and oozed pus. This must
> have been when her husband cast her off … Suicide was a common ending
> to such a story.   —Abraham Verghese, *Cutting for Stone* (2009)

After leaking begins, women with fistula—they are often framed as women now—
become outcasts, isolated, mistreated, and shunned by their kin and community.

They are divorced by their husbands (for whom the marriage was transactional), and live in dilapidated huts alone, somewhere outside the community. They are left to stew in their own psychological suffering and physical waste. Wild animals are often imagined to circle these huts, preying on the crippled bodies of small and helpless women. Apart from the occasional rotten leftovers thrown to them, the women are left to their own devices. In their isolation and abandonment they are driven to depression, even suicide.

This tightly scripted narrative can be found throughout the global media, including in several award-winning fistula documentaries, internationally renowned newspapers, and in the well-publicized biography of the cofounder of the first fistula hospital in Ethiopia, Catherine Hamlin (Hamlin 2001; Kristof 2003; Moylan 2016; O'Kane 1998; Salgo 2010; M. O. Smith 2007; Warner 2014). In this coverage, women suffering from fistula have been called "the most wretched people on this planet" (Kristof 2009). They are victims, confined so that "wild hyenas devour [their] tiny bod[ies] in the night" (Oprah.com 2005). Academic peer-reviewed articles on fistula in the disciplines of public health and medicine follow the same narrative (Brugière 2012) and parrot its vocabulary of suffering (see, Castille et al. 2014; Harouna et al. 2001; Kabir et al. 2003). For example, Anoukoum and colleagues aver that obstetric fistula is an "eternal nightmare, making a woman a ghost, shut out from society" (2010, 72). As evidenced in the quote above, the narrative has even permeated popular fiction.

Third Plot Device: Surgical Redemption

> Dr. James Marion Sims developed a surgical repair technique in the 1840s that is still more than 90% effective … It means that the only thing that separates a woman from escaping her living hell is a 170-year-old surgery that takes as little as 45 minutes.
> —Bryony Michaelson for Operation Fistula (2018)

Follow loss and isolation, a scientific, logical redemption beckons: the hospital, with its biomedical technologies, emerges as a place of physical healing and consequent social rebirth, emotional transformation, and religious renewal. There, the ailing woman is made continent by surgical intervention. Fistula surgery is reported to successfully "cure" women in the overwhelming majority of cases— 90 percent. Fistula surgeries are framed as effective, inexpensive, and rapid: they are often described as $300 surgeries that take no more than two hours, and often as little as twenty minutes (Clinton Foundation 2014; Engender Health 2014; Fistula Foundation 2014; IRIN Staff 2009; Kristof 2005; Menard-Freeman 2013; "Obstetric Fistula." [Wikipedia] 2014).[2] As phrased by Operation Fistula, "Fistula destroys lives. A simple surgery can bring a woman back from a fate many consider a fate worse than death" (Michaelson 2018).

DEBUNKING THE NARRATIVE

Although the fistula narrative is undeniably moving, it is at best reductionist and at worst, for some women, simply wrong. Surgeons and researchers acknowledge that fistula can occur during any birth, but the dominant narrative remains fixated on child marriage and first-time mothers. This emphasis does not trace meaningful causal relationships but reinforces semiotics of cultural failure. It is assumed that age is directly correlated with social value, leaving young parturient women unable to meaningfully advocate for their own health care. Also, as the thinking goes, the younger a woman is at marriage, the younger she will be at the onset of sexual activity and time of first pregnancy, and the smaller and more "immature" her pelvis will be at the time of her delivery. Thus, the more likely it is that delivery will become obstructed, resulting in obstetric fistula.[3]

While young age at pregnancy (and thus stymied physiological development) may account for small pelvic size, other factors that are not necessarily dependent on age—such as malnutrition during formative years of growth or inherited small stature—may also account for reduced pelvic size. And although women in Niger are often married before the age of 16,[4] the connection between age and the development of obstetric fistula is tenuous at best. First, women develop fistula throughout their reproductive lives, with a wide range of ages and parities. Some women I knew developed fistula during their first labor, and others during their twelfth. They ranged in age from 13 to 54 at onset.

And many women all over the world begin sexual activity in their midteens. The United States, for example, has a relatively high number of teenage pregnancies each year. Yet obstetric fistula is very rare in the United States because these teenagers typically deliver at a hospital and have access to emergency care in the event of birthing complications (Kabir et al. 2003; Mosher, Chandra, and Jones 2002). Obstetric fistula is not a function of age but of a lack of access to quality emergency obstetric care.

Additionally, in Niger, marrying young does not necessarily lead to early pregnancy. Women who are married young often experience an extended period of sexual abstinence after marriage. Frequently, the women I spoke with claimed that as young brides they continued to live with their parents until they were deemed "ready," a subjective and individualized state typically determined by their parents. This was not necessarily tied to physiological indicators of maturity such as menarche or breast development.[5] For example, Roukaya (age 21, Zarma), who was married at the age of 14, did not become pregnant until she was 20 years old. She explained, "If a girl is married young, the husband must wait before approaching her. The elders say that if he sleeps with her too early, it can bring on problems. So [my husband] waited until I was big enough, then he approached me." Youth marriage in Niger takes place within a context of social conventions that regulate young women's sexuality, protecting them until they are thought to be prepared for sex, pregnancy, and motherhood. These local cultural realities are lost in the dominant fistula narrative.

Once developed, fistula itself is not always as socially destructive as the dominant narrative leads us to believe. Women's experiences with the condition revealed not simply experiences of rejection and stigma, but also complex networks of care and support (as demonstrated in chapters 2 and 3). Although a handful of women admitted having experienced suicidal thoughts, these thoughts were fleeting, replaced with hope and faith in God. No woman I knew considered her incontinence a "fate worse than death." Women with fistula are not solely defined by their condition nor singly constituted by their suffering. Most are entangled in rewarding and intimate relationships with family, husbands, friends, and (for some women) children. As Marissa Yeakey and her colleagues stated in their study of 45 women with fistula in Malawi, many "remained married, supported, and fecund" (2009, 509). No woman I came to know lived completely alone, and none had ever lived in an isolated hut encircled by wild animals. Many managed relatively normal lives, and they continued to have pregnancies and children, often while concealing their fistulas from their communities, kin, co-wives, and sometimes husbands.

Finally, biomedical intervention was neither as physically nor socially transformative as the donor and media narratives portray. During my time in Niger, it became clear that surgical repair is often a protracted and ultimately disappointing process for women, as I discussed in chapter 5. Only 36 percent of the women I followed who actually received surgery left the clinic dry; the remaining 64 percent remained incontinent. The widely circulated surgical success rate for fistula repair procedures—90 percent—may thus reflect not actual surgical outcomes but an end point in a carefully constructed narrative. External pressures on clinics and practitioners to produce "better data" or higher rates of surgical success, along with the lack of international standardization of measurement or definition, result in wide-scale inflation and distortion of success rates. The international humanitarian marketplace shapes how data are produced and deployed, affecting how surgical success rates are translated from clinicians and researchers to material intended for public consumption—social facts unmoored from clinical practice.[6] This process of data construction has negative consequences for both the women seeking treatment and the centers competing for limited resources.

When I returned in the fall of 2010 from my first summer of pilot research in Niger, I was startled by these implications. I had gone to the field expecting to find heavily stigmatized women and girls navigating new corporeal and social realities after surgical transformations. Everything I had read prepared me for such encounters. But as I combed through my data, a different narrative—or, rather, different narratives—emerged. Yet when I presented my nascent findings to a senior researcher casually acquainted with the topic, she brushed them aside: "Senior scholars all agree, but you think you know better?"

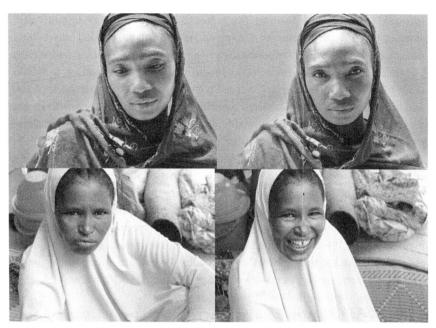

FIGURE 16. Which photograph of each woman would you choose to tell a story about oppression, pain, and poverty? And a story about resilience and strength? The portraits of two Nigérien women, taken seconds apart, illustrate the power of the storyteller to control a narrative through selective representation.

Once constructed by dominant voices, dominant narratives are resistant to change, even in the face of contradicting evidence. Over the years, I have diligently amassed a trove of data to construct alternative narratives. These data—the voices of the women, their kin, and the experts who provided their care—have structured this book. But for a moment let us linger not on these multiplicities of experience but on how women's experiences have been distilled and abstracted into a formula that has achieved narrative dominance, and on how social, economic, historic, and political forces enabled that process.

SUFFERING SUPERLATIVELY IN THE
HUMANITARIAN MARKETPLACE

The fistula narrative has been refined over time, through interactions between donor organizations, the media, and various publics who consume and respond to these stories. It is a story of archetypes, one that fits neatly into Western expectations and the demands of the capitalist marketplace within which humanitarian engagement must exist. The Global North's interaction with crises in the Global South demonstrates that compassion is not blind, and that victimhood is a status that must be earned—not through suffering or unjust persecution but through qualities that position the suffer as pure, innocent, depoliticized, abstractable, and nonthreatening. Groups and individuals are divided into discrete categories: those deserving of access to development and humanitarian assistance, and those who are not—worthy versus unworthy. The worthy victim, or, as Malkki (1996) calls her, the "exemplary victim," is imagined as helpless, in need of aid, and lacking in particulars. Through their innocence, young women with fistula are rendered visible—worthy, fundable, and capable of competing in an increasingly competitive marketplace of suffering.

In examining the media's coverage of famines in Africa, historian Susan Moeller critically examines how the media deploys children: "Starving children are the famine icon," she explains. "Skeletal children personify innocence abused" (2002, 36). This focus on children translates disasters that are geographically (and culturally) remote, complicated, and morally ambiguous into spectacles that are comprehensible to a lay Western audience. Children can be rendered as cultureless—they are not yet linked to their parents' culture, color, or political environment (or, at least, to Western stereotypes of these)—and they are thus legible and relatable (and fundable) for remote Western onlookers.

The girl with fistula plays into a Western preoccupation with the universal innocence of children and the moral panic that surrounds their sexuality, driving the need to protect them from predators (Manzo 2008; Ticktin 2017; Wark 1995). Yet the girl with fistula allows for the treatment of sexuality (certainly a favorite subject in the West) without conceptualizing the girls themselves as sexual subjects and thus unworthy victims. The fistula narrative's focus on "early" and "forced" marriage permits sexual engagement while still preserving a young woman's moral if not physical chastity; a focus on women at the other end of the spectrum— a mature woman who develops fistula after several intended pregnancies— would not have the same effect.[7]

However, the requisite threshold of suffering needed for a story to gain public traction in the Global North is ever-rising, and depictions of *human* suffering are being replaced by depictions of *superlative* suffering. As we mindlessly scroll through Twitter feeds, stream videos of ISIS beheadings, or half-listen to news of insurgencies or state-sponsored chemical attacks against its own people, we consume graphic and uncensored media, desensitizing many of us to the realities of suffering (see Kleinman and Kleinman 1996). As a result, a hungry child will no longer open wallets or capture readers' attention—now the child must be on the verge of death (recall Kevin Carter's Pulitzer Prize–winning photograph of a vulture stalking a Sudanese toddler who had collapsed from hunger). A girl child oppressed by regimes of patriarchy is rendered invisible until she is disfigured by an acid attack or close-range gunshots from the Colt .45 of an indurate terrorist.[8] A humanitarian crisis does not rouse the public until photographs of lifeless or bloodied toddlers go viral (and even then, the public's attention wanes quickly).[9] It is a race to the bottom of suffering. Young girls experiencing sexual violation, catastrophic labors, dead babies, broken bodies, and social rejection—the fistula narrative is competing intensely in this marketplace of victimhood.

Fistula narratives and fistula politics reflect a larger transformation in international development and humanitarianism and global health: the emergence of "philanthrocapitalism," or a market-based business approach to development that prioritizes efficiency, effectiveness, performance goals, and social returns on investments (Bishop and Green 2008). In turn, fundraising campaigns and development organizations more broadly have been restructured, favoring specific projects that have a measurable, direct impact rather than complex cross-cutting development agendas or governmental strategies whose impacts are systemic, hard to measure, and may take many years to yield visible results. In global health, organizations increasingly focus on disease-specific, technologically oriented interventions with measurable outcomes, which often rely on a reductionist understanding of disease causality. For fistula, philanthrocapitalism encourages rapid interventions that require few resources, are limited in scope, and can be performed by nonstate agents and organizations. Surgical intervention—framed as quick, inexpensive, highly effective, and executable by individuals—fits the bill, when what is really needed is systemic transformation of the basic infrastructure of maternal health provisioning.[10]

On Operation Fistula's website, potential donors are reminded that they can "change a life now for $100," that "$100 will make her smile again," and "bring her life back" (Michaelson 2018). Other organizations encourage donors to browse through patient photographs and profiles and fund part or all of "a life-changing surgery" for the woman of their choosing.[11] Thereafter, donors receive regular "progress" updates on "their" patient. The Fistula Foundation allows donors to enroll in the Love-A-Sister program, where $50 provides an anesthetist for one woman's surgery, $240 provides transportation for 12 women in need of treatment, and $450 fully funds one woman's fistula surgery. The majority of international nonprofits' websites now offer donors the opportunity to shop for specific interventions that they feel represent their personality, compassion, interest, or understanding of global need. The promise that an hour's time and the cost of a plane ticket to El Paso could pull an innocent girl, mistreated by her kin and culture, from the depths of suffering—that is compelling. It opens wallets and hearts in a way that longer-term, costlier approaches to the structural determinants of maternal morbidity simply do not.

Historical Narrative Continuity

Dominant narratives can be understood as resistant to fundamental change, undergoing only slight transformations over time to fit their contemporary contexts while retaining their essential outlines. And the Western dominant narrative of Africa has always been one of childlike or violent people in need of civilization, salvation, and intervention. Beginning with the writings of Herodotus in the fifth century B.C.E.—and continuing to today—Africa has been systematically depicted by explorers as a strange, dangerous land of monstrous races. The Africans themselves have been portrayed as subhuman, pseudo-human, and nonhuman exotics. Once Africans had been stripped of their humanity, their colonization, Christianization, enslavement, and slaughter along with the expropriation of their lands were justified by Europeans.

A kind of historical intransigence characterizes most oppressive narratives, such as those linking African Americans to criminality or immigrants with national threat: the narratives continuously adapt, but their gestalt does not.[12] Although the fistula narrative is subtler than these other oppressive narratives, it fits within existing and enduring narrative frames that pathologize the Other—the familiar narratives that have dominated Western readings of Africa for centuries.[13] The fistula narrative identifies unenlightened and often harmful culture as an intractable obstacle to a people's health and development—materially, socially, and spiritually. These logics have often served to justify imperialism and intervention.

The fistula narrative can therefore be read as simply a modern version of the same narrative contained in colonial medical texts, which often share a metanarrative of African cultural pathology and the shackles of "tradition" producing disastrous physical and social consequences. For example, Carol Summers (1991) describes the British reaction to a perceived crisis of population decline in Uganda in the early twentieth century, caused by epidemics of sexually transmitted infections. Ugandans were "diagnosed as immoral," and the cure was thought to be Christianity and mercury—"remedies" that caused the colonial disruption of African family structures. Dr. A. R. Cook, a prominent missionary medical authority, blamed both individuals and culture when he claimed of Ugandan syphilis patients that "the immense majority have fallen ill through immorality," that their illness was due to "the enormous influence of the evil surrounding them from birth, backed up by an hereditary tendency to do evil" (Cook 1908, cited in Summers 1991, 794).

As Megan Vaughan (1991) notes, during the British colonial period in East and Central Africa, the language of cultural difference as a causal factor for disease steadily supplanted a focus on economic and environmental causes. The cultural deterministic model, most explicitly held among Christian missionaries, was that "Africans got sick . . . because their societies were fundamentally sick" (Vaughan 1991, 201). Through the decades, the particular logics shifted, but the general position did not. For Western observers, Africa was "synonymous with disease, death, and uncontrolled sexuality. Africans, it seems . . . never get sick innocently" (Vaughan 1991, 205). The continent's contemporary public health crises, such as HIV/AIDS, diarrheal disease, or malnutrition, are still often framed using rhetorics of African promiscuity, ignorance, patriarchal abuse, or parental negligence.

The fistula narrative thus hooks into a historically salient theme of African cultural degeneracy, a contemporary manifestation of African transgressions of human rights carried out on the bodies of girls. Western interest in and intervention into fistula can be viewed as a *cause célèbre du jour*—today's cause in a long line of cultural interventions that reflect Western interest in passive female sexuality, male culpability, and Western biomedical/cultural potency in the Global South. The tropes of cultural deterioration, dangerous masculinity, and girl-child victimization typify the discourses around female genital cutting, sex trafficking, and fistula, illustrating the extent to which myths of African cultural primitivism retain their global currency. These perceived crises place the sexuality of the men and women of the Global South under critical public scrutiny and rest upon a stark binary opposition between good and evil—female innocence, purity, and passivity contrasted with male potency, brutality, and moral corruption.

Western interest in fistula may thus represent a repackaging of colonial messages about the "dark continent" as a barbaric, morally empty place that victimizes its most vulnerable and innocent: its girl children. In the 1990s, the popular Western version of this narrative focused on female genital cutting (FGC). In *Warrior Marks* (1993), Alice Walker's book about her filming of a documentary on female genital mutilation (FGM) and the "sexual blinding of women," Walker muses about why Senegalese people seem "joyless and oppressed."[14] She blames both Islam and genital cutting, expressions of male predation of powerless women:

> My beloved called to wish me Happy Valentine's Day, and it feels odd to think of a Valentine's Day kind of love here, where men have three and four wives, all of them poor, and even the mosque is forbidden to women until after menopause, when they are considered closer to being male. We strolled past the mosque one day, and it looked totally dead and boring . . . What has happened to these people, that they seem so joyless and oppressed? Is it Islam, as some suggest, which encourages passivity and desertification? Everything, including massive overgrazing of livestock, turning the fertile land into desert, is merely "the will of Allah"? I think genital mutilation plays a role. The early submission by force that is the hallmark of mutilation. The feeling of being overpowered and thoroughly dominated by those you are duty bound to respect. The result is women with downcast eyes and stiff backs and necks (they are of course beaten by fathers and brothers and husbands). And men who look at a woman's body as if it is a meal. (Walker and Parmar 1993, 69)

In this passage, echoing the semiotics of fistula, Alice Walker blames everything from environmental devastation to gender-based violence on Islam, in which men dominate and women submit. Walker sees "African men" as an uncomplicated whole—dominating and beastly, molding female bodies into submission by force—and "African culture and traditions" as harmful, coercive, and static. Walker frequently discusses men's role within their "mutilating culture," calling African men "backward" and "slave-masters" (among various other insults). Like fistula two decades later, female genital mutilation served as the embodied manifestation of a diseased culture, inflicting its wounds on the "female child of Africa," who in her "vulnerable loveliness" is rendered helpless, voiceless, and desperately requiring Western intervention (Walker and Parmar 1993).

The idea of culture as a cause of illness and mortality finds its contemporary expression in the notion of "harmful traditional practices." As global nongovernmental organizations (NGOs) increasingly become the principal agents for policing biomedical standards worldwide, this idiom has come to dominate many of their public health initiatives, especially in Africa and Asia. This discourse is highly gendered, focusing almost exclusively on the victimized bodies of women and girls and typically blaming brown-skinned men. As during colonial times, the gaze of the international audience is disproportionately fixed on the bodies of young women—on their reproductive capacity, their sexuality, and their genitals.

Early marriage, female genital cutting, obstetric fistula, even the recent humanitarian interest in menstruation's effect on school attendance are thematically linked. Westerners are positioned as the agents of change and salvation for a continent of young women oppressed by African men. Twenty-five years ago, Gayatri Chakravorty Spivak characterized British imperialism in India as "white men saving brown women from brown men" (1993, 93); the same dynamic plays out in global fistula interventions.

This impulse to make visible only certain bodies, certain conditions, is far from new. Nineteenth- and twentieth-century scientific Western discourse about Africans mediated ideas about race, gender, and vested social and political interests back home.[15] But the motivations to intervene on behalf of some and not others are complicated. As Martha Nussbaum writes, "the fascination with FGM contains at least an element of the sensational or even the prurient" (1999, 126). Altruism is often mixed with anger, and our interest may linger longer on narratives of sex, sexual abuse, and young women's bodies than, for example, stories of lower respiratory infections (although the morbidity and mortality rates are much higher).

Campaigns to eradicate fistula echo the previous calls to save African women—often from their own husbands and cultures—that have prevailed since Africa's colonization (Abu-Lughod 2002; Kapur 2002; Mohanty 1991). These colonial and postcolonial representations of Africa reified African male domination as "traditional" while ignoring the ways in which colonial intervention and economic transformation affected gender systems, oppressing both men and women of the Global South. This rhetoric at the same time indicts "African culture," Islam, and African men, a sentiment that is encapsulated in the closing words of a *New York Times* article on fistula, which quotes Dutch fistula surgeon Kees Waaldijk: "to be a woman in Africa . . . is truly a terrible thing" (LaFraniere 2005).

Gender and Narrative Construction

During the past 40 years, international interest has focused in on women and children in the Global South. In the 1950s and 1960s, women of the Global South were initially considered barriers to economic, political, and social development. However, by the mid-1960s, when economists realized that "development" was not progressing as hoped, the view of African women shifted; they were no longer seen as impediments but as victims—of their husbands, their cultures, and even of prior Western humanitarian impulses. Ester Boserup's 1970 study, *Woman's Role in Economic Development,* reported that not only were women not benefiting from development, but that many projects had actually deprived women of economic opportunities and status. Inspired partly by Boserup's work and partly by political trends in the United States, a new subfield in development emerged, "Women in Development." The United Nations declared 1976–1985 the Decade for Women and channeled funds into projects earmarked for women's rights, health, and empowerment. The United Nations Convention on the Rights of the Child then ushered in the 1990s, a decade that marked a high point in worldwide interest in issues affecting women and children—sometimes at the cost of blaming husbands and fathers for their wives' and daughters' peril.

The simultaneous erasure and villainization of African men, traced back to colonization and European imperialism, continues in post-1970s development movements. These movements' focus on women are based on the assumption that if African men were given money, they would buy drinks for their friends, go out, or invest in shows of wealth or status; women are thought to be both more adept at saving and investing wisely and more likely to channel resources to their children's health and education (Wilson 2008; Yunus 1994).[16] These gender assumptions mean that women (and girls) have become the flag-bearers of international development work. Their faces dominate fundraising materials and beneficiary rosters, and nearly every intervention integrates gender, focusing heavily on improving women's access to resources. Conversely, African men have become caricatures in the Western imagination; they are the fall guys for all bad things that befall African women and children. In this discourse, in the news and media consumed by Westerners, African men are either absent or depicted only as they hold guns, rape women, endanger and degrade their wives and daughters, participate in extortion and corruption, or join the growing ranks of religiously motivated extremists.

In Western engagement with sub-Saharan Africa, therefore, there is a strict gender divide. Suffering and victimhood belong to the continent's women, and perpetration and barbarity belong to its men. The implicit message of this approach is clear: African women are innocent; African men are not. Western anger and indignation is channeled to African men while compassion (and the resources that follow) goes to women and girls—girls' education, girls' business skills, women's health, and women's hygiene. But there are real consequences to forgetting men and boys. The "focus on women," which aims to empower, may in fact strip women of agency and naturalize women's place in the home as caretaker. The focus serves fundraising purposes because donor audiences infrequently respond to nuance—one is either a victim or a victimizer—but these programs overlook that families, communities, marriages, and businesses do not operate in the absence of half their members. It is hard to criticize development agendas that aim to increase the power and status of women in places largely defined by patriarchal hierarchies, but by framing African women as the victims of African men, the real victimizers—systemic inequalities and poverty—go unaddressed.

This dynamic is especially exaggerated when narrative subjects are Muslim women, as are the women with fistula in Niger. Muslim women are typically framed as triple victims: of patriarchal, cultural, and religious harm. This tendency of Western imperial power to construct Muslim women as "victims" has only increased after the events of September 11, 2001 (Abu-Lughod 2002, 2013). As Muslim men are derided, detained, and demonized in the post-9/11 landscape, narratives of Muslim women's oppression and their need for Western liberation have proliferated. Lila Abu-Lughod (2013) critiques the advocates for global gender justice like Nicholas Kristof and Sheryl WuDunn (in particular, their book *Half the Sky: Turning Oppression into Opportunity for Women Worldwide*, 2010), arguing that in their quest for gender emancipation, they are blinded by nineteenth-century orientalism. The narrative reliance on religious and cultural framings obfuscates regional specificity and historical context, and it inhibits meaningful exploration of local or global inequity. As Chandra Mohanty has asked in reaction to a book entitled *Women of Africa: Roots of Oppression*, "Is it possible to imagine writing a book entitled *Women of Europe: Roots of Oppression*?" (1991, 59). The heterogeneity, multivocality, and historical context afforded to people of the "West" are often absent in the flattened, reductionist dominant narratives about denizens of the Global South.

THE STORIES WE DO NOT TELL

Narratives about fistula as a symptom of cultural failure rather than a medical, socioeconomic, or political failure thus reinforce pernicious assumptions of African inferiority and inadequacy. Popular appeals to save women with fistula repeat colonialist discursive structures showing Africa as hobbled by dysfunctional beliefs and practices to justify Western intervention. And perhaps more importantly, when we tell these tired, harmful stories about cultural failings, Western intervention, and individual redemption, we shut out other stories. Historically shallow, contextually thin, largely apolitical, and without any meaningful reflexivity, the donor and media narratives about young women's health crises in sub-Saharan Africa ignore the structural failures, global priorities, and economic restructuring that have created these crises.[17]

The depoliticization that characterizes these humanitarian narratives can be seen in the Western treatment of famine in Africa. In *Famine Crimes,* Alex de Waal (1997) demonstrated that famine is a political issue that necessitates a political solution. But he pointed out that the narratives about famine neglect the systemic breakdowns such as vulnerability to environmental and economic shocks; instead, they present Band-Aid solutions such as food aid and short-term housing. According to de Waal, "most current humanitarian activity in Africa is useless or damaging and should be abandoned" (1997, xvi); de Waal argues that humanitarian involvement, by depoliticizing famine, framing it as the subject of a technocratic fix, tends to obstruct political reform aimed at addressing the causes of famine. Similarly, in his 1990 work *The Anti-Politics Machine,* which critiqued humanitarian interventions in Lesotho, James Ferguson argued that development discourse is self-serving—it screens out and ignores the political, historical, and structural contexts of poverty in the Global South to strengthen its own power and bureaucracy and maintain the demand for its industry.

Nigerian novelist Chimamanda Adichie (2009) warns of the West's single narrative about Africa: "Show a people as one thing, as only one thing, over and over again, and that's what they become." Adichie criticizes the "single story" of suffering and poverty told about Africa in the West, which obfuscates complexity, nuance, and the diversity of experience. She noted, "Stories . . . how they are told, who tells them, how many stories are told is really dependent on power. Power is the ability not only to tell the story of someone, but to make it the definitive story of that person . . . The single story creates stereotypes, and the problem with stereotypes is not that they are untrue, but they are incomplete. They make one story become the only story." This has happened with development narratives of Africa more broadly, and with the branding of fistula specifically.

The prevailing fistula narrative of exclusion and separation followed by the surgical "fix" has subsumed all other experiences with this injury. Fistula has become "single-storied." In the ethnographic accounts woven throughout this book, I have introduced an array of competing stories, attempting to take apart the narrative framework that has until now constructed fistula for international audiences. Yet just as there is no single true story of suffering and redemption, there is also no single alternative. Instead, as Clare Hemmings has suggested, there are only "ways of thinking stories differently" (2011, 22).

The humanitarian marketplace is currently spiraling downward in what I call a race to the bottom of suffering. Funding for humanitarian aid occurs in what Clifford Bob (2005) calls a "Darwinian arena"—a marketplace of suffering that functions shockingly similarly to the business world, producing better victims (more tragedy for your money) and increasingly cheap solutions. Humanitarian organizations must compete for donors, and reporters must compete for readers, but the fundraising strategies adopted by humanitarian organizations, which help them meet their short-term funding goals, are ultimately detrimental to their cause and to the people for whom they advocate. Attempting to rouse the public from their "compassion fatigue" (borrowing Susan Moeller's terminology), humanitarian and development agencies and media claim superlative states of suffering for increasingly pitiable victims. Their formulaic representation of distant suffering, with its sensationalism, its depiction of war and ravage, and its powerful images of the wretched, strips the sufferers of context and nuance while limiting the available roles to victim, villain, and redeemer.

Anthropologists have long problematized these types of narratives put forward by international NGOs.[18] Postmodernist theorists like Michel Foucault, Judith Butler, Jacques Derrida, and Gayatri Spivak, whose work recognizes individual subjectivity, the social construction of difference(s), and the limitations of knowing, have been integral in reshaping the field of (post)colonial studies and the resulting conversations around engagement in the development enterprise. Their work, and the work of countless others, has destabilized the ways that binaries of power, moral authority, and expertise between the West and Global South are being conceptualized. Within this vast corpus of critiques of development and humanitarianism, and of their totalizing narratives, humanitarian action is thought to perpetuate asymmetrical power relationships, contributing to what Didier Fassin (2007) called the "humanitarian reduction of the victim" to a passive recipient of aid. Carefully packaged media coverage, generalizations, and assumptions about naturalized states of violence and depravity in African and other resource-poor communities act to silence the victims, rendering them mute, ahistorical actors—a synecdoche for all the ravaged Global South. In many ways, the fistula narrative is the apogee of these portrayals. We are left to ask whether the "incredulity towards metanarratives" (proposed by Jean-François Lyotard as constituting the basis of postmodernism) can allow us to avoid this foreclosure of other narrative possibilities (1984, 5).

The public's interest in FGM and sex trafficking has waned, although girls continue to undergo genital cutting and young women continue to be trafficked into sex work. Perhaps this is an example of compassion fatigue, or perhaps editors (weary of dips in readership) or nonprofits (facing decreased donations) acted first to find a new crisis—fresh meat. And although fistula is the cause célèbre du jour, it will not continue to be so. Perhaps next month, or perhaps next year, fistula too will fade from the Western popular consciousness, only to be replaced by the next crisis—new brown-bodied girls who need saving. Many of today's young girls in the Global South will reach maturity in places with inadequate access to maternal health care, and they will suffer the consequences of poverty and inequality. But Western attention will be elsewhere, now moved on to the next crisis and its inevitable promise of quick solutions.

In the world of Western aid and nonprofit fundraising (where innumerable causes coexist and compete, where human suffering is displayed in various forms and manifestations, where a bold "donate" icon occupies the corner of nearly every NGO website), organizations fight tooth and nail for a limited pot of money. Humanitarian organizations championing fistula (and numerous other conditions, including cleft palate, HIV, and malnutrition) have begun to engage in a battle of the superlative pitiable, all making the same claims. Our victims are the most deserving. Our victims suffer the most. Such assertions are frequently followed by the promise of total redemption, of a quick and efficacious solution: a single pill, a simple surgery, a cheap bed net. But these kinds of appeals have consequences.

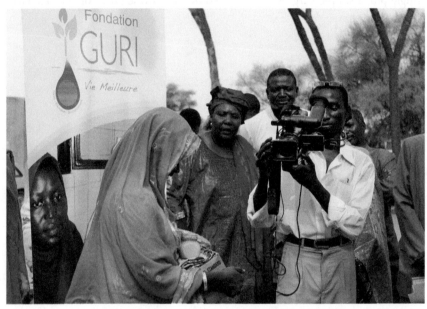

During a televised donation ceremony, a Hausa woman with fistula is filmed giving thanks

7 · COSTS AND CONSEQUENCES

The donor and media narrative—an imaginary of victims, villains, and redeemers—has very real consequences. It shapes how we think about Africa generally and African women specifically, and delimits the kinds of interventions we think possible. This narrative, in its potency and ubiquity, affects not only Western audiences' ideas about fistula but also local understandings. Fistula experts, local health agents, nonprofits working for women, caregivers, and even women themselves are all influenced by the myth of social loss followed by surgical redemption. The narrative affects how fistula care is envisioned and provisioned, sometimes in ways that are damaging to the women receiving care.

The dominant fistula narrative also encourages specious connections. Women with fistula are framed as "superlative sufferers"; the texture of their misfortune mirroring that of an iconic group whose diseased bodies resulted in their social death: lepers. The link between fistula and leprosy is repeatedly made in media accounts and humanitarian appeals. The comparison is powerful and likely facilitates fundraising, but, as Susan Sontag (1988) reminds us, metaphorical thinking can be both misleading and dangerous, reinforcing destructive taboos, propagating fear, reconfiguring regimes of treatment, and increasing the social marginalization of the ill. If the framing of women with fistula as the "new lepers" is both spurious and a barrier to effective treatment (and I argue it is), why is the link so readily made?

In this chapter, I first examine the logic of the connection between lepers and women with fistula. I show how leper colonies were constructed in large part for the benefit of Christian missionaries, whose continued need for a population receptive to religious conversion may explain their desire to create "new lepers". I then lay out the consequences to care that the comparison creates. Finally, I examine how centers' holistic care programs, which are modeled on the assumption that women with fistula are the modern day lepers with no social networks to which they can return, can actually damage women's wellbeing by requiring additional long absences from home and by "outing" the women who may have been successfully concealing their conditions. Influenced by compelling but deceptive narratives, the fistula centers actually cause some of the social consequences that they aim to address.

THE NEW LEPER

Within the global media and donor narrative, rhetorical links are frequently drawn between the woman with fistula and the iconic leper, capturing a specific form of social abandonment, spatial separation, stigma, suffering, and eventual salvation through setting apart. For example, Operation Fistula states, "Her community will nearly always ostracize her. In many cases, her husband will leave her or send her back to her family . . . The bright eyes and big smile that [a fistula sufferer] once had are replaced by the pain and loneliness that only a leper can know" (Michaelson 2018). Similarly, the CEO of the Fistula Foundation writes, "Women with fistula are often abandoned by their husbands and have been referred to as modern-day lepers, because they are treated as outcasts in their own communities" (Grant 2016). Reuters has reported that women with fistula live in poverty and are often abandoned—"the modern day equivalent of lepers who were ostracized and isolated" (Lazareva 2017).

Ostracized, outcast, isolated—but *are* women with fistula the "new lepers"? And why is this parallel so consistently drawn? Whose interests does this conceptual linkage serve? To understand the contemporary potency of this framing and its unintentional consequences, we must understand the history and social construction of leprosy—particularly how the leprosarium in Muslim sub-Saharan Africa was strategically constructed by evangelical Christians as a place of religious transformation.

Banishment and Salvation

In the biblical book of Leviticus, leprosy was seen as a physical manifestation of transgressions against God.[1] Those with leprosy, characterized as "defiled" and "unclean," were destined to live away from their communities, or "without the camp" (Numbers 13:44–46). Infecting, deforming, polluting, and threatening to social order, leprosy evoked fear and disgust. In the New Testament, however, people with leprosy were met with pity rather than revulsion, and the textual emphasis shifted away from diagnosis and segregation and toward treatment.

People with leprosy were the recipients of Jesus Christ's love and divine salvation. This led to a long-standing privileged relationship between leprosy and Christians. Those with leprosy became "special objects of divine compassion," and loving them was "a sign of sanctity" (Edmond 2006, 1; Vongsathorn 2012, 8). This relationship between leprosy and Christians was particularly evident throughout colonial Africa.[2] For example, in their 1928 annual report, the British Empire

Leprosy Relief Association wrote, "It is a Christian duty to help provide for lepers. Never let it be forgotten that the one particular class of sick people singled out by Jesus Christ for special attention, were the lepers. He Himself, when He was here, 'touched' the lepers and healed them, and He it was Who gave the distinct command: 'Cleanse the lepers'" (BELRA Annual Report 1931, LEPRA, 13–14, cited in Vongsathorn 2012, 8).

However, Christian missionaries' interest in leprosy was not entirely altruistic. The historical ostracizing and cultural marginality (real or imagined) of lepers made them attractive and accessible to missionaries across the Sahel. Unlike other types of medical care, such as setting broken bones or administering antibiotics, the treatment context for leprosy—long-term care that separated patients from social networks—made the patients especially receptive to spiritual transformation and conversion. The treatment typically required between 5 and 12 years of (rather ineffective) intramuscular injections, which kept the patients at centers for years and thus made them captive listeners for the Gospel. The leprosarium was an ideal terrain for Christian evangelism, providing missionaries with a vulnerable population who had nowhere else to go (Cooper 2006, 305).

Particularly in colonial settings, the sufferers lived in highly racialized, unremitting segregation: Foucauldian "exile-enclosures" (Bashford 2004).[3] According to Megan Vaughan, "leprosy offered to the missionaries the possibility of engineering new African communities, isolated from, and expunged of, all those features of African society which they saw as impeding the development of Christianity" (1991, 79). According to historian Barbara Cooper, colonial governments initially attempted to curb the power of leprosy centers to proselytize, but the missionaries were unambiguous about their objectives: "'No evangelism, no leprosy work'" (Turaki 1993, 180, as quoted in Cooper 2006, 304).

The Danja Fistula Center, located approximately 700 kilometers east of the capital near the city of Maradi, is run by the secular organization the Worldwide Fistula Fund, but it shares a campus and some administrative power with a missionary-run health center, CSL-Danja (Centre de Santé Léprologie de Danja, or the Danja Leprosy Health Center), which is run by SIM (Serving In Mission). SIM was originally established "to return to the 'pure' activity of preaching, converting, and establishing churches"—an intentional departure from the "service-based" or "social" missions that focused on doing good works such as providing health care and education (Cooper 2006, 6). As described by historian Rosemary Fitzgerald (2001), although medical humanitarian work was initially understood as counterproductive (or at least unrelated) to the primary goal of "saving souls," most missionary organizations increasingly envisioned medical work as an entry point to evangelization precisely because the patients were vulnerable to proselytizing: "Pain and suffering, the uncertainty of living and the threat of death were seen as transformative experiences that made the human heart open, soft and malleable. The intimate and probing nature of the medical encounter, when the patient's capacity for mental and physical resistance was at its lowest, was held to offer matchless evangelistic opportunities" (Fitzgerald 2001, 120–121).

SIM's initial interest in leprosy was purely evangelical. Medical work, health promotion, and the relief of suffering were never conceptualized as ends in themselves; rather, SIM missionaries in Niger (and throughout the Sahel) recognized the power of health centers to create Christian converts, who had proven difficult to produce in strongly Muslim areas like Niger. Medical ministries, mostly composed of basic hygiene and sanitation interventions, sought to, as David Hardiman (2006) puts it, "bring health to the 'native' by cleansing their bodies with soap and their minds with the Gospel" (11).

The leprosarium in Danja opened in 1956, and patients were required to submit to a "Gospel message" before receiving treatment. The lengthy stays required for leprosy treatment facilitated a Christian community life that SIM missionaries hoped would foster a sustained commitment to Christianity (Cooper 2006, 308). And indeed, Danja's leprosarium was a fruitful birthplace of new Christians, who—along with their Christian descendants—settled in a town abutting the center. The mission's success was due in part to converted patients' increased access to resources, and in part to the lack of their options back home, which continued to shrink as time passed at the leprosarium.

Making of the New Lepers

After successful multidrug therapy for leprosy was introduced in the early 1980s, patients went from spending their lives at Danja's leprosarium to spending several years and then only months; eventually, they were treated as outpatients. As treatment improved, the leprosarium's capacity to convert patients declined. In a 2006 analysis of SIM's medical work in Niger, Barbara Cooper explained that at this time many observers predicted that the mission would not be able to retain their medical institutions in Niger, which had become "unprofitable" (2006, 327).

So Danja adapted and expanded its services. The mission began offering basic medical care, a maternity ward, and specialized services often associated with (but not limited to) leprosy—burn care, rehabilitation, and prosthetics. Still, CSL-Danja struggled to turn a profit, either economic or in converted souls. A partnership with the Worldwide Fistula Fund offered economic incentives and promised to attract a new population considered to be "good material for proselytism": women who were stigmatized, socially isolated, vulnerable, and who were in need of long-term care (Hardiman 2006, 33). Women with fistula were packaged as a new kind of leper.

After the partnership, CSL-Danja changed its name to CSLF-Danja, or the Centre de Santé, Léprologie et Fistule (Danja Leprosy and Fistula Health Center). Along with the fistula operation theater and treatment ward, a hostel area with eight small houses—longer-term housing for fistula patients—was built at Danja. This "village" (as it is called) indicates the long-term access to women with fistula that SIM-Niger may have hoped to gain—access that was intended to off-set the losses they were taking on the leprosy side.

In 2013, SIM Niger's website highlighted the importance of the long-term treatment required in leprosy care to advance evangelical objectives, claiming that the relationship between the patients and staff has resulted in a "vibrant and growing Christian community." The site suggested that women with fistula require similar long-term care to leprosy patients, and thus might also provide an opportunity to accomplish their "main purpose": "to glorify God, and share the gospel through our work" (SIM Niger 2013). Similarly, a report written by the SIM Medical Advocacy Office highlighted the importance of the Danja Fistula Center to CSL-Danja's strategic future plan. The report stressed that, with the 93 percent drop in leprosy cases since 1993, CSL-Danja must redefine its medical and ministry role and function, and that women with fistula are central to CSL-Danja's future: CSL-Danja is a means to ministry first and a center of physical healing second.[4]

Many other organizations have also shifted their focus from leprosy to fistula, emphasizing the near-equation of the two populations in the zeitgeist. For example, Raoul-Follereau, a leprosy foundation based in France, recently began doing fistula work in Niger. I spoke with a project manager at the Niamey Raoul-Follereau office, inquiring if he believed women with fistula to be "the new lepers." He responded, "In truth, why we say that fistula women are the new lepers is so that people understand that fistula should not be neglected . . . Fistula can have the same social consequences as leprosy. People throw you out, put you aside. If you are with your husband and you leak urine or fecal matter, your husband sends you away—even women's own families send them away! That's why they have to find refuge in the centers—they find others like them, their sisters."

This answer, which ignores the most obvious difference between leprosy and fistula—fistula is not communicable, indicates how strongly the fistula narrative has influenced the perception of women with fistula. In its attempt to highlight the social isolation, exclusion, bodily impurity, and marginality that women with fistula are thought to endure, the donor and media fistula narrative has forged misleading links between fistula and leprosy, framing women with fistula as "new" or "modern-day" lepers. Yet this comparison may be apt in an unexpected way.

Although leprosy became a powerful metaphor for isolation, abandonment, and community revilement, the community stigmatization and isolation of people with leprosy is not, and never has been, universal. In colonial East and Central Africa, forced separation and isolation of people with leprosy was a colonial project, intended to protect public health (and aided by Christian missions with their own evangelical incentives; Vaughan 1991). Many people with leprosy who had been comfortably embedded in their communities were forcefully removed.

Silatham Sermrittirong and Wim Van Brakel (2014) have argued that "the general population did not tend to fear leprosy in the same way [as health officials] and resisted separation from their diseased family and friends" (2014, 8). Leprosy stigma, like fistula stigma, may have been produced by the compulsory segregation that uprooted people from their communities. The fear of leprosy may have paradoxically been due to the efforts to contain it.

The missionary-run centers focused on creating new identities and new ways of being for people with leprosy, but the social consequences of conversion to Christianity were often more significant than the disease. Christianization and confinement, not leprosy, resulted in social vulnerability back home. Although the isolation-in-community of people with leprosy was considered to be for humanitarian reasons not just for public health, these spaces of isolation, containment, and (ostensibly) healing were often no better than imprisonment. "Many of these early settlements were little better than Robben Island. African patients . . . were cut off from their kin, and often from their husbands, wives, and children—deprived, in fact of any social identity" (Vaughan 1991, 86).

In the cases of both leprosy and fistula, the sufferers' archetypal social isolation may be both less complete than portrayed and intensified by the isolating conditions of long-term treatment. Fistula organizations build fistula "colonies," "villages," or centers that isolate women, separating them from their families and communities throughout the lengthy treatment process. Yet women with fistula do have families and communities. Although (as discussed in chapter 6) the fistula narrative positions its archetypical sufferer as a complete exile, with nothing to go home to and nothing to lose, this was not true for the vast majority of women I met. Forty-four percent of the women I came to know had living children, 38 percent were married, and 36 percent were separated. The vast majority of women with fistula were socially embedded, but the long stays away from home threatened that connectedness. At the risk of cynicism, we must ask ourselves whether fistula centers do not recognize this risk of social disconnect—the possibility that they are actively creating the new lepers—or whether they perhaps see the construction of this social pariah as a benefit.

REEXAMINING "HOLISTIC CARE"

When women with fistula are likened to lepers, the long waits for treatment (as discussed in chapter 5) can be easily justified: clinicians and administrators believe that the women are social outcasts, and that waiting at the hospital is unequivocally better than returning to life without hope of the social redemption offered by surgery. When I asked administrators, clinicians, and center staff why women were kept away from home for so long, fingers were pointed elsewhere: bureaucratic inefficiencies, corruption, or mismanagement. But a more poignant social explanation also emerged. Administrators and clinicians frequently added that the women did not mind the long waits because being at the center was better than their alternatives. Some administrators spoke of the "sisterhood of suffering" that being at the center with other women with fistula offered—a sense of community that they could not feel in their marital or natal communities. Clinicians, fistula center staff, and nongovernmental organization (NGO) workers would say, "Women eat better here than at home," "Women like the city life," "Women get a break from hard work and mistreatment here at the center," and "These women, they have nowhere else to go."

While women at centers often felt less shame in leaking among other women who also leaked, less guilt about burdening their loved ones during their illnesses, and less pressure to do onerous physical labor such as farming, collecting water or firewood, or pounding millet,[5] for most women, the negative consequences of waiting far outweighed any benefits. However, the administrators' claims that the long center stays were an unmitigated good neatly deflects the clinic and health system's responsibility for the women's long stays. The centers' inability to deliver rapid care is reframed as a strength: providing a safe space, a refuge. The centers' responsibility to offer women timely access to surgical interventions is obfuscated when the long waits are seen not as clinical failures but as successes in offering social support. When global audiences hear of nine-month or year-long waits, there is no outrage; the unethically long waits are interpreted as time-intensive "holistic care" that results in social transformation for women who are otherwise alone and helpless. Although for Nigérien women with fistula, as noted by Julie Livingston, "Hospitalization, like serious illness more generally, is a process of social estrangement," the public is left to imagine the hospital as a site of restoration, recovery, and redemption (2012, 113). As Meryl Streep narrates in the documentary *Shout Gladi Gladi,* women with fistula are dependent on centers "not just for medical or economic help, but also [for] a sense of belonging and normalcy. A home" (Friedman and Kennedy 2015).

Fistula centers' donors and staff often believe that the social, emotional, and financial ruptures caused by fistula cannot be mended as easily or tidily as the anatomical holes that can be sutured shut inside women's bodies (although, as I note in chapter 5, these injuries are not always so easy to fix). Many fistula treatment centers focus on "holistic" treatment, including postoperative rehabilitative and reintegration assistance—programs, training, and services designed to improve the women's social futures. The centers educate women in sewing, embroidery, knitting, weaving, husbandry, life skills, and basic literacy and arithmetic (and sometimes religious education) to enable them to provide for themselves, gain social status, and rebuild their lives (figure 17). The rehabilitation and reintegration programs are frequently funded to run anywhere from several weeks to several months after a woman's fistula surgery and can cover "any experience that help

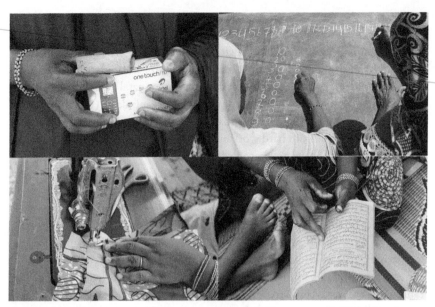

FIGURE 17. *Top left:* A woman holding 75,000 Franc CFA (approximately US$121) and a cellular phone, given as part of a reinsertion program. *Top right:* A woman learning to write numbers during a Danja Fistula Center literacy training. *Bottom left:* A woman learning to sew at a Niamey fistula center. *Bottom right:* Women at a Niamey fistula center teaching one another to read suras from the Qur'an.

improve women's lives after corrective surgery" (Lombard et al. 2015, 555). Although the programs at each center are run differently, the women stayed at the centers for extended periods of time, only half-learning skills. They frequently returned home still wet but with a brand new sewing machine, supplies for an income-generating activity, a new cell phone, or cash (often between 50,000 and 150,000 Franc CFA, approximately US$80 to $240).

Not only do these reintegration courses slow a woman's return home, but they also sometimes even hinder women from pursuing surgical treatment. The fistula center Dimol (which had no capacity to provide surgical interventions for women, but was funded primarily to run these reintegration courses) promised to pay women to participate in months-long training courses. Women with fistula were invited to Niamey from their villages (usually through word-of-mouth and radio advertisements) with vague promises, only to discover when they arrived at Dimol that they were being offered not surgery but some sort of life-skills training course. This happened to Zali (age 25, Hausa), who had lived with fistula for six years and had traveled hundreds of miles to Dimol in response to a radio advertisement. She explained, "After a failed surgery, I returned home until there was a radio message. I did not hear it myself, but my brother heard it and told me that even the transportation would be repaid. I did not know why they told me to come, but I assumed that it was for an operation. So I came here to Dimol. But when I arrived, they said it was for a training course."

When we met, Zali had been at Dimol for more than three months; she still had not been given any money, and she estimated that the center had only run five to seven total days of training since her arrival (during the months I regularly visited Dimol, I witnessed only two days of training courses). I asked Zali what she had learned. She responded, "Not so much. They told us to buy what we can to do some commerce. They told us that we can't let the goats we raise eat just anything like trash." Surprised by the apparent lack of substance in her training (or in her retention), I asked Zali if she thought it was worth it to come to all the way to the center. "Really, I don't know," she responded, looking frustrated. "When they called us here, I thought it was for an operation. Otherwise I would have stayed at home. I had to sell my things to raise the money for transportation here. I have nothing left and can't return home without money for the taxi."

Zali and many other women I met at Dimol opted to complete their training courses and then return home (a necessary step to receiving the promised money) rather than choosing to leave Dimol and move to the adjacent center (CNRFO, which offered fistula surgeries, however infrequently). At CNRFO, many reasoned, they might not being selected for surgery and ran the chance of surgical failure even if they were selected; in other words, at CNRFO they risked returning home both wet and indebted. Perversely, Dimol called back already reintegrated women for further training, encouraging them to leave their homes, their husbands, and their families for an indefinite period of time to participate in an amorphous—and not particularly useful—training program.[6]

Although these courses are largely well intentioned, and some are more useful to women than others, they are born from a particular perception of the social lives to which women with fistula will return. Rather than tacking reintegration programs onto all fistula initiatives, we must examine whether the value women gain from these courses outweighs the harm done by prolonging their absence from home. For some women, the answer will certainly be yes, but for others the reinsertion courses may do more harm than good.[7] Some women are anxious to return home after surgery to their loving husbands, supportive families, and young children, while others need additional support to find strategies to successfully reintegrate into their communities.

CONCEALMENT AND "PASSING"

My research complicates the dominant fistula narrative that frames women with fistula as modern lepers: exposure, abandonment, and isolation until social (if not corporeal and religious) transformation through Western biomedical intervention. Unlike leprosy, which tends to mark the body in visible (and permanent) ways, fistula and its symptoms can be concealed; its stigma can be reduced or eliminated by "passing," an activity that is impossible for most people with leprosy. However, when centers buy into the dominant fistula narrative, they may never consider the possibility that a woman's community might not know about her condition. Unintentionally, fistula centers undermine women's ability to "pass," thus reducing their capacity to return home and reintegrate successfully into their own communities.

Obstetric fistula is often portrayed as an eminently visible marker of a woman's identity, but most of the women I knew in Niger had invested significant resources of their time, energy, and finances into acts of concealment—hiding fistula's symptoms and maintaining control over the information others had about their health. These efforts turned fistula into a largely invisible condition, preventing easy observation.

After the development of her fistula when she was 18, Tshara (40, Hausa) continued to live happily with her co-wives and husband, birthing eight more children, four of whom survived. With the exception of her mother, Tshara concealed her fistula from everyone including her husband for over a decade. "In the beginning, people knew that I was sick," she explained. "I went to the hospital, and when I came back, I wore pads to hide the leak. And now people don't think that I have it anymore. They don't understand why I am back at the hospital now." She explained that because most people in her village were too polite to ask her directly about such an intimate part of the body, she was not often in a position where she had to directly lie about her health status: "If you go to a baptism, people will look at you. Those who visit you stare at you, looking at your feet and your back to see if you are wet or not. And, really, no one but my husband would ask me directly if I was healed. It isn't a polite question. But if they asked, 'How is your health?' I would say 'I have health!' (*Lahiya lau*). Then it is done." Admitting that her deception was sometimes more direct than indirect, Tshara laughed, "As for my husband, when he's asked, I just tell him that I'm healed. *Alhamdulillah* [Praise Allah], I say."

Women's concealment strategies help them to avoid social stigma. Concepts of social stigma (discussed in chapter 2) elucidate why some individuals are valued and others are devalued, considered dangerous or even grotesque. Defined by sociologist Erving Goffman (1963) as a socially undesirable difference, discrediting attribute, behavior, or reputation resulting from a process whereby one's identity is "spoiled" by the reactions of others, stigma acts as a social regulatory mechanism of abnormality. As I elaborated earlier, stigma can be separated into enacted or external stigma (actual experiences of discrimination) and perceived or internal stigma (shame and internalization of stereotypes). Goffman situated "passing" as "the management of undisclosed discrediting information about self" (1963, 42). In order to manage, mitigate, or resist social stigma, one who passes "presents himself as what one is not" (Rohy 1996). Passing is performative, a cultivation of self through routinized everyday acts. Those who engage in passing work know that it is illusory. This selective revelation (and obscuration) leads to a persistent fear of discovery.

Women with fistula often explicitly tried to "pass" as whole (non-fistulous) and sometimes even altogether healthy (generally "well" or "normal"). They employed strict forms of self-management to hide any incriminating evidence of leaks, smells, or other indications of incontinence from neighbors, friends, and some kin. For some women whose conditions had been previously acknowledged within their communities, this meant concealing surgical failure, and thus passing as "healed". Others who were able to conceal from the onset of their conditions went a step further, not only concealing the specific nature and effects of their conditions, but hiding that they were sick at all. A surprising number of women with whom I spoke explained how through ingenuity and discipline they had been able to elude the suspicions of their communities, friends, families, co-wives, and—most impressively—husbands.

Seventy-four of the 100 women I came to know had attempted to conceal the evidence of their incontinence and manage the information about their condition; many of whom were quite successful in their efforts. Fifty-five women hid their fistulas from all or most of their social contacts. For 36 women, only their immediate family or closest contacts knew about their incontinence and its cause. Incredibly, 15 women were able to successfully conceal their fistulas from even their husbands, 11 women claiming that he was still unaware of her condition at the time we initially spoke.

As described in chapter 2, to pass, women with fistula engaged in dual strategies of concealment: (1) quotidian changes in behavior, dress, and hygiene to disguise incontinence, and (2) systemic relational changes, whereby women modified the ways in which they engaged with their families, friends, husbands, households, and communities. Women's days were often dominated by their efforts to conceal as they carefully tended to fabric pads, diligently bathed, selectively fasted, tightly controlled circulating information, and heavily relied on perfumes to cover odors. Women also engaged in a spectrum of self-isolation behaviors, including both physical and social distancing, in order to limit their risk of leaking publically (and thus "outing" themselves). They left their homes less often, opted out of social commitments and reciprocal relationships, accepted marital separations to avoid close proximity to co-wives, and even relocated, moving from rural villages to larger urban towns or cities where they could enjoy relative anonymity.

Although women have conceived of many innovative management solutions to incontinence, the most ubiquitous strategy—used by nearly all of the women I came to know—was the use of fabric pads. Yet, most of the women lacked experience managing constant vaginal flows because they had historically experienced light menstruation or elongated periods of amenorrhea (due to pregnancies, lactation, and sometimes malnutrition), and thus they had little existing knowledge about the use of pads at the onset of their fistulas. Fabric pad construction, utilization, and hygiene was taught and learned among the women in centers, sometimes through direct teaching by clinic staff, but most often informally, through junior women's observation of more experienced women's daily management routines while women lived and bathed in close quarters. In places with limited resources, the women innovated solutions, creating their own appropriate technologies for incontinence management and concealment. The women used rags, towels, and foam stripped from couch upholstery to make pads, and plastic sheeting or crocheted plastic bags to sleep or sit on or to make water-resistant protective garments, depending on the severity of their incontinence.

Many women dressed to conceal their wetness, wearing their skirt wrappers, which customarily end at the ankles, extra long so that they cover the feet as well to conceal any stream of urine that might be visible on their skin. This was the method used by Zaynab (30, Zarma). "In the village there is dirt and dust everywhere. Our feet become grey with it. When the urine runs, the stream is clear on my legs, on my feet. People might stare. So I cover myself," she explained. As well as changing the way she wore her skirt wrapper, Zaynab also switched from the more popular chest-length *hijabi* to a more conservative floor-length *hijabi* to hide any visible wetness on her behind.

Many women also attempted to diminish the flow by controlling their intake of liquids. A'i (17, Hausa) explained, "I try not to drink water when the sun is up. I try to live a normal life. So my friends don't know. No one knows that I leak. At home, the secret is shared only between me, my mom, and my husband." A'i coupled the reduction in her intake of liquids with protective garments, investing much of her money in extra clothing; she wore two skirt wrappers over two pairs of underpants that she had purchased with saved money in urban markets.

To limit their risk of leaking in public, most women with fistula in Niger reduce the time they spend outside their home to a minimum, and they generally avoid social events. Rather than being discriminated against by their communities, as is frequently suggested in the donor and media narratives, most of the women I spoke to retreated from society of their own accord. When I asked Rachida (37, Songhai) if she felt that she was confined to her home because of her fistula, she responded, "No, it is my choice. I don't leave the house because I don't want people to look at me. But it is my choice." Raha (55, Hausa) explained that she rarely left the house and when she did, she went mostly into the bush where there were no people. "I don't want to be around them. I don't want them to look at me and ask each other, 'Is she wet? Does she smell?'" The women felt most comfortable when they were able to socially and physically distance themselves from community members and sometimes even kin. As they explained, staying home and self-isolating provided them some distance from the anxiety, shame, and humiliation they might experience if others saw their bodies out of control.

Nearly every woman I knew made some attempt to conceal her fistula (with the exception of the women with newly developed fistulas or the women who had not yet returned home).[8] Yet as ubiquitous and as important as I found concealment work to be in the lives of women, it is absent in the dominant conceptualization of fistula. It is also largely overlooked in the extant corpus of fistula literature; even the literature that does recognize women's investment in self-regulation focus not on concealment, but on "coping" strategies, where afflicted individuals attempt to mediate the negative externalities of their conditions.[9] Although the concepts are similar, "coping" overlooks women's intention not only to reduce community mistreatment or personal shame, but to *pass*. Concealment efforts—women's refusal to disclose—allowed women to at least publically embody whole (non-fistulous) and healthy (normal) identities. Although some women I came to know did seem to "cope" more than "conceal"—attempting only to manage their leaking and its accompanying smell—a stunning number of women's efforts far exceeded this. Their efforts were not just regulatory but transformational.[10]

These coping and concealment strategies were aimed at managing internal stigma as well as external stigma. Although the fistula narrative focuses largely on external stigma—the treatment women are subjected to by others, as explained in chapter 2—most women's narratives of suffering focused largely on the internal (experienced as shame, loss of identity, and valuelessness). When the women recounted their experiences, they talked about their embarrassment, the shame they felt, and the constant worry about whether they would ever get better.

Outed

Just as fistula centers create and shape women's separation from home and family, they also replicate the leprosy sufferer's public rejection by outing the women with fistula who had been able to conceal their conditions from their home communities—women who had *passed*. Outing is thus another real-world consequence of the fistula narrative. In an effort to increase public awareness of an organization (with the hopes that funding will follow), donation ceremonies become publicity events. Fabric (often emblazoned with the word "fistula"), soap, perfume, and other goods are given out to women with fistula. On donation days in Niamey, typically one or two women are asked to publically offer thanks to the organization, which is broadcast on television stations throughout Niger. At one particular donation ceremony in Niamey, organized by the First Lady's organization "Guri, for a Better Life," a Guri administrator eyed the woman who volunteered, telling a center nurse, "No, she won't do. We need someone younger and more beautiful." Eventually a stunning young woman with a child was chosen as requested. The woman was not asked for her consent, nor were the implications of her participation explained. She had been concealing her fistula from her community for two and a half years.

My research assistant would often excitedly tell women at the center that she had seen them on television the night before. The women were frequently surprised to hear it. One morning after a local student-run group had come to a center and given each woman five pieces of soap, a small bag of detergent, and half a box of powdered milk (a donation that was televised), my research assistant joked with the woman who had been chosen to give public thanks that she was now a television star. The woman was deeply concerned about her visibility; she had been hiding her fistula from everyone but her close family for two years, and although there was no electricity in her village, she was worried that someone would see the broadcast in town. The other women who were featured on the broadcast (including women who were not asked to give public thanks but were filmed nonetheless) expressed similar anxiety.

The gift of fabric (*pagne*, or *zane*) with fistula-related logos is a double-edged sword (figure 18). When organizations offer women fabric publicizing the fistula center, an international fistula organization, or fistula-related awareness campaigns, most women are not in a position to refuse. Women with fistula are often plagued by a perpetual scarcity of fabric due to their heavy use of cloth pads and the acidity of their urine that rapidly degrades their skirt wrappers. For example, Mariama (50, Hausa), who had lived with fistula for over 30 years, complained that she was constantly in need of more fabric to make pads: "Because of the urine, the fabric is quickly ruined. I have a difficult time getting enough fabric. Sometimes I have to use my husband's clothing for pads. When he goes out for the day, I will use a pair of his pants or a shirt to manage the urine. Before he returns home, I will wash and dry his clothing and put them back." For women like Mariama, the gift of fabric is a welcome resource. Yet, as no woman I interviewed was literate; the women may not be aware that these sartorial choices will advertise, or at least associate, them as women with fistula once home.

The women's confidentiality is also jeopardized when they are accompanied back home by clinic staff after postsurgical reintegration courses. For some women, outing might be a cause of increased shame, embarrassment, or mild social tensions. For other women, particularly those who found themselves socially vulnerable before the development of their fistulas, community or household/spousal knowledge of their conditions can be a cause of significant social harm. Aïshatou (27, Zarma) was healed of fistula. Yet, she had a precarious position within her household before the development of her fistula. The entire time she leaked, Aïshatou had hidden her fistula from her community members. However, after a successful repair surgery she was accompanied back to her village by health officers, who publically acknowledged that, like Aïshatou, women who leak can be fixed; such "community awareness" interventions are a common prevention strat-

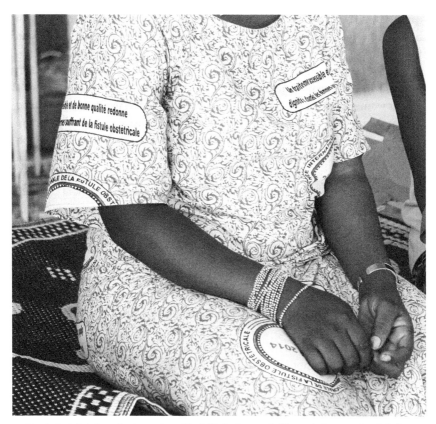

FIGURE 18. A fistula patient wearing gifted fabric that reads "Journée International de la Fistule Obstétricale 2014" (International Obstetric Fistula Day 2014). The fabric also advertises "accessible treatment with dignity for all women" along with other fistula-related phrases.

egy integrated into many fistula reintegration programs. Aïshatou recalled, "[The center staff person] called a village meeting to tell everyone about fistula. She pointed to me and said that because of my fistula I shouldn't be mocked or treated differently. I returned home, but for a month after I didn't leave my house because I was so ashamed. I wish she had not said anything about it." This public outing— driven by the center, whose staff could not imagine that someone might not know about the condition that plagued Aïshatou—did lasting damage to her social life. Aïshatou eventually returned to the fistula center—this time as a refuge—because of the outing's social repercussions and her deeply felt shame.

When I broached the subject of "accompaniment" at an international fistula conference held in Niamey in October of 2013, very few fistula experts acknowledged that women might not want to be accompanied home.[11] In a small working group, I suggested that accompaniment converts women into martyrs for the cause; it used them to raise community awareness about fistula but stripped them of the choice to reveal (or conceal) their own health status. A middle-aged man from eastern Niger who had worked with a fistula NGO for many years was indignant at my suggestion—his NGO's specialty was reinsertion programs that culminated in accompaniment back home. "Everyone in the community knows [about women's fistulas]!" he cried, raising his hands in the air. The room seemed to split among those who believed that women could conceal their conditions and those who did not. A middle-aged woman who worked in health administration chimed in, disagreeing with the NGO worker: "I knew of a woman who had fistula for 18 years and no one knew!" One particularly outspoken female obstetrician/gynecologist from the city of Maradi stood up: "For us, [accompaniment] is good. It offers us the opportunity to sensitize those who are otherwise hard to reach. But it serves us more than the women. And the woman accepts because she cannot tell the health agents no." After several hours of debate, the group came to an uneasy recommendation that the practice of accompaniment be discontinued. In the full session, dozens of participants challenged this recommendation, asking, "Why would you get rid of this? It is about holistic care!" and protesting, "This is also an opportunity for us to get the word out, and to follow up with other women who've been healed!"

This discussion revealed the prevalence of the assumption that fistula is an all-defining trait that cannot be concealed—a result, perhaps, of dominant donor and media narratives of fistula. Although sometimes contested, this assumption leads to fistula policy and programming that unintentionally threatens women's identities as "well" once home. This is not an indictment of the devoted practitioners and advocates for women's health, who fight with very limited resources to improve maternal health. Rather, it is evidence that women's concealment practices are still quite poorly understood, even among many of those working in the field of fistula prevention and treatment.

In discussions of female incontinence in the Global North, the focus is on the ethos of the sufferer—her struggle to redefine her identity, her feelings of shame and betrayal by her own body—not the reaction of her social contacts.[12] The same is not true of women with fistula in Niger, where the discourse surrounding fistula tends to focus on forces external to the women: mistreatment from husbands and rejection from communities, often due to a perceived corrupted culture that valorizes only the reproductive capacity of women. Yet, this persistent focus on the external fails to capture the daily struggles of Nigérien women with fistula. Women's quotidian reality of fistula was dominated by internal battles of identity, emotional isolation, anxiety about passing, fear of outing, and social alienation resulting from prolonged absences. These existential struggles are obfuscated by a dominant narrative that echoes the plight of the leper: visibility, rejection, and social abuse.

For women with fistula, likened to lepers and thus treated as such, their interface with the institutions mediating fistula care was not altogether salutary. Torn from the social fabric of their communities by their quest for care, women with fistula struggled to make sense of their social realities. Many became entangled in interventions that were designed for a different kind of woman, a woman who through her superlative suffering could benefit the centers and their staff. Women were kept at centers too long, their alibis for treatment-seeking were jeopardized by clinics, and their efforts at concealment and self-management were continually undermined; this is the cost of the hyperbolic donor and media fistula narrative.

There is a complicated relationship to truth in what Agustín (2007) terms the "rescue industry," where hyperbole is exchanged for compassion. Too often, these semifictionalized narratives occlude or obscure *truths* in the service to a greater *Truth*—the gestalt of a crisis, the intense need for intervention. But truth matters, and when we overlook specificities, particularities, and discrepancies, we risk doing more harm than good.

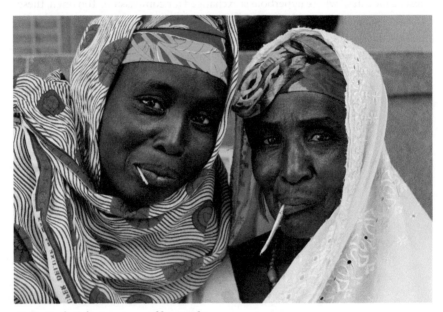

Portrait of a Fulani woman and her mother

8 · THE THRESHOLD OF CONTINENCE

A YEAR LATER

In the fall of 2014, several months after my departure from the field, I returned to Niger. During my brief visit in Niamey, I was able to speak to about two dozen of the women I had come to know the year before, adding another time slice to their rich life histories.[1]

When I returned to Niamey, I found Fana (43, Tuareg), the first woman I wrote about in this book, who had been healed of fistula seven years before we met. I initially went to Fana's father's house, but there I was told that two months before she had married her fourth husband and had moved into his home. With directions from her stepmother and her new cell phone number, I eventually found Fana and her young daughter Safi in a neighborhood on the edges of Niamey. Narrow, tortuous dirt paths were framed by tall gates that concealed houses in various states of disrepair. Fana's new home was decidedly nicer than her last. Still, with only two small, windowless rooms, a dirt floor, and mud walls, it was the house of a family with few means.

Over tea, Fana explained that after a year living in a small space with her ill father, his wife, and their children, money became tighter than ever, resentment intensified, and tensions reached a crescendo. She knew that her living situation was untenable. But because her mother was so poor and lived in a politically unstable region of Mali, she reckoned that she could not safely return. When Fana took stock of her options, she reasoned that there were few and none was particularly desirable. She conceded that marriage was her only realistic choice, and when Aboubakar came along, she reluctantly accepted his proposal:

> I didn't know his family, and I didn't know him. And I was sitting there when he came and said, "I am looking for a marriage." And I said, "So, you didn't hear about me? . . . I have my own problem, so tomorrow if you marry me, you won't say that I hid something from you? You won't say that I deceived you?" . . . And he said, "I

don't mind. But I am a poor man, so you must be patient with me. Sometimes I have, but sometimes I don't. So if I have, we can eat, but if I don't have, we must wait." . . . And so our marriage was celebrated. I didn't know anything about him, and he didn't know anything about me.

Fana's marriage to Aboubakar was neither a family marriage nor for love. She did not see her husband as a companion, a friend, or an ally; he was just her only option. She, a divorcée with little social capital and a dismal health record; he, destitute and unable to regularly provide for a family. The trade seemed even, they reckoned. Fana had long abandoned romantic ideas of marriage.

Powerlessness, Fana explained, was the curse of women: "I really thought that I would never get a husband again in this world . . . In my first marriage, my husband divorced me because of the urine. My second husband . . . it was because of my co-wife . . . The third, when he came to ask to marry me, I told him that I couldn't because I had the urine sickness, and he said he didn't care about that. He insisted, and finally I accepted, but only about one, two, or three weeks later he said he couldn't live with Safi and the urine . . . He said, 'Okay, take your stuff and leave my home.'" Remarking upon gender asymmetries in Niger, Fana accepted that patience was gendered: "It's a woman who has patience because if she has to leave, she doesn't know where to go, but a man—when it is a woman who has a problem, the man will throw her out, and replace her with another one." "Women here," she concluded, "have to get by. They have to trust in Allah. They must be patient." And with patience, she had scraped by for many decades, jumping from marriage to marriage after each husband had thrown her out.

Hoping for a happy—or at least tolerable—ending to her story, I asked Fana if she was satisfied with her marriage with Aboubakar. Fana gazed at her daughter, "I'm still here. Life is going. But I'm not feeling good. I'm really not feeling good. Sometimes we eat, and sometimes we don't. It's been since yesterday evening that we ate; we didn't have anything until now. I am not going to say I am happy in my marriage." Seeing the disappointment in my face—I had longed for a better future for Fana—she almost apologetically added, "Telling the truth is better than not."

As we chatted, swapped stories, and looked through photos I had taken, Fana's husband walked into the room. Fana's jaw stiffened. She refused to make eye contact with him. The pitch of her voice changed, and she snapped at him, asking him for money. He said he had none and left the room, taking with him the last bowl of rice in the house.

Fana had confided in me that her new husband looked at her daughter with anger and impatience; she feared that he would hit the little girl, or decide that he did not want her in his home anymore despite his promises, just as her third husband had. Fana also explained that since the marriage she had been experiencing gynecological pain. Although she initially suggested that perhaps something had gone wrong with her cesarean scar (then the same age as Safi, four years old), the more we discussed it, the clearer it became that Fana suspected that her husband had given her a sexually transmitted infection. Its diagnosis alone was far beyond her financial means, to say little of its treatment.

Although Fana had been healed of her incontinence for eight years, fistula continued to place constraints on her life—both financial and social. Fistula had reduced her fertility, added to the number of divorces behind her, and increased the years between her and a stable married life. This, in her estimation, drastically reduced her social value, leaving her with few marriage options. So she had to settle for Aboubakar, a man she mistrusted and disliked. Her fistula had continued to imprint itself on her marriage, her body, her child, and her future—even after she was healed and her continence was restored. Fistula's persistent power was mediated by several converging factors: the absence of Fana's mother in her daily life, which left her socially unprotected; her lived poverty, which constrained her marital options; and gender inequalities, which left Fana, and women like her, disproportionately vulnerable at all life's stages. So Fana waited vigilantly, expecting that one day Aboubakar would tire of her and she would be forced to move on again, a guest in another fickle man's home.

I had returned to Niamey during the tail end of the rainy season. Because of the chronic nature of fistula, many women's treatment-seeking behaviors look a lot like seasonal migration. Fistula centers' numbers often rise and fall along with the need for labor at home and in fields. During Niger's dry season, when there is little work to be done in the fields or with food preparation in the villages, women head to the centers. Their numbers peak during the "hungry season," the period between harvests when stored grains run out and there is little left to eat. During these periods fistula centers in Niger are overcrowded, with women sometimes sleeping two to a bed and in outdoor shaded areas, which are always covered with mats. But I returned during the rainy season in the fall of 2014, and very few women were at either CNRFO or Dimol. They were said to have returned home where their labor was essential to the next year's harvest. I was told that they would return to the centers after the rain.

With so few women, the centers felt particularly static and the remaining women seemed listless. The six women's dorm rooms at CNRFO had all been in use for the majority of my fieldwork; during the rainy season of 2014 one had been converted into storage, and another was being used as an office for female personnel. Many of the beds were empty, and the center's atmosphere was languid. The usual six or seven groupings of women (ordinarily divided by ethnicity and then again by age) had been consolidated to three—the Hausa and Tuareg women spent their time on mats under a newly constructed tin-roofed hangar while the Zarma women congregated around the large neem tree in the central courtyard. The remaining women lounged on their beds in their rooms, spending time with their roommates or occasionally joining the two groups. Only a handful of women were left at Dimol.

I learned that since I left many of the women I had interviewed had undergone one or two additional surgeries. Some had returned home for a few months in between surgeries; some had not. Most claimed to be no better. In the year that had passed, little to no progress appeared to have been made in determining how to care for complex and potentially incurable cases. The women like Nafissa, whose case files were scribbled with words such as "very difficult," "no urethra," "extensive scarring," and "huge fistula," were disproportionately still at the centers. Not only were many of these women with the most complex, difficult-to-repair fistulas still at the centers when I returned a year later, they also still had not been told anything about their cases, nor had they been given a timeline for their care. When I asked them how long they had been at the center, many shrugged; "forever," one woman responded.

Most women I spoke to this time were still incontinent, still waiting for answers, still searching for solutions. However, this small sample was certainly unrepresentative. Among the women whom I did not speak with—those who were lost to follow-up, were no longer at the centers, could not be reached by phone, or had simply disappeared—were likely those who had successfully attained continence. Probably they had resumed their lives, severing their connections with the fistula centers and only infrequently (if at all) returning for follow-up consultations or for gynecological care.

Most of the women who left the centers and did not return left behind a contact number. Some women had come to centers with cell phones; the rest were given one from donor reintegration funding. However, in mid-2013, the Nigérien government began to require that Nigériens register their numbers with their cell phone companies using photo identification. Those with preexisting numbers who did not go to one of three major cellular phone carriers' offices had their SIM cards and phone numbers cut off. Many rural people, particularly women, have no forms of identification, no money for transport to telecommunications headquarters, and no knowledge of changes in policies. As a result, the contact numbers women had given me the year before often were no longer in service. Fewer than a dozen of the 100 women were reachable by phone. Each attempt I made to call was met with the same high-pitched, atonal French recording informing me that the number was unavailable.

Still, through the grapevine I heard that some of these women were now dry (or drier). Many women were said to have returned home, several had remarried, and a few had even birthed children. During my time in Niamey, I witnessed the cesarean delivery of a woman whose fistula had been successfully closed two years before. She gave birth to her first living son. After her five stillborn children, this child was her opportunity for a renewed future. Her husband had not made the trip down to see her give birth, he had not sent money, and he had not called. But her mother waited anxiously outside her hospital room, reluctant to leave her daughter's side during the operation. As the woman recuperated from her cesarean, she stroked her infant's forehead and ruminated about their future. "Everything has changed," she said, laughing. For this woman, her son represented so many transformations: the possibility of renewed warmth with her husband, equality with her co-wife, protection in her old age, and a new identity for herself—no longer a woman with the "sickness of urine" or a *wabi,* but a mother of a healthy boy.

I was able to reinterview one other young Zarma woman who might otherwise have been lost to follow-up. One Sunday while I was in Niamey, four of her friends from Dimol placed her things above their heads and ceremoniously moved her five blocks away to her new home. Two years before, she had arrived at Dimol with a fresh fistula, and there she waited many months before finally walking across the street to CNRFO where she eventually received her first operation. Luckily, she attained continence with that first surgery. In the months that followed, she met an honest young man in the neighborhood and became his second wife. We sat down to catch up three days after her wedding. Her girlfriends were still packed into her small room—it was customary for them to stay close to her for her first week of marriage to ease her transition into married life. Her hands and feet were covered in the deep browns and bright reds of ceremonial henna that festoon the toes and fingers of all new Nigérien brides. Her husband's name was dyed in the center of her palm. It was clear that she too had begun again.

Of the 16 women I was able to reinterview during this follow-up visit, 12 were still wet, and only four were dry. Eleven were at either Dimol or CNRFO; only five were at home. Three of the women had undergone two additional failed surgeries each during the previous year; each of these three women had at this point undergone a total of seven failed surgeries. They now waited at the center for their eighth operations. I was also surprised to see three women at the center who I had previously counted as dry; I learned that since I had left Niger their repairs had broken down, and they had all begun to leak again. As if to balance out this sad news, I learned that three other women had remarried in the capital, and two others had given birth to children. Of the 84 women I did not speak with again, I cannot say how many of them had stories of success and renewal to tell. Some, I imagine, were given an opportunity to start anew, and some were not.

REIMAGING FISTULA WORK

Much of this book has highlighted surgeries that fail, representations that mislead, and interventions that might actually harm—in short, what is not working in the realm of fistula care. The stories of these 100 women, women like Fana, Laraba, or Hasana, may leave us feeling frustrated and even a bit cynical. Some readers may experience this work as undermining the project of fistula intervention. They might ask, if the consequences of fistula on women are not as bad as we thought, does their suffering still merit all of this attention? Perhaps, the money could be better spent elsewhere? Does intervening do more harm than good? Others who are less willing to altogether abandon fistula intervention might instead wonder about the specific allocation of resources. If surgical outcomes are poorer than is commonly claimed, should treatment be financially deprioritized? Is it ethical to send women home with sewing machines or sums of money, or invest resources into reintegration programs when basic maternal care is so poor? Should fistula care be rationed? If so, how many repeat surgeries should be attempted on women who are (according to the data) unlikely to achieve continence, when a backlog of women wait at centers for first-time surgeries? These are all questions that I have heard; some I myself have asked, and they deserve discussing.

How do we move forward, and where exactly is "forward"? A widely quoted passage from Michel Foucault gives us direction on how we can make the experiences of these 100 women impactful: "My point is not that everything is bad, but that everything is dangerous, which is not exactly the same as bad. If everything is dangerous, then we always have something to do. So my position leads not to apathy but to a hyper- and pessimistic activism" (1983/2003, 104). The discourse surrounding fistula can indeed be dangerous; as I have shown, it has both conceptual and concrete consequences, shaping how we think about intervening in Africa generally and with fistula specifically. But we should not turn away from fistula because of this danger. A heightened awareness of the problems, in the words of Foucault, gives us "something to do." Armed with data, we can become advocates for thoughtful innovation of current practice.

Born of a "hyper- and pessimistic activism," in this book I have begun to imagine how fistula programming might be improved. Although anthropologists are trained to critique—artfully problematizing and relentlessly scrutinizing—we often stop short of offering solutions. Still, translating women's lived experiences into research and then translating research into action, change, and reform are essential. We must become more attentive to the complexity of experience, and more cautious with our conclusions. We must be ever more vigilant to uphold the ethics surrounding the provision of fistula care and to transform knowledge gained from ethnographic endeavors into more insightful, targeted interventions.

Most fistula interventions endorse a three-pronged approach, focusing on prevention, treatment, and reintegration, so in the remainder of this chapter, I offer some ideas of how to constructively move forward in all three levels of care in ways that will best benefit the women with fistula I came to know and the thousands of other women like them. Although the suggestions I offer are specific to fistula work in Niger, many may also be relevant to fistula care elsewhere in the Global South. They offer us a place to start.

The right to health is not only the right to treatment, but the right to prevention. Thus, current interventions to prevent fistula—which often place blame on victims and focus on "changing culture" rather than changing structures—must be reimagined. Committed action to reduce the incidence of fistula (and all other preventable maternal morbidities and mortalities) should refrain from pathologizing local norms, practices, or people, but instead target poorly performing health services, female disempowerment, regional poverty, and the global systems that promote such inequity. Admittedly, the scope of structural transformation is lofty, long-term, some may say impractical, and incompatible with current funding mechanisms on which most interventions rely. Still, we are a part of a global system, and how we vote, where we put our money, what policies we promote, and which media we consume matters. Health inequities are political and through inaction we are all complicit.

If we think smaller-scale and shorter-term, there is still room for a significant retooling of our approach to fistula prevention. By intervening into the base of Niger's health care system pyramid, which currently fails many rural women, we can work to reduce third-phase delays—the delay women experience in receiving quality care once at a health center. Prevention-focused interventions must increase the quality of emergency obstetric care at all levels, its accessibility, and the public trust in it. Specific strategies may include the improvement of referral systems during problematic labors (incentivizing referrals that are rapid and vertical) and strengthening the professionalism and caliber of training of low-level health care providers. Yet the improvement in the quality of care will not translate into better outcomes if women cannot access it; so financial and transportation barriers must be addressed through the continued elimination of user fees, the increased availability of low-cost or free essential medicines, and the expansion of free ambulance services in rural areas. Finally, patients' will not access biomedicine often or promptly enough if they have reason to mistrust it. Women's confidence in the health care system must be supported, both through improved clinical communication and increased accountability of providers and clinics for medical malpractice.

A committed attention to prevention may help to stem the tide of obstetric catastrophes, leading to fewer women who develop fistula in the future. Yet, as essential as prevention proves to be in the fight against fistula, it does little for the women who already have it. For those women, the findings of this research can reshape the ways in which fistula clinics and their funders envision care. Interventions must increase the accessibility of fistula repair surgeries, ensure that surgical treatment is faster and less disruptive to women's lives, and endorse a broader and more comprehensive approach to fistula treatment. Additionally, donors should reexamine funding paradigms for treatment that may unintentionally discourage the rapid provision of care.

Poor clinician-patient communication and the lack of coordinated responses in health centers all along the referral chain mean that too many women have fistulas for months or years before they enter an appropriate fistula care center. To address this, clinicians and administrators at all low- and mid-level health centers in Niger should be trained in basic detection and diagnosis of fistula. If providers throughout the health care pyramid could identify the condition, were aware of treatment possibilities, and had the current contact information for fistula centers as well as the dates for upcoming surgical missions, women could be rapidly referred to the appropriate centers—reducing the financial, social, and emotional burdens for women living with untreated fistula.

Once the women arrive at the centers, practitioners should work to improve their communication with them. Many women are not told that they have fistula until they arrive; even so, they rarely understand what fistula is, how they developed it, what its consequences are for them, or when or if they are likely to find a cure. Although some centers already do this, all of them should organize regular counseling sessions where women can ask questions, voice their concerns, and be advised by center staff on the cause of their injuries and the potential options for closure and continence. Importantly, women should be given realistic information about their likely surgical outcomes so that they can make individual and informed decisions regarding if or when to stop pursuing surgical treatment.

Generally, the prospects of surgical success could be improved. Coordinated efforts should be made to increase surgical expertise and local capacity by encouraging more collaborative work among experts and facilitating intracontinental training for Nigérien fistula surgeons. An investment must be made in building the capacity of and retaining local surgical experts; however, there also must be more aggressive control of who operates on women. First-time operations sometimes take place in regional hospitals or by inexperienced visiting medical missions, and it is not until these operations fail that women are referred to specialized fistula surgeons. As a woman's best chance for surgical success is during her first operation, fistula surgeries should be exclusively performed by highly-trained fistula repair surgeons in centers with strong oversight.

A woman's chance of obtaining continence is not solely determined by the skill of her surgeon or the complexity of her condition; the prospects of closure and continence are often mediated by postoperative care. Activities of daily living—coughing, sleeping on one's stomach, sweeping, or defecation, for example—increase abdominal pressure, which can cause surgical breakdown (known as operative dehiscence). Researchers such as Yves-Jacques Castille and his colleagues (2013) have shown that physiotherapy—the management of abdominal pressure and pelvic floor training—in conjunction with health education sessions dramatically improved the odds of recovery for postoperative women, both increasing the chances of surgical success and decreasing the chances of residual stress incontinence.

While fistula centers should strive to offer physical therapy for women, on an even more basic level, women must be continuously cared for by a trained nursing staff. Although women at the Danja Fistula Center received both physical therapy and constant monitoring by highly trained practitioners, nowhere else in Niger was this the case. Women at other centers were obligated to care for themselves or their roommates following surgery. Unassisted, women got up to go to the bathroom, to sweep their floors, or to get food. It is unclear how many surgeries broke down because of these demands of daily living. When I asked a visiting Sudanese fistula surgeon about success rates, he explained: "In my experience, if the center is well equipped and has good staff, the cure rate is always raising. The problem is that people think that the failure or success depends only on the surgeons . . . But in truth, outside of the operation room, 50 percent of the operations fail." Clearly, when envisioning improvements to treatment, we must look beyond the surgical table.

Given that many women experienced repeated surgical failure and continued incontinence, surgery cannot be seen as the only solution. Fistula centers should begin to institute contingency plans in the case of surgical failure, including improving strategies for living with chronic fistula. More money and research should focus on how women can manage fistula with safe, affordable, accessible, and discreet technologies. Currently, most women improvise their own strategies using the limited materials available to them to cope with and sometimes conceal their incontinence. With dedicated research, better devices and technologies could be designed; with dedicated funding, the technologies that exist could become more widely available. Urethral plugs, modified silicone menstrual cups, and pads and garments fashioned from innovative absorptive materials, for example, have been shown to be effective tools for some women to comfortably manage incontinence (Russell 2016). Simple, low cost technologies such as these are an essential component of a comprehensive fistula treatment strategy. The benefits they provide women must not be underestimated. When we accept that surgery is not a magic bullet, we can reimagine innovative management of incontinence as the key to enhancing the quality of life for the women who may live with some degree of leaking for decades.

Additionally, we must prioritize the organization of a surgical committee to evaluate "incurable" or "inoperable" cases in Niger. Women with complex cases, who often wait at centers for years without much hope of attaining continence through surgery, should be shifted into an alternative treatment paradigm, such as training in the techniques and technologies for chronic incontinence management. Leaving these women waiting for surgeries in hope of a successful repair is a gross violation of their dignity and rights.

Women who cannot or will not receive timely care should not be kept at centers while their social lives at home slowly degrade. The long wait times at centers must be dramatically decreased. To do this, fistula care should rely less on foreign missions, whose visits are irregular and infrequent, for surgical interventions. Instead, the centers could strengthen intercenter collaborations to pool their resources and decrease wait times for operations. For example, Dimol (with many patients but no surgeons) could send women to Danja (with the capacity to operate but not enough patients to fill beds); Danja could then send the postoperative women who wanted reintegration training back to Dimol. National standards should be set; if surgeries cannot be provided within one month, women could have the choice to return on a given date for surgery rather than waiting at centers for indeterminate periods of time. Scheduled appointments would minimize the time women spend at centers and maximize their time at home, reducing the social consequences caused by long absences.

These long waits cannot be addressed if women's waiting translates into profit for fistula centers. Women with fistula must not be seen primarily as sources of revenue. Ethical interventions can only take place when women are viewed as clients entitled to the highest quality, most efficient services. In too many centers the patients currently act as "employees" of sorts, simply by filling the beds; they are providing income for the centers because large multinational agencies pay the women's room and board. These findings are thus of concern not only to centers: funders must examine whether these funding schemes disincentive rapid care and thus jeopardize women's social health.

For women who finally regain continence (or at least are preparing to return home, perhaps still incontinent), reintegration interventions should be reimagined to better meet their needs. Programming that would benefit the majority of women with fistula would integrate maternal health modules. Women with fistula have high rates of stillbirths with their subsequent pregnancies (as shown in chapter 3), and the women should be taught to recognize and act upon the signs of problems early in their pregnancies and to identify and avoid infection.

Importantly, reintegration interventions should be crafted to respect women's privacy. The interventions must acknowledge that many women conceal their fistulas, and they must respect the women's choice to "pass" by not calling their husbands or family members and by not insisting on accompanying the women home. Women should also be able to opt out entirely from reinsertion programming. For some women, the most effective way to reduce fistula stigma is to reduce the time they spend away from their homes in the pursuit of treatment, so reintegration courses should not be compulsory or tied to surgical benefits. This means that we must question the business model of centers such as Dimol that do not offer medical treatment and thus are incentivized to hold women with fistula indefinitely.

As a question of human rights, women must not be denied their papers or stopped from leaving the centers when they wish—a practice that often forces women to wait months to be released after their initial requests to leave. For women who have no supportive networks to return to, alternate solutions—such as apprenticeship programs in cities—should be envisioned and enacted.

My final suggestion concerns the way we tell stories. I have focused, in part, on the harm done by the dominant fistula narrative—cherry-picked stories twisted to suit a certain agenda, stories that subordinates truth to Truth. In conservation biology, the somewhat pejorative term *charismatic megafauna* describes a group of large animals that have widespread popular appeal: elephants, lions, Bengal tigers, giant pandas, bald eagles, great white sharks, gorillas. Due to the disproportionate interest the public has in these particular animals, conservation activists often leverage these "charismatic" animals to achieve larger ecological goals. For example, by raising public awareness about the environmental pressures and shrinking natural habitat of the giant panda (their iconic animal), the World Wildlife Fund (among many other organizations) galvanizes the public to donate their money, time, and political capital toward the protection of the panda—and, by extension, the entire ecosystem to which the panda belongs. The trickle-down conservation philosophy behind these efforts has been called the *umbrella effect,* where preserving one iconic animal can "save less-glamorous species that thrive in its shadow" (Marris 2013).

The girl with fistula achieves for humanitarian aid organizations, feminist activists, and concerned journalists what charismatic animals achieve for conservationists. Women with fistula—or "superlative sufferers," as I have called them—can be understood as charismatic victims. They are more captivating than the millions of other women who suffer from poor quality maternal health care. But just as within conservation biology where the trickle-down effect of the charismatic animal has been questioned, the charisma of the superlative sufferer may do little to change the maternal health landscape as a whole. Conversely, her suffering may eclipse the suffering rendered "ordinary" of millions of women in the Global South whose bodies bear witness to the everyday violence of a health system that has failed them.

How can we tell stories of suffering that neither exploit the sufferers nor trivialize their trials? How can anthropologists affect the way that stories of suffering are told outside our purview, on the opinion pages of the *New York Times* and in the fistula aid organization brochures? I suggest that increasing the readability and accessibility of ethnography, the tool of the anthropologist, is one answer.[2] Neither reductionism nor obfuscation, ethnography's only goal is to capture women's words and actions and to place them in context. Ethnography captures the rich variety and texture of life, rather than reducing many voices to one that fits tidily into a 700-word column. In listening to women in Niger, I have heard stories of incredible strength and determination in the face of hardship. Through decades of fistula concealment or dogged quests for treatment, women demonstrate agency despite myriad constraints. Women's fistula narratives so often expose vulnerability and shame, and a deep sense of loss for stillborn children, broken marriages, and shattered womanhood. Yet still there is hope—a fiercely loving mother, a new boyfriend who does not care about a woman's incontinence, a community does not mistreatment a woman with fistula.

In an ancient Hindu parable, a group of blind men attempt to "see" an elephant by touching a single part of its body—a tusk, a tail, a trunk, a torso, but their partial experiences mislead them. For the man touching the elephant's trunk, a giant snake stands before him. For the man groping the leg, a tree trunk takes root. The man touching the elephant's side imagines himself standing in front of a great wall. None of the men can envision the elephant because its parts are felt in isolation. Similarly, when we hear a single story of a woman with fistula, we may believe that she represents the totality of truth; two stories—the proverbial trunk and tail—can then feel irreconcilable. In isolation, we cannot decipher the true shape of the problem. To begin envisioning better solutions, we must step back, take the time to gather data, share knowledge, and accept the multiplicities of experience.

APPENDIX

TABLE 4 Demographic characteristics by ethnic group of 100 women with fistula

Characteristic	Hausa N (%)	Zarma N (%)	Tuareg N (%)	Fulani N (%)	Other* N (%)	Total** N (%)
No. of women	41 (41)	31 (31)	14 (14)	8 (8)	6 (6)	100 (100)
Age at time of interview (years)						
12–19	5 (55.6)	3 (33.3)	1 (11.1)	0 (0.0)	0 (0.0)	9 (9.0)
20–27	11 (30.6)	10 (27.8)	6 (16.7)	4 (11.1)	5 (13.9)	36 (36.0)
28–35	12 (42.9)	12 (42.9)	4 (14.3)	0 (0.0)	0 (0.0)	28 (28.0)
36–43	5 (41.7)	4 (33.3)	2 (16.7)	0 (0.0)	1 (8.3)	12 (12.0)
44+	8 (53.3)	2 (13.3)	1 (6.7)	4 (26.7)	0 (0.0)	15 (15.0)
Average age	31.7 (±12)	29.3 (±7.3)	30.5 (±13.1)	35.2 (±14.3)	26.3 (±7.8)	31.0 (±10.6)
Education						
No education	36 (41.4)	24 (27.6)	14 (16.1)	7 (8.0)	6 (6.9)	87 (88.8)
Primary	2 (22.2)	6 (66.7)	0 (0.0)	1 (11.1)	0 (0.0)	9 (9.2)
Secondary	1 (50.0)	1 (50.0)	0 (0.0)	0 (0.0)	0 (0.0)	2 (2.0)
Average years	0.4 (±1.6)	1.0 (±2)	0 (±0)	0.2 (±0.6)	0 (±0)	0.5 (±1.6)
Age at first marriage (years)						
10–13	12 (60.0)	3 (15.0)	0 (0.0)	2 (10.0)	3 (15.0)	20 (20.6)
14–17	19 (32.2)	22 (37.3)	9 (15.3)	6 (10.2)	3 (5.1)	59 (60.8)
18–21	7 (41.2)	5 (29.4)	5 (29.4)	0 (0.0)	0 (0.0)	17 (17.5)
22–25	0 (0.0)	1 (100.0)	0 (0.0)	0 (0.0)	0 (0.0)	1 (1.0)
Average age	14.9 (±2.7)	16 (±2.5)	17.0 (±2.0)	15.0 (±1.2)	13.8 (±1.2)	15.5 (±2.5)
Marital status at initial interview						
Married	14 (36.8)	12 (31.6)	10 (26.3)	2 (5.2)	0 (0.0)	38 (38.0)
Divorced	11 (47.8)	5 (21.7)	1 (4.3)	2 (8.7)	4 (17.4)	23 (23.0)
Separated	15 (41.7)	14 (38.9)	1 (27.8)	4 (11.1)	2 (5.6)	36 (36.0)
Widowed	1 (33.3)	0 (0.0)	2 (66.7)	0 (0.0)	0 (0.0)	3 (3.0)

*Including the Mossinke and Kanuri ethnic groups.

**Some totals do not add up to 100 or 100 percent due to rounding or missing data.

TABLE 5　Reproductive history and health characteristics of 100 women with fistula by ethnicity

Characteristic	Hausa N (%)	Zarma N (%)	Tuareg N (%)	Fulani N (%)	Other N (%)	Total* N (%)
No. of women	41 (41.0)	31 (31.0)	14 (14.0)	8 (8.0)	6 (6.0)	100 (100.0)
Age at first birth (years)						
12–15	10 (58.8)	3 (17.6)	1 (5.9)	0 (0.0)	3 (17.6)	17 (17.9)
16–19	21 (35.6)	19 (32.2)	8 (13.6)	8 (13.6)	3 (5.1)	59 (62.1)
20–23	5 (29.4)	7 (41.2)	5 (29.4)	0 (0.0)	0 (0.0)	17 (17.9)
24–27	0 (0.0)	2 (100.0)	0 (0.0)	0 (0.0)	0 (0.0)	2 (2.1)
Average age	17.0 (±2.3)	18.5 (±2.6)	18.4 (±1.8)	17.1 (±1.1)	15.7 (±1.4)	17.6 (±2.4)
Total no. of pregnancies						
0	2 (100.0)	0 (0.0)	0 (0.0)	0 (0.0)	0 (0.0)	2 (2.0)
1	9 (26.5)	12 (35.3)	6 (17.6)	3 (8.8)	4 (11.8)	34 (34.0)
2–4	10 (34.5)	8 (27.6)	6 (20.7)	4 (13.8)	1 (3.4)	29 (29.0)
5–7	10 (45.5)	9 (40.9)	3 (13.6)	0 (0.0)	0 (0.0)	22 (22.0)
8+	10 (76.9)	1 (7.7)	1 (7.7)	1 (7.7)	0 (0.0)	13 (13.0)
Average no.	4.7 (±3.4)	3.2 (±2.4)	3.3 (±2.5)	2.9 (±2.3)	1.5 (±0.8)	3.7 (±2.9)
No. of living children						
0	22 (40.7)	16 (29.6)	4 (7.4)	6 (11.1)	6 (11.1)	54 (54.0)
1	9 (52.9)	5 (29.4)	3 (17.6)	0 (0.0)	0 (0.0)	17 (17.0)
2	2 (18.2)	3 (27.3)	5 (45.5)	1 (9.1)	0 (0.0)	11 (11.0)
3 or 4	6 (50.0)	5 (41.7)	1 (8.3)	0 (0.0)	0 (0.0)	12 (12.0)
5+	2 (33.3)	2 (33.3)	2 (33.3)	0 (0.0)	0 (0.0)	6 (6.0)
Average no.	1.1 (±1.6)	1.2 (±1.6)	1.7 (±2)	0.6 (±1.2)	0.0 (±0)	1.1 (±1.6)

*Some totals do not add up to 100 or 100 percent due to rounding or missing data.

TABLE 6 Fistula history characteristics of 100 women with fistula by ethnicity

Characteristic	Hausa N (%)	Zarma N (%)	Tuareg N (%)	Fulani N (%)	Other N (%)	Total* N (%)
No. of women	41 (41.0)	31 (31.0)	14 (14.0)	8 (8.0)	6 (6.0)	100 (100.0)
Duration of labor leading to fistula						
<24 hours	4 (66.7)	2 (33.3)	0 (0.0)	0 (0.0)	0 (0.0)	6 (6.2)
1–2 days	14 (38.9)	13 (36.1)	2 (5.6)	3 (8.3)	4 (11.1)	36 (37.1)
3–4 days	17 (44.7)	10 (26.3)	8 (21.1)	3 (7.9)	0 (0.0)	38 (39.2)
5+ days	4 (23.5)	5 (29.4)	4 (23.5)	2 (11.8)	2 (11.8)	17 (17.5)
Average duration (days)	2.7 (±1.6)	2.9 (±2)	4.0 (±2.1)	2.9 (±1.8)	3.1 (±2.4)	3.0 (±1.9)
Age at fistula onset (years)						
<20	16 (34.8)	13 (28.3)	8 (17.4)	4 (8.7)	5 (10.9)	46 (46.0)
20–29	11 (36.7)	12 (40.0)	4 (13.3)	2 (6.7)	1 (3.3)	30 (30.0)
30–39	10 (52.6)	6 (31.6)	2 (10.5)	1 (5.3)	0 (0.0)	19 (19.0)
>39	4 (80.0)	0 (0.0)	0 (0.0)	1 (20.0)	0 (0.0)	5 (5.0)
Average age	25.5 (±10)	22.6 (±6.5)	20.6 (±5.8)**	25.0 (±10)	17.0 (±2.4)	23.4 (±8.4)
Time living with fistula						
<7 months	4 (30.8)	7 (53.8)	2 (15.4)	0 (0.0)	0 (0.0)	13 (13.0)
7–23 months	8 (47.1)	5 (29.4)	2 (11.8)	1 (5.9)	1 (5.9)	17 (17.0)
2–6 years	18 (43.9)	10 (24.4)	8 (19.5)	3 (7.3)	2 (4.9)	41 (41.0)
>6 years	11 (37.9)	9 (31.0)	2 (6.9)	4 (13.8)	3 (10.3)	29 (29.0)
Average years	6.8 (±8.4)	5.0 (±6.5)	7.1 (±3.4)	10.3 (±8.8)	7.9 (±9.1)	6.7 (±8.6)

*Some totals do not add up to 100 or 100 percent due to rounding or missing data.
**Including two cases of recidivistic fistula, the average age increases to 21.5 (± 6.1) years.

TABLE 7 Surgical history and outcomes of 100 women with fistula by ethnic grouping

Characteristic	Hausa N (%)	Zarma N (%)	Tuareg N (%)	Fulani N (%)	Other N (%)	Total* N (%)
No. of women	41 (41.0)	31 (31.0)	14 (14.0)	8 (8.0)	6 (6.0)	100 (100.0)
No. of women looking for surgery	37 (43.0)	29 (33.7)	9 (10.5)	6 (7.0)	5 (5.8)	86 (86.0)
No. of women who underwent surgery	28 (46.0)	19 (31.1)	8 (13.1)	2 (3.3)	4 (6.6)	61 (61.0)
No. of previous fistula surgeries						
0 or 1	14 (35.9)	14 (35.9)	7 (17.9)	2 (5.1)	2 (5.1)	39 (39.0)
2 or 3	17 (60.7)	6 (21.4)	3 (10.7)	1 (3.6)	1 (3.6)	28 (28.0)
4 or 5	8 (40.0)	6 (30.0)	1 (5.0)	3 (15.0)	2 (10.0)	20 (20.0)
6+	2 (15.4)	5 (38.5)	3 (23.1)	2 (15.4)	1 (7.8)	13 (13.0)
Average no.	2.7 (±2.5)	3.5 (±2.1)	2.2 (±2)	4.4 (±2.9)	3.3 (±2.7)	2.8 (±2.2)
Time waiting at clinic at initial interview (months)						
1–2	12 (38.7)	10 (32.3)	6 (19.4)	3 (9.7)	0 (0.0)	31 (39.7)**
3–6	12 (41.4)	11 (37.9)	1 (3.4)	3 (10.3)	2 (6.9)	29 (37.2)
7–12	6 (46.2)	5 (38.5)	1 (7.7)	0 (0.0)	1 (7.7)	13 (16.7)
>12	0 (0.0)	2 (40.0)	1 (20.0)	0 (0.0)	2 (40.0)	5 (6.4)
Average months	3.5 (±3.2)	5.2 (±5.6)	3.4 (±3.8)	2.4 (±2.4)	21.3 (±27.3)	5.3 (±9.3)
Surgical outcome by continence						
Wet (incontinent)	16 (41.0)	12 (30.8)	5 (12.8)	2 (5.1)	4 (10.3)	39 (63.9)
Dry (continent)	12 (54.5)	7 (31.8)	3 (13.6)	0 (0.0)	0 (0.0)	22 (36.1)

*Some totals do not add up to 100 or 100 percent due to rounding or missing data.
**Only the women who were looking for surgery were counted. Eight women could not estimate how long they had been at the center, so their data were left out of the calculations.

TABLE 8   Demographic information of all women quoted in the text

Pseudonym	Age at Interview	Primary Ethnic Affiliation	Age at Fistula	Age at First Marriage	Marital Situation at First Interview*	Age at First Birth	Total Pregnancies	Pregnancy That Led to Fistula	No. of Living Children	No. of Previous Surgeries	Surgical Outcome at End of 2013*
A'i	17	Hausa	13	12	S	13	1	1	0	3	NS/RH
Abou	23	Zarma	19	19	M	19	1	1	0	1	NS/SW
Adama	29	Hausa	27	15	S	17	3	3	1	1	Wet
Ade	26	Zarma	19	15	D	18	2	1	0	5	NS/SW
Agaicha	29	Hausa	25	14	D	NA	0	NA	0	1	NS/NL
Aishatou	27	Tuareg	18	15	S	18	1	1	0	3	NS/NL
Aminatou	45	Hausa	45	20	W	22	12	11	5	4	Dry
Amira	40	Hausa	21	20	S	21	1	1	0	5	NS/INC
Arantut	30	Tuareg	30	19	M	22	4	4	2	0	NS/CATH
Asma'u	25	Zarma	22	17	S	21	1	1	0	6	NS/SW
Balkissa	27	Hausa	16	14	M	16	5	1, 5	3	1	Wet
Baraka	37	Hausa	18	15	D	18	5	1	1	9	NS/INC
Bibata	28	Hausa	23	14	M	16	3	2	0	2	NS/SW
Binta	30	Hausa	30	12	S	14	5	5	3	1	Dry
Fana	42	Tuareg	16	15	D	16	4	1	2	1	NS/NL
Fatouma	32	Tuareg	18	15	M	18	8	1, 4	1	2	Wet
Gomma	25	Hausa	20	20	S	20	1	1	0	2	Wet
Habiba	49	Fulani	19	13	D	19	3	1	0	7	Deceased
Habsu	20	Kanuri	16	14	D	15	1	1	0	1	Wet
Hadiza	32	Hausa	32	15	M	17	6	6	0	0	NS/RH
Hadjo	18	Zarma	17	14	S	17	1	1	0	1	Dry
Hagera	27	Zarma	16	15	S	16	3	1	0	4	Wet
Halima	21	Hausa	21	15	M	18	2	2	1	0	NS/SW
Hasana	20	Mossi	14	13	S	14	1	1	0	4	NS/NL

TABLE 8 (continued)

Pseudonym	Age at Interview	Primary Ethnic Affiliation	Age at First Fistula	Age at First Marriage	Marital Situation at First Interview*	Age at First Birth	Total Pregnancies	Pregnancy That Led to Fistula	No. of Living Children	No. of Previous Surgeries	Surgical Outcome at End of 2013*
Hassia	20	Hausa	17	15	D	NA	0	NA	0	1	Dry
Indo	50	Hausa	48	12	M	14	8	8	0	1	Dry
Jamila	16	Hausa	14	13	S	14	1	1	0	5	Wet
Jeka	33	Hausa	29	18	S	18	4	4	1	2	Wet
Ju'mai	47	Hausa	17	14	D	17	9	1	0	2	Dry
Kadi	22	Fulani	16	14	D	16	1	1	0	3	NS/NL
Kadigya	28	Zarma	20	20	S	20	1	1	0	3	Wet
Kaltumi	45	Songhai	18	16	D	18	7	3, 7	4	1	NS/SW
Karima	26	Tuareg	19	17	M	19	2	1	1	4	NS/NL
Kouloua	33	Zarma	33	16	M	17	7	7	5	1	Dry
Ladi	35	Hausa	15	13	M	14	5	1, 2	0	11	NS/NL
Lahiya	22	Hausa	20	15	D	17	2	2	0	2	Wet
Laraba	27	Kanuri	17	14	D	15	3	3	0	8	Wet
Mairi	27	Kanuri	18	16	D	18	1	1	0	4	Wet
Maou	35	Hausa	35	18	M	20	10	10	4	2	Dry
Mariama	50	Hausa	16	10	M	15	8	1, 2	1	3	Wet
Nafissa	35	Songhai	15	14	S	15	1	1	1	2	NS/SW
Naio	29	Zarma	28	14	M	17	6	6	4	1	Wet
Nana	56	Hausa	35	DK	S	DK	5	3	1	2	Wet
Rabi	32	Zarma	32	15	S	20	6	6	3	0	NS/SW
Rachida	37	Zarma	30	15	M	18	6	2, 6	3	7	Wet
Raha	55	Hausa	54	20	M	DK	12	12	0	0	NS/RH
Rahila	25	Tuareg	17	15	W	17	1	1	0	6	NS/RH

(continued)

TABLE 8 (continued)

Pseudonym	Age at Interview	Primary Ethnic Affiliation	Age at Fistula	Age at First Marriage	Marital Situation at First Interview*	Age at First Birth	Total Pregnancies	Pregnancy That Led to Fistula	No. of Living Children	No. of Previous Surgeries	Surgical Outcome at End of 2013*
Roukaya	21	Zarma	20	14	M	19	1	1	0	1	Dry
Sa'adé	23	Fulani	19	17	M	18	4	2, 4	0	4	Wet
Sadata	45	Fulani	35	16	S	18	8	8	3	8	Wet
Sakina	22	Fulani	16	15	S	16	1	1	0	5	NS/RH
Salamatou	41	Kanuri	16	13	D	16	1	1	0	2	NS/SW
Samira	55	Fulani	45	12	S	16	1	1	0	0	NS/RH
Saouda	30	Zarma	28	21	D	24	4	4	0	1	Wet
Souweiba	30	Hausa	30	D/K	S	18	7	7	4	1	NS/INC
Talata	19	Hausa	18	16	S	18	1	1	0	1	NS/RH
Tamoutan	40	Hausa	38	12	S	14	8	8	0	2	Dry
Tandahamad	20	Tuareg	20	19	M	20	1	1	0	1	Wet
Tshara	40	Hausa	18	15	M	18	9	1	4	4	Wet
Yaha	30	Hausa	25	12	D	16	5	5	1	4	Dry
Zali	27	Hausa	17	14	D	17	4	1	0	4	NS/RH
Zara	27	Zarma	21	11	D	21	1	1	0	4	Dry
Zeinabou	30	Zarma	30	18	S	19	5	5	2	1	Wet
Zina	37	Hausa	36	15	M	17	10	10	4	3	Wet
Zuera	26	Hausa	23	12	S	17	3	3	1	3	Wet

*Marital status abbreviations: D, divorced; M, married; S, separated; W, widowed.

**Of the 65 women quoted in the text, 36 underwent surgery; 24 of whom were still wet and 12 were dry. Table abbreviations: CATH, treated with catheter only, no surgery; D/K, did not know age at first birth; INC, classified as incurable or inoperable; NA, not applicable; NL, not looking for surgery; NS, no surgery; RH, returned home without surgery; SW, still waiting for surgery at fistula center by end of research period.

ACKNOWLEDGMENTS

Lately, when I sign on to Facebook, my news feed is populated by grainy images of early ultrasounds: "Baby's first photo!" Friends pose in bikinis, showing off pregnant bellies, blooming. I follow impassioned exchanges: "Natural or epidural?" I read about birth-plans and doulas and "like" photos of baby showers and nurseries, elaborately decorated and unselfconsciously public shows of certainty: This baby is coming home healthy. For many women in resource-rich countries, once they are pregnant, the future can feel predetermined. Although maternal mortality rates in the United States are increasing—particularly among African American, native American, low-income, and rural women, who are at disproportionate risk for poor reproductive outcomes—birthing in the United States is generally considered safe. Few seem overly concerned about the threat of obstetric complications, which has made miscarriage and stillbirth taboo, sometimes shameful, often unspoken subjects. When I worry about my own reproductive future, I fixate on questions of work–life balance, childcare costs, school districts, and how to raise a kid who isn't a jerk. It is telling that my perpetually anxious mind skips past the perinatal period.

Each and every day in Niger I was reminded that for so many women neither healthy babies nor safe outcomes were ever assumed. Once she becomes pregnant, the future for a woman is unknown, mapped with danger and uncertainty. I am still overcome not only by the injustices of these embodied global inequalities but also by the graciousness with which women who had lost so much continued to give.

My deepest gratitude is reserved for the women in Niger who opened up their hearts and lives to me, who chose to trust me with their intimate secrets, disappointments, and joys. Anthropologists have little to offer back to our informants, yet we have so much to gain from the depths of their narratives and the richness of their experiences. For their generosity of time, trust, honesty, vulnerability, and friendship, which I can never fully reciprocate, I am forever indebted and truly thankful to these women in Niger. My research, this book, and the significant personal and professional gains from which I have benefited are thanks to these generous and courageous women.

I am also grateful to the many people in Niger who facilitated my research—the government employees who helped me navigate the tortuous process of attaining research approval, my three research assistants who worked long and taxing hours, the fistula center staff who answered every question I asked, no matter how inane, the friends who kept me sane after long days of emotional work, and the

Nigériens I met every day whose kindness permeated my soul and reminded me why I continue to return to the Sahel. I especially thank the Nigérien Ministère des Enseignements Moyen et Supérieur et de la Recherche Scientifique and the Nigérien Comite Consultatif National d'Ethique, the U.S. State Department, Niger's Réseau d'Eradication de la Fistule, SIM-Niger, and LASDEL (Laboratoire d'Etudes et de Recherche sur les Dynamiques Sociales et le Développement Local)—institutions that facilitated my research. Although I can only name a few, countless individuals in Niger were essential to my success: Rahmatou Tahiru, Soumana Mamoudou, Lucien Djanikbo, Ahmed Mamane, Hauwa and Thomas Shelwah, Itengré Ouédraogo, Ganda Oumarou Sanda, Issoufou Maarouf, Sarah Burgess, Caroline and Kaocen Agalheir, Mark Shaker, Bert and Elaine Haaga, Steve Schmidt, Sue Rosenfeld, Eric Schmidt, Salamatou Traoré, Rahina, Hanna-tou, and Dorfaye.

Writing a book often feels like screaming into a void. Without the careful feedback of my colleagues, friends, and mentors, my work would be much poorer. I am grateful to my peers and mentors at Washington University in St. Louis where this project was conceived. Glenn Stone closely mentored and inspired me, and he, Shanti Parikh, Leonard Lewis Wall, Jean Allman, Rebecca Lester, Bret Gustafson, Paul Stoller, and Nancy Pope invested countless hours in carefully reading my work and adding to its depth and clarity. My colleagues Andrew Flachs, Elyse Singer, Natalie Mueller, John Willman, and Joe Orkin made my work stronger and made the working feel less arduous.

I am lucky to have the support of my department, college, and enthusiastic colleagues at the University of Maryland College Park. I couldn't have found a better academic home.

Over the years I have been fortunate to accrue mentors who have helped guide me and sharpen my ideas, particularly Adeline Masquelier, Barbara Cooper, and Lenore Manderson. I cannot express enough appreciation to Lenore Manderson, who has been giving me brilliant advice since my first summer in Niger. Lenore's brilliance, kindness, and intellectual generosity have shaped me, my work, and this book directly, as its meticulous series editor.

I am deeply grateful for the dedicated editing of Heath Sledge, whose sharp eye and thoughtfulness are reflected in each page of this manuscript. Kim Guinta moved this book with efficiency and grace through each stage of the publishing process. Additionally, the beauty of the peer-review process is the complexity that comes from the perspectives of many minds. My work is so much stronger due to the careful review of dedicated readers.

I am thankful for my time at the School for Advanced Research, where as a Vera Campbell Fellow I had the opportunity to transform my dissertation material into a book manuscript. Michael Brown, Paul Ryer, Maria Spray, and my cohort of fellows gave me invaluable feedback and support.

This research was made possible due to generous funding from the National Science Foundation, the Fulbright-Hays Program, and the Wenner-Gren Foundation, which I am humbled to have received. I give additional thanks to the Olin Fellowship, P.E.O. International, the Worldwide Fistula Fund, the Washington University Graduate School of Arts and Sciences, and the Department of Anthropology, the School for Advanced Research, and the University of Maryland College Park for their generous financial support.

I also thank my dear friend and collaborator, Dana Sacco, for venturing into the field and reintroducing me to the art of teamwork. I am also grateful for my collaboration with Anita Hannig, beginning as "team incontinence" when we both newly emerged from the field.

To my family of birth and my family of choice: thank you for always caring for my heart, which nourishes my mind. Your names are too numerous, but thank you to the Galvins, Hellers, Busches, Hajaris, Doves, and Cases. To Kim, John, Annie, James, Sarah, Dana, Amie, Chris, Doron, Jason, Blaine, Scott, Matthew, Julia, Asa, Ben, Maren, Justine, Natalie, Torri, Alec, Sam and so many others—when I have been lost in the process, you've known when to pluck me from it; you've filled me with love and recharged my soul.

Finally, thanks to my closest companion, Adam Hajari. Being the spouse of an anthropologist is in itself worth acknowledging—it requires patience, understanding, and some sacrifice. An anthropologist's partner must allow their loved one to fade away into a crackling voice, a dropped call, a mere handful of pixels over a poor Skype connection for months at a time. Adam's support over the past nine years has been unending—a cascade of confidence and love. Not least of all, this project has benefited from the sharp mind, generous editing, and patient statistical guidance of this physicist-cum-data-scientist, without whom my forays into statistical testing may have been of questionable validity.

NOTES

CHAPTER 1: INCONTINENCE AND INEQUALITIES

1. The large span reflects a deep division within the community of fistula experts over the incidence and prevalence of the condition, which is notoriously difficult to measure. Some scholars have suggested that the most commonly cited numbers surrounding fistula (2 million women living with fistula and 50,000 to 100,000 new cases a year) are overestimated, based on "surgeon's estimates" rather than robust epidemiological methods (Adler et al. 2013; Stanton, Holtz, and Ahmed 2007). These widely cited numbers can be traced to a two-page paper written in 1993 by Dutch fistula surgeon Kees Waaldijk, who extrapolated fistula's prevalence based on his personal clinical experience in northern Nigeria (Waaldijk and Armiya'u 1993). Other scholars believe that these numbers understate the problem, arguing that women with fistula are difficult to access and thus have been missed in many measurements (see Wall 2006). These numbers, which have clear implications on funding and the allocation of resources, are political and politicized.

2. Many clinics throughout sub-Saharan Africa are newly established, but the Hamlin Fistula Hospitals have existed for decades; they were founded in Ethiopia in 1974.

3. In *A Better Woman: A Memoir of Motherhood* (2003), Australian novelist Susan Johnson describes her own experience with fistula after birthing complications. This memoir provides a rare example of fistula experienced, imagined, and portrayed outside the Global South.

4. According to Islamic law, if a man can financially, and equitably, support his wives, he is permitted to marry up to four women at any given time.

5. I received an update from the head surgeon at Danja Fistula Center in February of 2017, who reported that Jamila had undergone a total of nine surgeries, had somehow developed a rectovaginal fistula, but was now dry. Jamila was permanently living at the fistula center as a nurse's aide.

6. For example, see Barageine et al. (2015), IRIN Staff (2009), Lavender et al. (2016), Moylan (2016), Mselle and Kohi (2015), M. O. Smith (2007), Warner (2014), and Yeakey et al. (2009).

7. As part of the dominant fistula narrative, female genital cutting (often described as female genital mutilation) and early marriage (often described as child or forced marriage) are often thought to play a part in fistula development. However, this is physiologically inaccurate. See chapter 3.

8. Among the 100 women whom I came to know, 85 had vesicovaginal fistulas, 11 had vesicovaginal fistulas *and* rectovaginal fistulas, and 4 had only rectovaginal fistulas. With a vesicovaginal fistula, the tissues between the vagina and the bladder are destroyed during labor, resulting in urine running uncontrollably through the vagina. With a rectovaginal fistula, a hole forms between the tissues of the rectum and the vagina, leading to the uncontrolled passage of feces or gas through the vagina.

9. For the majority of Nigériens, this religious invigoration has resulted in a redefining and strengthening of their relationship to Islam. However, as Barbara Cooper (2006) has demonstrated, a small but important minority has turned to Christianity, typically Protestantism.

10. Although conscious acts of visible piety have been on the rise in Niger, not everyone displays the same interest or commitment in Islam. Some Nigériens, particularly women, often secretly cling to relationships with the powerful spirit world and actively participate in *bori* spirit possession cults (Masquelier 2009).

11. Niger has one of the world's lowest rates of both contraceptive use and unmet need for contraception because desired family size exceeds actual family size (Sedgh, Ashford, and Hussain 2016). Fewer than 1 percent of women want only two children; 80 percent want more than six (INS and ICF International 2013).

12. In addition to relying on triangulation to better comprehend women's daily experiences with fistula, I used triangulation to estimate quantitative data. For example, birthdays are not typically celebrated by Nigériens, and age is not diligently recorded, so often I had to triangulate to estimate women's current ages or their ages at important life events using historical events, guesstimates, and typical age at menstruation.

13. SIM was founded in 1893 as the Soudan Interior Mission to evangelize in sub-Saharan Africa. In the 1980s, the Asian, South American, and African ministries came together to form the Society for International Ministries (SIM). In 2000, SIM adopted the name Serving In Mission.

14. Outside of CSLF and Danja village, Christians represent only 1 to 2 percent of the region's and the country's population. See Cooper 2006 for a historical examination of Danja.

15. Although it is still popular in rural areas, scarification has largely been abandoned by urban dwellers, who tend to adopt more cosmopolitan beautification rites such as eyeliner and lipstick.

16. For an in-depth look at the rise of the Izala movement, see Masquelier 2001b.

17. The hundred women came from across Niger's eight regions: 25 percent from Tilabéri (versus 16 percent of the national population distribution), 23 percent from Maradi (20 percent nationally), 21 percent from Dosso (12 percent nationally), 7 percent from Tahoua (19 percent nationally), 6 percent from Zinder (21 percent nationally), 4 percent from Niamey (6 percent nationally), 4 percent from Diffa (3 percent nationally), and 1 percent from Agadez (3 percent nationally). Areas close to the four fistula centers were overrepresented as compared with national population distributions (particularly the Tilabéri and Dosso regions near Niamey); regions far from centers were underrepresented (such as Tahoua and Zinder).

18. In a systematic review, Thom and Rortveit (2010) have estimated postpartum urinary incontinence to be 33 percent. In the South Australian Health Omnibus Survey in 2004, urinary incontinence was estimated at 28 percent (Avery and Stocks 2016). In a study of 379 Saudi women, 41 percent experienced urinary incontinence, with the risk increasing for women with parity greater than five, increased age, and menopause (Al-Badr et al. 2012). Urinary incontinence was found to affect 34 percent of female respondents between the ages of 10 and 90 years old in the People's Republic of China (Li, Low, and Lee 2007), and 37 percent of female respondents in the United States (Diokno et al. 2004).

19. As coined by *The Economist* editor Matthew Bishop in 2006, philanthrocapitalism refers to the infusion of philanthropy within capitalist practice to demonstrate the economic structure's benevolent potential through innovation, competition, and strategic or high-performance donations (see Bishop and Green 2008).

20. To name a few, see Biehl (2013), Bornstein (2012), Escobar (1995), Fassin (2012), Ferguson (1990, 2006), Hunt (1999), Mosse (2005), Nguyen (2010), Redfield (2006, 2013), Ticktin (2011, 2017), and Vaughan (1991).

LARABA'S STORY

1. Families tend to arrange first marriages and often do not consult the young brides, although women have more choice in subsequent partners (Bovin 1988; Prost 1970). Because the bride and groom are absent during the religious ceremonies, young brides may not even know that they have been married until the ceremonies have been concluded (see Bornand 2015).

2. The causal link between child marriage and obstetric fistula is a component of the dominant media and humanitarian narrative, but marrying young is not necessarily a risk factor for fistula.

3. Global health interventions offer condition-specific quick-fix solutions, leaving large gaps in strained postcolonial health care systems. Only certain ailments and certain bodies are rendered legible. Patients of these fragmented systems must negotiate their own visibility, demanding recognition by the gatekeepers of crucial services. As Alice Street (2014) demonstrates in hospitals in Papua New Guinea, the politics of visibility are paramount when access to medical interventions and essential drugs is limited. Patients struggle to make themselves visible to the medical gaze, without becoming socially invisible at home. The women I came to know were forced to identify as women with fistula at hospitals, and were often engaged in what Nguyen (2010) calls therapeutic citizenship through confessional testimony. Yet most women distance themselves from these identities at home, masterfully concealing their conditions.

CHAPTER 2: FISTULA STIGMA

1. Expanding on Goffman's work, others have theorized stigma to understand where it is located and how it is assigned, reproduced, reinforced, and resisted. See Jenkins and Carpenter-Song 2008; Jones et al. 1984; and Major and O'Brien 2005.

2. Theorists have problematized monolithic categories and proposed theories of stigma that accommodate complex social contexts, individual agency to resist, and dynamics of power and exclusion. See, for example, Castro and Farmer 2005; Link and Phelan 2001; Parker and Aggleton 2003; Rhine 2009; Schoepf 2001; Shih 2004; and Yang et al. 2007.

3. This is less true of rectovaginal fistula and fecal incontinence, which women generally believe to be the result of an infection.

4. Female urinary incontinence affects around 30 percent of women worldwide and increases in prevalence with age and parity (see note 17 in chapter 1). As Nigérien women have the highest fertility in the world, some degree of incontinence is common, and women with non-fistula-related heavy urinary incontinence (such as Samira) may be locally diagnosed with the illness of leaking urine, thus shouldering the same social consequences as women with fistula.

5. After fistula surgery, a woman's fistula may be closed, yet she may still leak urine. In these cases, many women may be counted as having been successfully repaired yet remain wet or incontinent. Persistent transurethral urine loss can be caused by many factors: loss of bladder capacity, compliance, sensation, or motor innervation; loss of coordination between the bladder and sphincter; diminished urethral length; or disruption or destruction of the sphincter (Arrowsmith, Barone, and Ruminjo 2013; Wall and Arrowsmith 2007). During my research period, several women who had under gone successful surgical repairs (but also experienced some form of residual incontinence) did report some improvement; they explained that they were now capable of holding their urine for between a few seconds to a few minutes, which gave them time to make it to a toilet, which greatly improved their quality of life. However, many others whose fistulas were closed experienced persistent incontinence that was so troublesome that there was no significant change in their quality of life. Many of these women did not learn that their fistulas were considered cured until I consulted their clinical file.

6. In social psychology or sociology, stigma is considered a latent construct—having theoretical variables that cannot be directly observed or measured. Even when direct linguistic correlates exist, stigma must be deconstructed into its measurable components.

7. In an attempt to standardize these imperfect measurements, I also integrated two scales. I adapted the Participation Scale, which measures perceptions of limitations in social participation (van Brakel et al. 2006), and the HIV/AIDS Stigma Instrument (HASI-P), which

measures stigma using proxy measurements of verbal abuse, negative self-perception, social isolation, fear of contagion, health care neglect, and workplace stigma (Holzemer et al. 2007).

8. The original HASI-P, used to measure HIV/AIDS stigma, returned similar results. In their measurement of HIV/AIDS stigma in five sub-Saharan African countries, Holzemer et al. (2007) found that highest reports of stigma were in the domains of negative self-perception (with an average of 0.95, significantly lower than my measurement for women with fistula), verbal abuse (0.65), social isolation (0.64), and fear of contagion (0.27).

9. Scores from the stigma survey were normalized. All 11 external stigma questions and all seven internal stigma questions were multiplied by three (the greatest possible points for each question), giving a total of 33 possible points for external stigma and 21 for internal. The women's total scores for each category were divided by the possible points for that category and multiplied by 100. For example, a woman who responded once or twice (scored as 1 point) to each external stigma question would have an external stigma score of 33.3: $(1 \times 11)/33 \times 100$. Sixty-six women reported high (between 51 and 75) or very high (75 and 100) rates of internal stigma, and only 15 women reported no (0–25) or low (1–25) internal stigma.

10. On a perceived external fistula stigma scale of 0 to 100, these seven women averaged 63; the remaining 93 women had an average score of 11. The seven women's average for internal stigma, 72, was also higher than the remaining 93 women at 58, although the difference did not reach statistical significance.

11. This difference was statistically significant ($P=.029$). These numbers were calculated among the 94 women who knew how many co-wives they either currently had (for married or separated women) or had at the point of divorce or their husband's death. Only three of the seven women with high external fistula stigma were currently married or separated, and these women had an average of 1.7 co-wives each; the remaining 69 married or separated women had 0.7 co-wives each, a difference that was statistically significant ($P=.016$).

12. Additionally, women who lived with their mothers and stepfathers (in the case where parents divorced and then mothers remarried) also reported higher rates of mistreatment than women who lived with their mothers and fathers, indicating (not surprisingly) that when children are not raised within supportive family environments, they are more susceptible to mistreatment in the face of illness.

13. Such dynamics are not unique to West Africa; studies demonstrate that children in the United States living with stepmothers receive markedly less food, education, and health care than those who lived with their biological mothers (Case and Paxson 2001).

14. Three women were left out of the statistical calculation because they could not estimate their age at marriage. Using an unpaired two-tailed t-test, the age of marriage for women without mothers is statistically significantly younger than the age of marriage for women with mothers ($P=.042$).

15. Other studies have also demonstrated that women without family support experienced greater challenges in seeking treatment (such as Yeakey et al. 2011).

16. The relationship between fathers and daughters in Niger is complex in the context of divorce. Men often spend very little time at home, and the relationships between co-wives can be riddled with jealousy and resentment. Co-wives are often engaged in a silent but strategic war that can continue for decades over scarce resources, status, and a husband's preference. When disputes between co-wives erupt (or myriad other conjugal problems), divorce or separation is common. Children are considered the property of the father, so when women leave their husband's home they are obligated to leave behind their older, weaned children. If a young woman's mother is gone and she is left living with her father, his remaining wives often lobby for him to send the girl away to live with a relative elsewhere (to reduce the competition for resources).

17. In line with Fana's perception of fistula stigma and poverty, Mselle et al. (2011, 10) noted how existing issues in inequity help define the experience of fistula: "The vast majority of women affected by obstetric fistula in this study constituted a socially weak group even before their birth injury . . . As documented in this work, the women's physical and social disability due to the injury pushes them further into marginalization, making them vulnerable to social exclusion and discrimination."

18. Quoted by Al-Ghazali (1967), the Shafiʻi jurist who died in 1111 (Al-Ghazali 1967, 1, 170; quoted in Rispler-Chaim 2006, 19).

19. Two of these 21 women were healed during the research period (and were reinterviewed after their repair); nine were healed of fistula before I came to know them (but returned to centers to be treated for other health complaints, to receive prophylactic cesarean deliveries, to participate in center trainings, or to collect money). Ten others were wet at the time of the interview but had been previously healed of a fistula (all these women had recidivistic fistula).

20. In Niger, compliments are thought to attract the attention of the evil eye or bad spirits. Overt compliments are thus avoided, particularly about young children and babies, who are thought to be especially vulnerable.

CHAPTER 3: LIMINAL WIVES

1. Women are typically granted divorces by religious leaders or state authorities when their husbands refuse to grant them.

2. According the Demographic and Health Surveys for all West African countries, less than 8 percent of Nigérien women are currently unmarried—the lowest rate in West Africa (the highest is 33 percent in Ghana) (DHS Program 2018).

3. Cross cousins are children of a parent's opposite-sex sibling; parallel cousins are children of a parent's same-sex sibling. For example, a maternal cross cousin would be the child of a person's mother's brother.

4. High rates of divorce are not universal and may have increased over time (Antoine 2002; Masquelier 2005). Adeline Masquelier (2005) noted that among Hausa women in the Dogondoutchi region, divorce was historically infrequent due to its dramatic consequences—the stripping of membership to the lineage.

5. Polygamy, which refers to a marriage in which more than one person share a common spouse, can encompass both polyandry (the sanctioned marriage of a woman to multiple men) and polygyny (the sanctioned marriage of one man to multiple women). Polygyny is the most common form of polygamy. Some scholars believe West Africa's high rates of polygyny (compared with the rest of sub-Saharan Africa) can be attributed to the African slave trade. More male slaves were exported in the trans-Atlantic slave trade from Western Africa whereas more female slaves were exported via the Indian Ocean from East Africa. The resultant prolonged period of abnormal sex ratios in West Africa is thought to have encouraged polygyny (see Dalton and Leung 2011).

6. Additionally, three women were widowed.

7. In examining fistula in Niger and Mali, Maulet, Keita, and Macq (2013) observed that fistula led to marital rupture at three notable points: immediately after an incontinence diagnosis, later when care-seeking took longer than expected, and finally when the irreversibility of the incontinence was diagnosed or feared (527).

8. Men in Niger can divorce wives without much effort or justification through a unilateral verbal pronouncement of talaq in the presence of three witnesses (Callaway 1984; Izugbara and Ezeh 2010). Wives cannot appeal a marriage dissolved through talaq, but men can divorce and take back their wives up to three times. Religious law prohibits them from going back on the

decision a fourth time; after the third divorce, a woman must remarry and divorce another man before she can return to her previous husband (Prost 1970).

9. Although divorce is notoriously easy, culturally accepted, and common in Niger, it is poorly tracked. Countrywide surveys tracking currently divorced women often underestimate divorce rates because women remarry rapidly. For example, we know that 2.3 percent of Nigérien women between the ages of 15 and 49 are currently divorced, but there are no reliable data about lifetime rates of divorce or rates of remarriage (INS and ICF International 2013).

10. If men initiate the divorce, women are entitled to keep their bride-wealth; if a woman initiates divorce, she must repay it. In an effort to retain the bride-wealth, men may push women to initiate divorce through calculated neglect or verbal abuse (Prost 1970). Regardless of who initiated the divorce, a woman must leave behind her older children (who are likely to be placed in the care of her former husband's other wives or his mother or sisters).

11. In Hausaphone northern Nigeria, Solivetti (1994) found that 86 percent of divorces were initiated by women. This is far more than in other parts of West Africa. For example, Wittrup (1990) found that only 20 percent of divorce cases among the Mandinka in the Gambia were initiated by women.

12. In a cohort study of 120 women with fistula in Niger and Mali, Maulet et al. (2013) noted that 13 women were married during the study period, including seven who remained married while still incontinent, revealing that some marital and sexual bonds were maintained despite fistula and incontinence.

13. Because so many women develop fistula from their first labors (51 percent), this proportion might be higher than the proportion of women in family marriages in the population at large, although Manvell (2006) found that in two rural Hausa villages the family marriage rate was around 60 percent.

14. This is, of course, a generalization. Mothers-in-law sometimes act as advocates for their daughters-in-law (regardless of familial relationships), encouraging their sons to be patient and support their wives through the illness. In some cases, mothers-in-law even accompanied their daughters-in-law to fistula treatment centers.

15. Among the women I came to know, the average age at first marriage was 15.1 years old (ranging from 10 to 23 years)—0.2 years less thank the national average. Yet, in contrast to much of the discourse on "forced" marriage in sub-Saharan Africa, the *type* of marriage was independent from *age* at marriage. While 58 women were married by the time they were 15 years old, only 26 women considered their marriages forced. There was no statistically significant dependence between the age of first marriage and whether a woman considered her marriage forced (P=.256). Being forced into marriage was independent from age.

16. The divorce rates were lowest among the women with family marriages (10 percent) and love/family marriages (7 percent). Family marriages as a whole (including both co-categorized love/family and forced/family marriages) had a divorce rate of 15 percent. Rates of continued marriage were also highest for the family marriages (52 percent) and love/family marriages (43 percent). The divorce rates were highest for love marriages (34 percent) and family/forced marriages (29 percent).

17. Twenty-four women were divorced, and three other women had been absent from home for so long that they did not know how many (if any) co-wives they had.

18. These findings are in line with previous studies that found that women who remained married after the development of fistula frequently had to accept another co-wife into their households (see Maulet et al. 2013).

19. Among married Hausa women (and to a lesser extent, among Fulani and Kanuri), female seclusion—*auren kulle* or *purdah*—is a cultural norm, although it is practiced with varying levels of rigor. Between marriage and menopause, women may be expected to not leave their

houses without a male kin escort—or sometimes never at all—except to celebrate occasional ceremonies or seek medical help (Calloway 1984; Cooper 1997). In reality, strict adherence to locked-in marriage is often reserved for the wealthier families. In rural communities, there is often only a cultural nod to such practices, and a *hijabi* may stand for a type of portable seclusion.

20. For example, women nearing menopause are often more receptive to the prospect of expanding their households to accommodate a new wife than women in their early reproductive years. Similarly, women with more economic autonomy are less vulnerable to the potential inequities of polygyny, and they may particularly benefit from a reduction in household responsibilities, an increase in free time, and greater independence. Position also affects women's relationships with their co-wives. First or senior wives are considered to be more respected, although perhaps less loved, by husbands (Ware 1979). First wives who have solidified their position in the household through reproductive success may even encourage their husbands to take a second wife to enjoy the social respect and deference of the younger bride and to command greater managerial power within the household. For more information about what factors affect co-wife relationships, see Borgerhoff Mulder 1992; Bove and Valeggia 2009; Jankowiak, Sudakov, and Wilreker 2005; Tabi et al. 2010; and Wittrup 1990.

21. Performed in the company of only married women, this playful, although often acrimonious, ritual allows co-wives to transgress boundaries of propriety and senior wives to mourn the loss of their status. In this highly scripted ritual, senior wives accuse junior wives of stupidity, mendacity, immodesty, madness, arrogance, and infertility. In response, junior wives call senior wives "cow dung" and accuse them of jealously, sexual undesirability, and madness.

22. Generally, Nigérien rates of child death are markedly high. According to the 2012 Demographic and Health Survey, Nigérien women aged 15 to 49 had birthed an average of 4.2 living children but only 3.4 were still living at the time of interview, indicating a 20 percent mortality rate. The rate was higher for women 45 and older, who lost 28 percent of their children (INS and ICF International 2013).

23. In Hausa, the words *bora* and *mowa* refer to the least favored and the favorite wife, respectively. (They are commonly employed in the proverb *Ba a mowa sai da bora,* or "one does not have a favorite wife unless he has a least favorite.")

24. Thirty-seven women had had between two and five pregnancies, 25 women had experienced 6 to 10 pregnancies, and two women had had 11 or 12 pregnancies (with a sample average of nearly four pregnancies per woman; see the appendix).

25. In a cross-sectional study of women with fistula in Tanzania, Mselle et al. (2011) highlighted the relationship between treatment-seeking and marital tension. According to these authors, "Women stayed in the hospital seeking treatment for a long time. When they returned home, they found their husbands already remarried" (7).

SIX BEDS, SIXTY MINUTES

1. Favoritism, clientelism, and nepotism are frustrating realities in the provision of health care in Niger (and West Africa generally), where who you know often determines the care you get. This is reflected in the term *mon passe* in French: someone who has a standing relationship with the practitioner and thus is protected when she seeks care. She is seen to first and is given reduced rates (see Jaffré and Olivier de Sardan 2002). For this reason, the importance of networks is paramount when seeking care.

2. Niger's maternal mortality rate is 40 times larger than that of the United States, and Nigérien women bear an average of 7.6 children over their lifetimes compared with U.S. women's average of 1.9 children each, which amplifies the lifetime risk for Nigérien women.

CHAPTER 4: THE "WORST PLACE TO BE A MOTHER"

1. The sleeping fetus or sleeping embryo is a legal construct in Islam, primarily aimed at protecting women who commit adultery (*zina* in Hausa) who could otherwise be subject to stoning under Sharia law. Using the theory of the sleeping fetus, pregnancy is not proof of adultery. According to the *mazhab* Maliki, women can carry pregnancies for up to five to seven years after a divorce or the death of a woman's husband. These children, dormant during the extended postmarital period, may still be considered as belonging to the woman's previous or late husband (Miller 2006). The related concept *kwantacce* (literally "lying down" in Hausa) is sometimes used to explain infertility. When women have *kwantacce,* their pregnancies go into dormant periods, and fetal development is thought to pause or stop permanently (see Wall 1988).

2. In Save the Children's State of the World's Mothers report (2012), Niger, which was indexed at number 165 of 165 countries, was called the worst place to be a mother due to scores on multiple indicators, including maternal mortality, education, contraceptive use, women's income relative to men's, primary school enrollment, and child malnutrition, which were all considered "among the very worst in the world" (Save the Children 2012, 51). However, Niger has made some progress; in the 2015 report, Niger was indexed at number 175 of 179.

3. Women typically do not give birth alone during their first births or if they have a history of birthing complications. Other categories of women locally perceived as high risk may also be advised not to give birth alone: women who have birthed many children or women who are considered ill or weak, for example. When birthing alone is not possible, for these or other reasons, an older family member such as an aunt or close family friend is often (but not always) preferred to a local midwife or *ungozoma,* due to the midwife's perceived limited skill-set and the concern over her discretion. Similarly, when women fail to deliver quickly, they may call an older female relative (typically a maternal aunt) or a midwife to intervene.

4. The silence, secrecy, shame, and solitude that surrounds pregnancy and childbirth in West Africa has also been documented by Gertie Janssen (2007) among the Zarma-Songhai; Lise Østergaard (2015) among the Mossi, Bissa, and Fulani in Burkina Faso; Paul Riesman (1992) among the Fulani in Niger, and Carolyn Sargent (1989) among the Bariba in Benin.

5. There has been a dramatic increase in the use of health centers because of the increased focus on interventions promoting birthing in health clinics (such as the reduction or elimination of user fees for most maternal health services); in just six years, Niger has seen the percentage of health center births jump from 8 percent of births to 21 percent (DHS Program 2018).

6. These figures come from the most recent Demographic and Health Surveys of Benin, Burkina Faso, Chad, Mali, and Cameroon. Nigeria was an exception, but Nigeria has vast regional differences in birthing alone. In the southwest region, only 1.3 percent of women give birth alone, but in the northwest zone, primarily inhabited by the Hausa ethnic group who are also present in Niger, 27.8 percent of women give birth alone (DHS Program 2018).

7. This is unlike many places in sub-Saharan Africa where midwives and traditional birth attendants (TBAs) play an important role in assisting women with birth and recognizing (and referring) emergencies. It is also distinct from some Hausaphone areas of Nigeria, as demonstrated by *Baba of Karo* (M. F. Smith 1954) where local midwives like Baba are competent and relied upon by laboring women.

8. An *ungozoma*'s service might continue throughout the 40-day postpartum period. She may come every day to a woman's house to prepare hot water infused with special herbs for the woman to bathe in, and serve the woman a medicinal porridge to fortify and protect her body, which is weakened and vulnerable to spirits.

9. Amulets, commonly written prayers encased in darkened leather, hang visibly from the necks, wrists, hair, ankles, or bellies of young children across Niger. Less visible are the amu-

lets adults attach to themselves. Stowed in pockets or hidden underneath clothing, many women rely on these amulets' protective powers. During labor, amulets are commonly used to encourage the safe passage of a child, particularly in the face of obstetric complications. When a woman's labor fails to normally progress, an amulet may be dropped into a calabash of water that is then drunk by the laboring woman. The ritual act is intended to catalyze contractions and successful delivery. Prayers are also written on handheld chalkboards and then washed away. Intended as a protective act, the prayer is harnessed by the water, collected, then ingested by the laboring woman.

10. The delay in diagnosis and treatment of obstetric fistula has been called by Ruder, Cheyney, and Emasu (2018) as the fourth delay.

11. I am reluctant to define this category as cultural as it suggests a naturalized, monolithic entity of Nigérien culture, overlooking the vast diversity, dynamism, and heterogeneity that exists within Niger. Instead, I note locally held meanings, values, and practices, which while not homogeneous, can influence health-seeking behaviors.

12. The brutality and venality of the Nigerian Joint Task Force paramilitary teams of police and soldiers are well-known; they are as feared as Boko Haram insurgents in some parts of northern Nigeria. Government forces have viciously attacked civilians, burning down villages and gunning down people as they ran from their homes.

13. Three women did not develop obstetric fistula during labor, but as the consequence of a local treatment for an ethno-medical gynecological abnormality known as *gurya*. *Gurya* exists predominantly among the Hausa ethnic group of Niger (although similar concepts exist among the Nigérien Zarma and Hausa of Nigeria, known as *haabize* and *gishiri*, respectively). Gurya is an umbrella condition covering perceived pathological sexual behaviors and desires (particularly a woman's refusal of her husband) as well as genital pathology (vaginal narrowing or growths that obstruct vaginal penetration). Treatment includes a genital cutting procedure to open up the vagina performed by the *wanzami* (local barber/surgeon), which may inflict unintentional damage to the urethra and cause a fistula. The fistulas were therefore not obstetric in nature, and none had ever had sexual intercourse.

14. Women labored an average of 1.6 days (range: 0 hours to 7 days) at home before seeking care. Once they reached a health care facility, women labored for an average of 1.4 more days (range: < 1 hour to 8 days). Eighty-four percent of women eventually sought biomedical intervention, 40 percent of them within 12 hours of beginning the labor that caused their fistula. Eighteen women spent no time laboring at home at all, going to the hospital directly at the start of their contractions. The average length of labor for women who went to clinics immediately after their labors began was 2.6 days (range: 12 hours to 7 days). On the other end of the spectrum, 16 women never made it to clinics, laboring entirely at home. The average length of labor for these women was 2.3 days (range: 4 hours to 7 days).

15. These findings mirror the data gathered by United Nations Population Fund (UNFPA) and Niger's Ministry of Health, which revealed that of all the women entering fistula repair centers in Niger in April 2013, only 16 percent gave birth at home and 84 percent birthed in state-run health centers (Doudou 2013).

16. Rates of referral are quite low. Of all patients consulted in Niger's state-run health system in 2016, approximately 1.5 percent were referred to another health center (République du Niger 2017).

17. This practice is similar to (although not the same as) fundal pressure, sometimes called the Kristeller maneuver, where a clinician applies pressure to the top of a woman's uterus during contractions. Although 80 percent of institutions in the United States reported the use of fundal pressure in 1990, studies have found no confirmed benefits of the practice (Matsuo et al. 2009, 781). In fact, it may be harmful, particularly when used during cases of shoulder dystocia

(Hofmeyr et al. 2017). Due to the lack of evidence supporting its use, it remains controversial and is practiced with decreased frequency in U.S.-based biomedical births.

18. A partogram is a graphical record of key maternal and fetal data during labor (with indications for normal birth progression measured through markers such as cervical dilation, fetal heart rate, duration of labor, and vital signs of the mother). The partogram is intended as a low-cost, low-technology rubric for detecting delays or deviations from normal labor progression to facilitate the rapid detection and treatment of obstetric complications.

19. Practitioner abuse of birthing women has been well documented by numerous scholars, including Moyer et al. (2014) in Ghana, Van Hollen (2003) in India, Janevic et al. (2011) in the Balkans, Mselle and Kohi's (2015) in Tanzania, and Okafor, Ugwu, and Obi (2015) in Nigeria.

CHAPTER 5: THE INDETERMINABLE WAIT

1. Although women came from all of Niger's neighboring countries, Hausa women from Nigeria commonly visited Nigérien centers. After undergoing one or more failed surgeries in Nigeria, often at one of the 13 facilities in Dr. Kees Waaldijk's well-known Nigeria National Fistula Program, many Nigerian Hausa found their way north. Similarly, after unsuccessful surgeries in Niger, women frequently migrated south in hopes of better outcomes. These movements mirror larger patterns of mobility of Hausa communities, divided between the artificial Niger-Nigeria border (Miles 1994).

2. The Nigérien health care system is shaped by global forces; it was never intended to serve the rural poor during French colonialism, and then it was slowly dismantled over half a century of neoliberal policies that encouraged the retreat and decentralization of the state (see Arzika 1992; Körling 2011; Masquelier 2001a).

3. Women at Danja had waited an average of 1.9 months (from two weeks to three months); women at Lamordé averaged 3.8 months (two weeks to eight months); women at CNRFO averaged 5.2 months (one week to two years); and women at Dimol averaged 11.6 months (two weeks to six years).

4. Staff at Dimol accused the government and high-level staff at CNRFO of recognizing the value and potential profitability of fistula intervention, and thus deciding to enter the fistula market through the theft of Dimol's center. Dimol staff believed that that this theft was justified by the government under completely false pretenses. They claimed that the state had quickly built a surgical building on the grounds to complicate Dimol's legal challenge (even if Dimol had won, it would likely be on the condition that Dimol repay the government for the costs of construction—an insurmountable barrier for the small organization). With ongoing legal challenges, the animosity between Dimol and CNRFO grew, and the possibility of compromise or collaboration withered.

5. A few women had been sent to Burkina Faso for surgeries by Dimol, but women were similarly met with long waits and were unable to secure interventions there. Met with growing unrest at the center, Dimol staff had asked many of the women to lie to the other women upon their return to Niger, to suggest that they had been operated on. Generally, the only medical solution offered to women with fistula at Dimol was catheterization. Dimol staff placed a Foley catheter in most women upon their arrival (leaving the catheter in place for up to several months at a time). Although there is evidence that catheterization for small, fresh fistula may be an effective treatment and close some fistula, prolonged catheterization may also result in infection and discomfort for women.

6. And by the time I wrote this book, this surgeon had already left the DFC, leaving the center in a state of limbo.

7. These rumors were not unfounded. For example, during the summer of 2011, I witnessed a visiting Worldwide Fistula Fund (WFF) board member (and Christian pastor) perform an exorcism on a Fulani patient experiencing uterine spasms (screaming, "Send the devil back to the bush"). When it came to daily operations, SIM and WFF were frequently at odds regarding the role of evangelism within the clinic.

8. Niger struggles less with corruption than many of its sub-Saharan African neighbors; it is ranked 101th of the 176 countries included in the Corruption Perception Index in 2016, which includes 30 other countries in sub-Saharan Africa ranked between 101 and 176 (on the Transparency International website in 2017; https://www.transparency.org). But cases of graft and the misuse of public funds do sometimes make international news. For example, in 2013, 20 Nigérien doctors were arrested for embezzling funds from a Bill and Melinda Gates Foundation initiative for vaccinations (Reuters Staff 2013).

9. Adler et al. (2013) and others call into question existing estimations of fistula incidence and prevalence. See note 1 from Chapter 1.

10. Fistula centers also provide for women's non-fistula-related health care while at the center, regularly providing women with medications for malaria, respiratory infections, and (as women often fall in the slick tiled or paved showers at centers) broken bones.

11. Practitioners were forced to engage in acts of everyday corruption to supplement salaries and/or look to the nonprofit sector as a more reliable source of income.

12. In an important contribution to the human rights of fistula patients, Lewis Wall (2014) proposes a Bill of Rights for patients with obstetric fistula. Included are the rights to dignity, competent care, privacy, the refusal of services or inclusion in research studies, self-determination, and informed consent; however, Wall omits the right to timely care.

13. Rather than hard facts, statistics are better thought of as an end result of a long series of choices about what to count and how to count it, often mediated by the interests of those who do the counting. I argue that the widely cited 90 percent success rate of fistula surgery may not reflect actual surgical outcomes, but are instead the end point in a carefully constructed narrative (see Heller 2018).

14. Of the 86 women who were seeking surgery, 25 women (29 percent) did not receive surgery during my year-long research period (61 women, or 71 percent, did). According to a UNFPA study reported on by Issoufou and Tassiou (2013), between 2009 and 2012, only 71 percent (2,205 out of 3,122) of all identified cases of obstetric fistula were operated on, making the findings from my sample representative of Niger as a whole. As an ethnographer, with some distance from women's clinical experience, I did not have access to all the women's clinical diagnoses and cannot confidently report on closure rates (which require a surgeon's diagnosis). Instead, my metric for success was directed by the women's self-evaluations, whereby continence was the sole criterion for success. Although there is a difference in the future prognosis of fistulas that cannot be closed and postrepair incontinence (which may be diagnosable and treatable through future surgical interventions), I have categorized all postsurgical incontinence together. For my purposes, I define surgical success as a binary: wet (incontinent) or dry (continent). I defined incontinence using the previous International Continence Society (ICS) definition as an involuntary loss of urine that is a social or hygienic problem (see Abrams et al. 2010). With the understanding that some degree of incontinence may be normal after pregnancy, labor, or aging, women were counted as wet only if their leakage was both persistent and subjectively reported as problematic. In this way, women with mild urge or stress incontinence were not included.

15. These confirm the findings of Holme, Breen, and MacArthur (2007), where new cases were significantly more likely attain continence than old cases (P=.045). I could not ascertain thorough clinical information about each woman, and with a lack of consensus regarding the

classification of simple versus complex fistula, I could not delimitate the simple cases from the complex cases.

16. See Heller 2017. Dimol's outcomes are not considered as Dimol did not conduct or oversee operations.

17. Shrime, Sleemi, and Ravilla (2015) argue that fistula surgeons are not considered experts until they have performed 300 fistula surgeries, which for short-term missions, given the lapses in time between operations, takes years. Complicated obstetric fistula surgeries are best performed at high-volume, specialized surgical hospitals. These do not exist in Niger, although Danja Fistula Center has the potential to become one.

18. In 2013, the United Nations Population Fund (UNFPA) and Niger's Ministry of Health conducted a study of the demographics of fistula cases in Niger, sampling all 176 women at the six state-run fistula repair centers in Niger in April 2013. The study revealed that only 24 women (13 percent) had never undergone fistula surgery; 47 women (26 percent) had undergone one previous failed surgery, 33 women (19 percent) had undergone two previous failed surgeries, and the largest proportion, 74 women (42 percent), had undergone between 3 and 10 previous failed surgeries (Doudou 2013). In presenting these data at an international fistula conference, Dr. Hassane Doudou criticized the quality of fistula care, nothing that women had "often experienced many interventions without success . . . The multiple operations indicate the need to ameliorate the quality of interventions at the centers" (2013).

19. The remaining nine women were not looking for surgeries at the time of the interview (they had come to the centers for various reasons: other health care, cesarean deliveries with subsequent pregnancies, for training, to collect money, etc.). Three women were categorized as incurable (and thus were not operated on), two women were treated with catheters, and one woman died at the center of unknown causes before receiving surgery.

20. These figures vary dramatically across the various centers: 96 percent (22 out of 23) of the women looking for surgery at Danja received it during the research period, but only 67 percent (32 out of 48) of the surgery-seekers at CNRFO/Lamordé did. Given the politics of Dimol, it is unsurprising that only 47 percent (7 out of 15) of the women seeking surgeries were able to receive one. See the appendix for more demographic information on the women's waits by center and ethnicity.

21. Longer waits for complicated cases are not necessarily a matter of preference. On-staff surgeons may lack the expertise to operate on complicated cases, so women must wait for surgeons with specialized surgical techniques to pass through, as was the case with the Danja Fistula Center. With no standardization regarding the definition or treatment of women who are incurable or inoperable, these most difficult and often unpromising cases are often left in uncertainty for years at fistula centers.

22. Five women (16 percent) were healed after their second surgery, four (13 percent) were healed after their third surgery, five (16 percent) were healed after their fourth surgery, one (3 percent) was healed after her fifth surgery, and one woman (3 percent) was healed after her seventh surgery.

23. Long wait times and prolonged stays at fistula centers are not unusual in Niamey. Harouna (2001) noted that only 20 percent of patients were at the Niamey hospital for less than six months, while 45.5 percent waited between six months and one year, and 34.5 percent of patients stayed for over a year.

24. Approximately 81 percent of Niger's population lives in rural areas, and only 5 percent of rural households have electricity (INS and ICF International 2013; World Bank 2018). Although 44 percent of rural households have a cell phone, access to electricity or money to buy credit to recharge the phone may be difficult to come by (INS and ICF International 2013).

Additionally, women often would lose the phone numbers of their family contact during their prolonged absences.

ARANTUT'S STORY

1. Despite the *brassage*, or cultural and ethnic blending or hybridity, that defines ethnic identity in Niger (see chapter 1), there are still some important differences in marriage practices and meaning within Niger's main ethnic groups. Tuareg women, like most women from nomadic traditions (including Fulani, Toubou, and Arabs in Niger), have historically had high status and independence. Tuareg women traditionally own herds and enjoy freedom of movement, the right to self-represent in litigation, and the ability to initiate divorce (Rasmussen 1994). However, as Tuareg communities have moved toward sedentarization, women have experienced a gradual loss of autonomy, status, and economic independence, and they may no longer have their own tents or herds—and thus they are increasingly dependent on their husbands' homes and incomes. Still, compared with other ethnic groups in Niger, social interaction between Tuareg men and women is significantly more egalitarian. Tuareg women may travel, visit men, and flirt before (and even after) marriage (Rasmussen 2004). In contrast, Hausa gender norms and marriage traditions for women tend to be significantly more restrictive.

CHAPTER 6: SUPERLATIVE SUFFERERS

1. See, for example, the work of Hannig 2017; Heller and Hanning 2017; Landry et al. 2013; Maulet, Keita, and Macq 2013; Mselle et al. 2011; Phillips et al. 2016; Sullivan, O'Brien, and Mwini-Nyaledzigbor 2016; and Yeakey et al. 2009. Although it is uncommon for media and donor representations to the acknowledge the demographic diversity of women with fistula, such nuances are beginning to emerge in some academic literature. For example, in a large-scale cohort study of 1,354 women with fistula in five countries, Landry et al. (2013) state that fistula affects women across all age groups, not just young women; fistula does develop among women with higher parities; and not all husbands and families abandon women with fistula—only a very small minority live alone (15). However, the presence of work that contradicts the hegemonic fistula narrative does not, as Clare Hemmings put it, make a dent in the relentless persuasiveness of the presumed (2011, 20).

2. An 85 to 98 percent success rate for fistula repair surgeries is commonly reported (Mselle et al. 2011; Nafiou et al. 2006; Ndiaye 2009). High surgical success rates are only reported in donor and media narratives but also appear in some academic literature (see Miller et al. 2005). For example, in an epidemiology dissertation on fistula prognosis, Veronica Frajzyngier (2011) introduces fistula by claiming that "the majority (80–95 percent) of fistulas can be closed surgically" (6). In a review piece on obstetric fistula, Semere and Nour (2008) write, "About 80 percent to 90 percent of women with VVF [vesicovaginal fistula] can potentially be cured by simple vaginal surgery" (196). Such claims are common.

3. The reasoning is that during pregnancy a girl's body will direct all additional energy away from her own physical maturation and to the development of her fetus. A young woman whose body has not developed to maturity is at a higher risk of obstructed labor because the fetus may be too large to pass through the available space in the immature maternal pelvis (Wall 1998).

4. The average age of first marriage in Niger (for women aged 20 to 49) is 15.8, dropping to 15.6 for rural women, and 15.5 for the poorest quintile of women (INS and ICF International

2013). Among the 97 women I came to know for whom I had data, the average age of first marriage was 15.5.

5. Nafissa (mid-30s, Zarma) explained that in her village there is a local custom dictating that grooms migrate for work after marriage, allowing their young brides time to mature. "In my village, if a girl is young when she is married, the husband goes away for two years, then they sleep together when he returns." Samira (55, Fulani) was married by choice before menarche, probably at around 13 years old. She was not sexually active until three years after her marriage and did not get pregnant until she was 16, delivering when she was 17. Habiba (49, Fulani) was married at 13 and lived with her mother-in-law for two years before deciding to divorce her husband, at which point she and her husband had still never consummated their marriage.

6. There are myriad methods commonly deployed to manipulate data and inflate success rates. One: Inflate successful cases by (1) defining success as closure, not continence, and (2) defining success after surgery, not at follow-up. Two: Deflate the number of total cases by (1) defining the total as the number of women who have left the centers over a stated period, not the number of women or operations; (2) defining the total as the number of women, not the number of operations; and (3) excluding the operations that are most likely to fail. For more on this process of data manipulation to inflate success rates, see Heller 2018.

7. Similarly, as Miriam Ticktin notes of victims of sexual violence—who before the 2000s were not considered compelling humanitarian subjects—the medicalization of gender-based violence has allowed women to be abstracted from their political contexts, rendered blameless, and treated (2017, 582). Although women's entry into such a conceptual space of innocence has brought important advantages, Ticktin argues that it has been less helpful insofar as it has worked to depoliticize the larger gendered inequalities that lead to such harm (2017, 582).

8. Here I reference the widely covered attack on Malala Yousafzai, a Pakistani girl who in 2012 survived being shot in the hand, arm, and face by a member of the Taliban in retaliation for outspoken support of girls' rights to education.

9. This is in reference to the Syrian humanitarian crisis and the respective photographs of Alan Kurdi (of a three-year-old boy who downed along with his mother and brother in an attempt to flee the conflict; his body washed up on a Turkish beach and was photographed) and Omran Daqneesh (of a five-year-old who was rescued from the rubble of a bombed Aleppo building, dazed and bleeding; his photograph became emblematic of the widespread violence and state-sponsored terrorism in Aleppo).

10. There are notable exceptions to this statement. Many organizations work to address the structural impediments to health. However, the philanthrocapitalist environment in which these organizations are forced to compete works to discourage these holistic and structural approaches.

11. A similar strategy, whereby potential funders can browse through pictures and profiles of brown-skinned sufferers, has been adopted in various humanitarian charity campaigns. See, for example, Erica Bornstein, "The Value of Orphans" (2010).

12. Alexander's The New Jim Crow (2010) and DuVernay's documentary 13th (2016) demonstrate how a system of racial caste has been maintained in the United States for nearly four centuries, often by situating criminality as a pathology of the black subculture. This narrative has resulted in policies leading to slavery, then Jim Crow laws, and then a law-and-order rhetoric that disproportionately inflicts mass incarceration on African Americans as a form of racialized control. Similarly, immigrants have been linked with both an existential threat to cultural (and often racial) national identity and to physical safety. Who qualifies as an immigrant, as nonwhite, as Other, and as a national threat has shifted through time: from Western Europeans and Jews, to Chinese and Japanese, to Mexicans, to Arabs and other Muslims, for example. But the rhetoric has been consistent.

13. The Western condemnation of culture or tradition in the Global South is not limited to Africa. The discourse that indicts culture or tradition in the development of fistula in Africa resembles the discourse surrounding *sati* (widow-burning) in India, foot binding in China, or veiling and *purdah* (wife seclusion) throughout Islamic societies.

14. In Walker's novel *Possessing the Secret of Joy* (1992), the main character Tashi's dysfunctional sex life, painful childbirth, deformed child, malignant marriage, and profound unhappiness are all attributed to female genital cutting.

15. For example, the "Negro" came to represent a rapacious sexual appetitive, a primitiveness—the "incarnation of a genital potency beyond all moralities and prohibitions" (Fanon 1952/2008, 136).

16. In a critique of the focus on women's agency, Wilson (2008) argues that the positioning of women as altruistic, efficient, and responsible has become an integral part of development orthodoxy, marginalizing the analysis of oppressive structures in the advancement of neoliberal economic agendas.

17. Additionally, when we focus so singly on the moral imperative to intervene, to save the innocent, we overlook the powerful drive to witness, to act—to become a savior—and the associated consequences (Abu-Lughod 2013; Ticktin 2017).

18. Although there are too many to name, see, for example, Abramowitz, Marten, Panter-Brick (2014); Butt (2002); Fassin (2012); James (2010); Kleinman, Das, and Lock (1997); Malkki (1996), and Ticktin (2017), who critique representational practices of NGOs, which often unintentionally commodify images of faraway suffering, erase local voices, dehistoricize indigenous accounts, and lead to ineffective or counterproductive interventions.

CHAPTER 7: COSTS AND CONSEQUENCES

1. Scholars have long considered mycobacterial leprosy or Hansen's disease—modern leprosy—as the condition in the Bible referred to as *tzaraat*. However, it is now recognized that *tzaraat* was a general category covering a group of diverse skin diseases, not one particular condition. Consensus is building among scholars that the condition once believed to refer to leprosy in the Bible bears no resemblance to modern-day Hansen's disease, particularly as evidence suggests that the Hebrew Bible (Old Testament) was written before the introduction of mycobacterial leprosy to the lands inhabited by the Hebrews (see Grzybowski and Nita 2016).

2. According to historian Shobana Shankar, Islam and Christianity were thought to have separate medical spheres, and treatment for leprosy was labeled as Christian. See Shankar 2006, 281.

3. Edmond (2006) argues that leper colonies represented spaces of what Agamben termed "bare life," life that does not deserve to live (and can be terminated without consequence). In spaces of bare life, people are separated from others and denied the rights associated with human existence.

4. Shared through personal email communication by CSL staff. The letter is addressed to CSL-Danja's Hospital Director.

5. Some women, even those previously healed of fistula, do use the clinics as sites for economic and social growth because they become eligible for a host of goods and services that are otherwise unavailable to them back home. They can obtain items intended for income-generating activities such as sewing machines, cell phones, cash, and foodstuff, and services such as training, microcredit lending activities, and free health care, often for conditions unrelated to fistula. Additionally, at the centers women have the opportunity to expand their social support systems through the relationships they cultivate with other women with fistula, and by

establishing relationships with center staff (an urban, highly educated, middle-class sector of the population who are otherwise inaccessible to these poor, rural women). Some women use the centers not only for acute and short-term physiological intervention but as life-long sites of opportunity. The centers may act as a recourse from difficulties at home and a space of refuge from undesired marriages or persistent mistreatment. They may also present women with opportunities to transform their lives, often through marriage or employment in the city. Some women use the centers strategically to build status back home through the cultivation of urban habits and knowledge. Others see the centers as providing opportunities to ease financial strain through the participation in training courses.

6. At the time of my research, several organizations were working to craft better reinsertion programming. The reinsertion program at Danja provided an excellent model for appropriately tailored postoperative courses. Women at Danja were allowed to opt in to the three-month, highly structured training course (and were not pressured to do so nor punished if they opted out). Women who opted out of the training course (largely due to impatience to return home) still participated in weekly hygiene and health courses as well as regular activities. Women enrolled in the training program attended courses five days a week and learned a variety of skills, including knitting, embroidery, sewing, soap and lotion making, and basic literacy skills. When I left the field the Danja reinsertion program was still in its nascent stages, but the center planned to provide small groups of neighboring reintegrated patients with centrally located cooperatives (equipped with the necessary tools for a small shared business, such as a sewing machine). This plan, however, required clusters of at least five reintegrated women; due to the relatively small number of ex-patients and their geographic diversity, no clusters had been established by the time I left the field.

7. While some studies have demonstrated that rehabilitation after repair was an important component of fistula care (see Donnelly et al 2015; Landry et al. 2013; Mohammad 2007), other scholars have disagreed, emphasizing that successful surgery is sufficient for reintegration and that there is no need for reintegration services (see Nathan et al. 2009; Yealey et al. 2012). Some scholars generally question the efficacy of rehabilitation services as they currently exist (see Donnelly et al. 2015; Velez, Ramsey, and Tell 2007).

8. Even women who claimed not to have actively hidden their fistula still attempted to control the outward evidence of their wetness.

9. Concealment, the refusal of disclosure, in conjunction with these coping strategies, was acknowledged among women in Ethiopia and Uganda, who hid their conditions from neighbors, relatives, and even husbands (Barageine et al. 2015; Gjerde et al. 2013). In a study of women with fistula in Tanzania, Watt and colleagues (2014) found that women went to extreme efforts to hide their conditions from their religious communities. Similarly, Anita Hannig's (2015) research with nurse aides in fistula hospitals in Ethiopia demonstrates the lengths to which these former fistula patients-cum-hospital-employees go to conceal their chronic incontinence from the patients with fistula they are treating in order to maintain their authority as a healer. For other studies examining these coping strategies, see Barageine et al. 2015; Blum 2012; Gebresilase 2014; Mwini-Nyaledzigbor, Agana, and Pilkington 2013; and Okoye, Emma-Echiegu, and Tanyi 2014.

10. I spoke with an administrator at the Danja Fistula Centre who translated for *New York Times* columnist Nick Kristof when he interviewed women with fistula a few months after I had left. Kristof originally spoke with one particularly young and beautiful girl, but when he asked her about rejection and humiliation back home, she insisted that no one, not even her husband, knew of her condition. Kristof aborted the interview and never used her story. As I have mentioned, the story Kristof ultimately wrote was about "humiliated women and girls" who were "sent away by their husbands" and "endured years of mockery and ostracism" (Kristof 2013).

The acts of passing that this young woman described and that Kristof rejected are quite usual—perhaps even the norm.

11. *Accompaniment* is the word used to describe the process whereby after surgery women would be taken back home by center staff and often reintroduced to the community as a healed woman.

12. For example, see Lagro-Janssen, Smits, and Weel 1992; Lose 2005; Manderson 2011.

CHAPTER 8: THE THRESHOLD OF CONTINENCE

1. Due to time constraints and concerns regarding Boko Haram (which had increased its activity over the Niger/Nigeria border), I did not return to Danja.

2. For an excellent example of public anthropology, see Paul Stoller (2016) who regularly blogs for the *Huffington Post*.

BIBLIOGRAPHY

Abramowitz, Sharon, and Catherine Panter-Brick. 2015. *Medical Humanitarianism: Ethnographies of Practice.* Philadelphia: University of Pennsylvania Press.

Abrams, Paul, Karl-Erik Andersson, L. Birder, L. Brubaker, Linda Cardozo, C. Chapple, A. Cottenden, et al. 2010. "Fourth International Consultation on Incontinence Recommendations of the International Scientific Committee: Evaluation and Treatment of Urinary Incontinence, Pelvic Organ Prolapse, and Fecal Incontinence." *Neurourology and Urodynamics* 29 (1): 213–240.

Abu-Lughod, Lila. 2002. "Do Muslim Women Really Need Saving? Anthropological Reflections on Cultural Relativism and Its Others." *American Anthropologist, New Series* 104 (3): 783–790.

———. 2013. *Do Muslim Women Need Saving?* Harvard: Harvard University Press.

Adams, Vincanne. 2012. "The Other Road to Serfdom: Recovery by the Market and the Affect Economy in New Orleans." *Public Culture* 24 (1): 185–216.

———. 2013. *Markets of Sorrow, Labors of Faith: New Orleans in the Wake of Katrina.* Durham: Duke University Press.

Adichie, Chimamanda. 2009. "The Danger of a Single Story." TED.com, July 2009, https://www.ted.com/talks/chimamanda_adichie_the_danger_of_a_single_story.html.

Adler, A. J., C. Ronsmans, C. Calvert, and V. Filippi. 2013. "Estimating the Prevalence of Obstetric Fistula: A Systematic Review and Meta-Analysis." *BMC Pregnancy and Childbirth* 13 (246): 1–14.

Aghanwa, H. S., F. O. Dare, and S. O. Ogunniyi. 1999. "Sociodemographic Factors in Mental Disorders Associated with Infertility in Nigeria." *Journal of Psychosomatic Research* 46 (2): 117–123.

Agustín, Laura María. 2007. *Sex at the Margins: Migration, Labour Markets and the Rescue Industry.* London: Zed Books.

Ahmed, Saifuddin, and Rene Genadry. 2013. "Défis de la prévalence de la fistule obstétricale au Niger." UNFPA Atelier de Réflexion Stratégique sur la Fistule Obstétricale au Niger/UNFPA Conference on a Strategic Reflection on Obstetric Fistula in Niger. Grand Hotel, Niamey, Niger, October 8, 2013.

Ahmed, Sarah, and S. A. Holtz. 2007. "Social and Economic Consequences of Obstetric Fistula: Life Changed Forever?" *International Journal of Gynecology and Obstetrics* 99 (Suppl. 1): S10–S15.

Alan Guttmacher Institute. 2002. "Sexual and Reproductive Health: Women and Men." 2002. New York: AGI, https://web.archive.org/web/20081127071604/http://www.guttmacher.org/pubs/fb_10-02.html.

Al-Badr, A., H. Brasha, R. Al-Raddadi, F. Noorwali, and S. Ross. 2012. "Prevalence of Urinary Incontinence among Saudi Women." *International Journal of Gynecology and Obstetrics* 117: 160–163.

Alexander, Michelle. 2011. *The New Jim Crow.* New York: New Press.

Al-Ha'iri, Ayatollah Hasan. 1972. *Ahkam al-Shi'a.* Kuwait: Maktabat al-Imam Ja'far al-Sadiq 'alayhi al-salam.

Alidou, Ousseina. 2005. *Engaging Modernity: Muslim Women and the Politics of Agency in Postcolonial Niger.* Madison: University of Wisconsin Press.

Alio, Amina, Lauren Merrell, Kimberlee Roxburgh, Heather Clayton, Phillip Marty, Linda Bomboka, Salamatou Traore, and Hamisu Salihu. 2010. "The Psychosocial Impact of Vesico-Vaginal Fistula in Niger." *Archives of Gynecology and Obstetrics* 284 (2): 371–378.

Al-Juwayni, 'Abd Allah b. Yusuf. 1994. *Al-Tabsira*. Beirut: Dar al-Kutub al-'Ilmiyya.

Al-Krenawi, Alean. 1999. "Women of Polygamous Marriages in Primary Health Care Centers." *Contemporary Family Therapy* 21 (3): 417–430.

Anderson, Connie. 2000. "The Persistence of Polygyny as an Adaptive Response to Poverty and Oppression in Apartheid South Africa." *Cross-Cultural Research* 34 (2): 99–112.

Anoukoum, T., K. Attipou, L. Agoda-Koussema, K. Akpadaz, and E. Ayite. 2010. "Aspects epidémiologiques, etiologiques et thérapeutiques de la fistule obstétricale au Togo." *Progrès en Urologie* 20: 71–76.

Antoine, Philippe. 2002. "Les complexités de la nuptialité: de la précocité des unions féminines à la polygamie masculine en Afrique." Paris: DIAL (Documents de Travail).

Arrowsmith, Steven, Mark Barone, and Joseph Ruminjo. 2013. "Outcomes in Obstetric Fistula Care: A Literature Review." *Current Opinion in Obstetrics & Gynecology* 25 (5): 399–403.

Arrowsmith, Steven, Catherine Hamlin, and L. Lewis Wall. 1996. "Obstructed Labor Injury Complex: Obstetric Fistula Formation and the Multifaceted Morbidity of Maternal Birth Trauma in the Developing World." *Obstetrical and Gynecological Survey* 51 (9): 568–574.

Arzika, Ayouba. 1992. "Colonisation et santé: action sanitaire Française et realités au Niger (1922–1958)." PhD diss., Université Paris VII.

Auyero, Javier. 2012. *Patients of the State: The Politics of Waiting in Argentina*. Durham: Duke University Press.

Avery, J. C., and N. Stocks. 2016. "Urinary Incontinence, Depression and Psychological Factors—A Review of Population Studies." *European Medical Journal Urology* 1 (1): 58–67.

Bangser, Maggie, Manisha Mehta, Janet Singer, Chris Daly, and Catherine Kamugumya. 2011. "Childbirth Experiences of Women with Obstetric Fistula in Tanzania and Uganda and Their Implications for Fistula Program Development." *International Urogynecology Journal* 22: 91–98.

Barageine, Justus, Jolly Beyeza-Kashesya, Josaphat Byamugisha, Nazarius Tumwesigye, Lars Almroth, and Elisabeth Faxelid. 2015. "'I Am Alone and Isolated': A Qualitative Study of Experiences of Women Living with Genital Fistula in Uganda." *BMC Women's Health* 15: 73.

Bashford, Alison. 2004. *Imperial Hygiene: A Critical History of Colonialism, Nationalism and Public Health*. New York: Palgrave MacMillian.

Bates, I., G. K. Chapotera, S. McKew, and N. van den Broek. 2008. "Maternal Mortality in Sub-Saharan Africa: The Contribution of Ineffective Blood Transfusion Services." *BJOG* 115: 1331–1339.

BBC. 2012. "Niger Worst Place to Be Mother—Save the Children." BBC News Africa, May 8, http://www.bbc.co.uk/news/world-africa-17984899.

Biehl, João. 2013. *Vita: Life in a Zone of Social Abandonment*. University of California Press.

Bishop, Matthew, and Michael Green. 2008. *Philanthrocapitalism: How the Rich Can Save the World*. New York: Bloomsbury Press.

Blanford, Justine, Supriya Kumar, Wei Luo and Alan MacEachren. 2012. "It's a Long, Long Walk: Accessibility to Hospitals, Maternity and Integrated Health Centers in Niger." *International Journal of Health Geographics* 11 (1): 24.

Blum, Lauren S. 2012. "Living with Obstetric Fistula: Qualitative Research Finding from Bangladesh and Democratic Republic of Congo." New York: USAID/EngenderHealth, https://cdn2.sph.harvard.edu/wp-content/uploads/sites/32/2014/05/LivingWith_FistulaCare_ResArt_2012.pdf.

Bob, Clifford. 2005. *The Marketing of Rebellion: Insurgents, Media and International Activism.* Cambridge: Cambridge University Press.

Booth, David, and Diana Cammack. 2013. *Governance for Development in Africa: Solving Collective Action Problems.* London: Zed Books.

Borgerhoff Mulder, Monique. 1992. "Women's Strategies in Polygynous Marriage: Kipsigis, Datoga, and Other East African Cases." *Human Nature* 3 (1): 45–70.

Bornand, Sandra. 2005. "Insultes rituelles entre coépouses. Étude du Marcanda (Zarma, Niger)." *Ethnographiques.org*, no. 7, http://www.ethnographiques.org/2005/Bornand.html.

———. 2012. "Voix de femmes songhay-zarma du Niger." *Cahiers Mondes Anciens*, no. 3, http://journals.openedition.org/mondesanciens/675.

———. 2015. "Faire Reconnaître Sa Vulnérabilité: Quand Les Épouses Zarma (Niger) Quittent le Foyer Conjugal." *Cahiers du Genre*, no 1: 113–133.

Bornstein, Erica. 2010. "The Value of Orphans." In *Forces of Compassion: Humanitarianism Between Ethics and Politics*, ed. Bornstein and Redfield, 123–147. Santa Fe, N.M.: School for Advanced Research.

———. 2012. *Disquieting Gifts: Humanitarianism in New Delhi.* Stanford: Stanford University Press.

Boserup, Ester. 1970. *Women's Role in Economic Development.* London: Allen & Unwin.

Bossyns, P., and W. Van Lerberghe. 2004. "The Weakest Link: Competence and Prestige as Constraints to Referral by Isolated Nurses in Rural Niger." *Human Resources for Health* 2 (1): 1.

Bourdieu, Pierre. 2000. *Pascalian Meditations.* Stanford, Calif.: Stanford University Press.

Bove, Riley M., Emily Vala-Haynes, and Claudia R. Valeggia. 2012. "Women's Health in Urban Mali: Social Predictors and Health Itineraries." *Social Science and Medicine* 75 (8): 1392–1399.

Bove, Riley M., and Claudia R. Valeggia. 2009. "Polygyny and Women's Health in Sub-Saharan Africa." *Social Science and Medicine* 68: 21–29.

Bovin, Mette. 1988. "'Mariages de la maison' et 'mariages de la brousse' dans les sociétés peul, wodaabe et kanuri autour du lac Tchad." In *Actes du Quatrième Colloque Méga-Tchad, 2: Les relations Hommes–Femmes dans le Bassin du lac Tchad.* ed. N. Echard, 265–329. Paris: ORSTOM.

Browning, Andrew. 2004. "Prevention of Residual Urinary Incontinence following Successful Repair of Obstetric Vesico-Vaginal Fistula Using a Fibro-Muscular Sling." *BJOG* 111: 357–361.

Browning, Andrew, W. Fentahun, and Judith Teng Wah Goh. 2007. "The Impact of Surgical Treatment on the Mental Health of Women with Obstetric Fistula." *BJOG* 114 (11): 1439–1441.

Brugière, Michel. 2012. "Obstetric Fistulas in Mali, Combating Maternal and Child Mortality" *Field Actions Science Reports*, Special Issue 5, http://factsreports.revues.org/2707.

Bruner, J. 1986. *Actual Minds, Possible Words.* Cambridge, Mass.: Harvard University Press.

Burgess, Sarah. 2016. "Creating the Next Steps to Care: Maternal Heath, Improvisation, and Fulani Women in Niamey, Niger." *Anthropology and Medicine* 23 (3): 344–359.

Butt, Leslie. 2002. "The Suffering Stranger: Medical Anthropology and International Morality." *Medical Anthropology* 21 (1): 1–24.

Callaway, Barbara J. 1984. "Ambiguous Consequences of the Socialisation and Seclusion of Hausa Women." *Journal of Modern African Studies* 22 (3): 429–450.

Cam, Cetin, Ates Karateke, Arman Ozdemir, Candemir Gunes, Cem Celik, Buhara Guney, and Dogan Vatansever. 2010. "Fistula Campaigns?—Are They of Any Benefit?" *Taiwan Journal of Obstetric Gynecology* 49 (3): 291–296.

Campaign to End Fistula. 2013. "Taking Stock: Ten Years Fighting Fistula in Niger." EndFistula.Org, November 13, http://www.endfistula.org/news/taking-stock-ten-years-fighting-fistula-niger.

Case, Anne, and Christina Paxson. 2001. "Mothers and Others: Who Invests in Children's Health?" *Journal of Health Economics* 20: 301–328.

Castille, Yves-Jacques, Chiara Avocetien, Dieudonné Zaongo, Jean-Marie Colas, James Peabody, and Charles-Henry Rochat. 2014. "Impact of a Program of Physiotherapy and Health Education on the Outcome of Obstetric Fistula Surgery." *International Journal of Gynecology and Obstetrics* 124: 77–80.

Castro, Arachu, and Paul Farmer. 2005. "Understanding and Addressing AIDS-Related Stigma: From Anthropological Theory to Clinical Practice in Haiti." *American Journal of Public Health* 95 (1): 53–59.

Clark, Shelley, and Sarah Brauner-Otto. 2015. "Divorce in Sub-Saharan Africa: Are Unions Becoming Less Stable?" *Population and Development Review* 41 (4): 583–605.

Clinton Foundation. 2014. "Obstetric Fistula in Mali: Women Living with Dignity, Commitment by IntraHealth International, Inc." Clinton Global Initiative, https://www.clintonfoundation.org/clinton-global-initiative/commitments/obstetric-fistula-mali-women-living-dignity.

Cohen, Ronald. 1971. *Dominance and Defiance: A Study of Marital Instability in an Islamic African Society.* Anthropological Studies 6. Washington, D.C.: American Anthropological Association.

Cooper, Barbara. 1997. *Marriage in Maradi: Gender and Culture in a Hausa Society in Niger, 1900–1989.* Portsmouth, N.H.: Heinemann.

———. 2006. *Evangelical Christians in the Muslim Sahel.* Bloomington: Indiana University Press.

Creanga, A. A., and R. R. Genadry. 2007. "Obstetric Fistula: A Clinical Review." *International Journal of Gynecology and Obstetrics* 99 (Suppl. 1): S40–S46.

Dalton, John, and Tin Leung. 2011. "Why Is Polygyny More Prevalent in Western Africa? An African Slave Trade Perspective." Working paper. Mimeo, Wake Forest University.

De Bernis, L. 2007. "Obstetric Fistula: Guiding Principles for Clinical Management and Programme Development, a New WHO Guideline." *International Journal of Gynaecology and Obstetrics* 99 (Suppl. 1): S117–S121.

Delamou, Alexandre, Bettina Utz, Therese Delvaux, Abdoul Habib Beavogui, Asm Shahabuddin, Akoi Koivogui, Alain Levêque, Wei-Hong Zhang, and Vincent De Brouwere. 2016. "Pregnancy and Childbirth after Repair of Obstetric Fistula in Sub-Saharan Africa: Scoping Review." *Tropical Medicine and International Health* 21 (11): 1348.

Demographic and Health Surveys (DHS) Program. 2018. STAT Complier. USAID, https://www.statcompiler.com.

De Waal, Alexander. 1997. *Famine Crimes: Politics and the Disaster Relief Industry in Africa.* Bloomington: Indiana University Press.

Diarra, Aïssa. 2012. "La prise en charge de l'accouchement dans trois communes au Niger: Say, Balleyara et Guidanroumji." Niamey, Niger: Laboratoire d'Etudes et de Recherche sur les Dynamiques Sociales et le Développement Local (LASDEL).

Diokno, Ananias C., Kathryn Burgio, Nancy H. Fultz, Kraig S. Kinchen, Robert Obenchain, and Richard C. Bump. 2004. "Medical and Self-Care Practices Reported by Women with Urinary Incontinence." *American Journal of Managed Care* 10 (2): 69–80.

Donkor, E. S., and J. Sandall. 2007. "The Impact of Perceived Stigma and Mediating Social Factors on Infertility-Related Stress among Women Seeking Infertility Treatment in Southern Ghana." *Social Science and Medicine* 65: 1683–1694.

Donnelly, Kyla, Elizabeth Oliveras, Yewondwossen Tilahun, Mehari Belachew, and Mengistu Asnake. 2015. "Quality of Life of Ethiopian Women after Fistula Repair: Implications on Rehabilitation and Social Reintegration Policy and Programming." *Culture, Health and Sexuality* 17 (2): 150–164.

Dorjahn, Vernon. 1988. "Changes in Temne Polygyny." *Ethnology* 27 (4): 367–390.

Doudou, Hassane Boukary. 2013. "Profil da la femme victim de FO au Niger." UNFPA Atelier de Réflexion Stratégique sur la Fistule Obstétricale au Niger/Conference on a Strategic Reflection on Obstetric Fistula in Niger. Grand Hotel, Niamey, Niger; October 8, 2013.

Ducrotoy, Marie J., Crawford W. Revie, Alexandra P. M. Shaw, Usman B. Musa, Wilson J. Bertu, Amahyel M. Gusi, Reuben A. Ocholi, Ayodele O. Majekodunmi, and Susan C. Welburn. 2017. "Wealth, Household Heterogeneity and Livelihood Diversification of Fulani Pastoralists in the Kachia Grazing Reserve, Northern Nigeria, during a Period of Social Transition." *PloS One* 12 (3): e0172866.

DuVernay, Ava, dir. 2016. *13th.* Sherman Oaks, Calif.: Kandoo Films.

Edmond, Rod. 2006. *Leprosy and Empire: A Medical and Cultural History.* Cambridge: Cambridge University Press.

EngenderHealth. 2014. "What Is Fistula?: Surgical Repair and Rehabilitation." Fistula Care Plus Project, https://web.archive.org/web/20160603230340/https://fistulacare.org/pages/what-is-fistula/surgical-repair.php.

Escobar, Artuto. 1995. *Encountering Development: The Making and Unmaking of the Third World.* Princeton, N.J.: Princeton University Press.

Essien, E., D. Ifenne, K. Sabitu, A. Musa, M. Alti-Mu'azu, V. Adidu, N. Golji, and M. Mukaddas. 1997. "Community Loan Funds and Transport Services for Obstetric Emergencies in Northern Nigeria." *International Journal of Gynecology and Obstetrics* 59 (2): 237–244.

Falandry, L. 2000. "Traitement par voie vaginale de l'incontinence résiduelle des urines après fermeture de fistule obstétricale: A propos de 49 cas." *Journal de Gynécologie Obstétrique et Biologie de la Reproduction* 29: 393–401.

Fanon, Frantz. 1952/2008. *Black Skin, White Masks.* London: Pluto Press.

Fassin, Didier. 2007. *When Bodies Remember: Experiences and Politics of AIDS in South Africa.* Berkeley: University of California Press.

———. 2012. *Humanitarian Reason: A Moral History of the Present.* Translated by Rachel Gomme. Berkeley: University of California Press.

Ferguson, James. 1990. *The Anti-Politics Machine: "Development," Depoliticization, and Bureaucratic Power in Lesotho.* Cambridge: Cambridge University Press.

———. 2006. *Global Shadows: Africa in the Neoliberal World Order.* Durham, N.C.: Duke University Press.

Fife, Betsy, and E. Wright. 2000. "The Dimensionality of Stigma: A Comparison of its Impact on the Self of Persons with HIV/AIDS and Cancer." *Journal of Health and Social Behavior* 41 (1): 50–67.

Filippi, V., C. Ronsmans, O. M. Campbell, W. J. Graham, A. Mills, J. Borghi, M. Koblinsky, and D. Osrin. 2006. "Maternal Health in Poor Countries: the Broader Context and a Call for Action." *Lancet* 368 (9546): 1535–1541.

Fistula Foundation. 2014. "Fast Facts and FAQ." http://www.fistulafoundation.org/what-is-fistula/fast-facts-faq.

Fitzgerald, Rosemary. 2001. "'Clinical Christianity': The Emergence of Medical Work as a Missionary Strategy in Colonial India, 1800–1914." In *Health, Medicine and Empire: Perspectives on Colonial India,* ed. Biswamoy Pati and Mark Harrison, 88–136. Hyderabad, India: Orient Longman.

Foucault, Michel. 1983/2003. "On the Genealogy of Ethics: An Overview of Work in Progress." In *The Essential Foucault: Selections from The Essential Works of Foucault 1954–1984,* edited by Paul Rabinow and Nikolas Rose, 102–125. New York: New Press.

Frajzyngier, Veronica. 2011. "Toward a Better Understanding of Urinary Fistula Repair Prognosis: Results from a Multi-Country Prospective Cohort Study." PhD diss., Columbia University.

Friedman, Adam, and Iain Kennedy, dirs. 2015. *Shout Gladi Gladi.* Documentary. [n.p.]: Vertical Ascent.

Gebresilase, Yenenesh Tadesse. 2014. "A Qualitative Study of the Experiences of Obstetric Fistula Survivors in Addis Ababa, Ethiopia." *International Journal of Women's Health* 6:1033–1043.

Gjerde, Janne L., Guri Rortveit, Mulu Muleta, and Astrid Blystad. 2013. "Silently Waiting to Heal." *International Urogynecology Journal* 24 (6): 953–958.

Goffman, Erving. 1963. *Stigma: Notes on the Management of Spoiled Identity.* New York: Simon & Schuster.

Good, Mary-Jo DelVecchio, Sandra Teresa Hyde, Sarah Pinto, and Byron J. Good, eds. 2008. *Postcolonial Disorders: Reflections on Subjectivity in the Contemporary World.* Berkeley: University of California Press.

Goody, Jack. 1976. *Production and Reproduction: A Comparative Study of the Domestic Domain.* No. 17. Cambridge: Cambridge University Press.

Grant, Kate. 2016. "Why Do a Million Women Still Suffer the Treatable Condition of Fistula?" *The Guardian,* May 23.

Grzybowski, Andrzej, and Małgorzata Nita. 2016. "Leprosy in the Bible." *Clinics in Dermatology* 34 (1): 3–7.

Hamid, Tengku Aizan, Minoo Pakgohar, Rahimah Ibrahim, and Marzieh Vahid Dastjerdi. 2015. "'Stain in Life': The Meaning of Urinary Incontinence in the Context of Muslim Postmenopausal Women through Hermeneutic Phenomenology." *Archives of Gerontology and Geriatrics* 60 (3): 514–521.

Hamlin, Catherine. 2004. *Preventing Fistula: Transport's Role in Empowering Communities for Health in Ethiopia.* Washington, D.C.: World Bank.

Hamlin, Catherine, and John Little. 2001. *The Hospital by the River: A Story of Hope.* Oxford: Monarch Books.

Hannig, Anita. 2015. "Sick Healers: Chronic Affliction and the Authority of Experience at an Ethiopian Hospital." *American Anthropologist* 117 (4): 640–651.

———. 2017. *Beyond Surgery: Injury, Healing, and Religion at an Ethiopian Hospital.* Chicago: University of Chicago Press.

Hardiman, David. 2006. *Healing Bodies, Saving Souls: Medical Missions in Asia and Africa.* New York: Rodopi.

Harouna, Y. D., A. Seibou, S. Maikana, J. Djambeidou, A. Sangare, S. Bilane, and H. Abdou. 2001. "La fistule vesico-vaginale de cause obstétricale: Enquête auprès de 52 femmes admise au village des fistules." *Sante Tropicale Médecine d'Afrique Noire* 48 (2): 55–59.

Heller, Alison. 2017. "Demographic Profile and Treatment Outcomes of 100 Women with Obstetric Fistula in Niger." *Proceedings in Obstetrics and Gynecology* 7 (2): 1, http://ir.uiowa .edu/pog/vol7/iss2/1.

———. 2018. "The Hidden Harm of Surgery." *Anthropology News* 59 (1): 6–10.

Heller, Alison, and Anita Hannig. 2017. "Unsettling the Fistula Narrative: Cultural Pathology, Biomedical Redemption, and Inequities of Health Access in Niger and Ethiopia." *Anthropology and Medicine* 24 (1): 81–95.

Hemmings, Clare. 2011. *Why Stories Matter: The Political Grammar of Feminist Theory.* Durham, N.C.: Duke University Press.

Hofmeyr, G. Justus, Joshua P. Vogel, Anna Cuthbert, and Mandisa Singata. 2017. "Fundal Pressure during the Second Stage of Labour." *Cochrane Database of Systematic Reviews* 3: CD006067.

Hollos, Marida, Ulla Larsen, Oka Obono, and Bruce Whitehouse. 2009. "The Problem of Infertility in High Fertility Populations: Meanings, Consequences, and Coping Mechanisms in Two Nigerian Communities." *Social Science and Medicine* 68: 2061–2068.

Holme, A., M. Breen, and C. MacArthur. 2007. "Obstetric Fistulae: A Study of Women Managed at the Monze Mission Hospital, Zambia." *BJOG* 114 (8): 1010–1017.

Holzemer, W. L., L. R. Uys, M. L. Chirwa, M. Greeff, L. N. Makoae, T. W. Kohi, and P. S. Dlamini. 2007. "Validation of the HIV/AIDS Stigma Instrument—PLWA (HASI-P)." *AIDS Care* 19 (8): 1002–1012.

Hörbst, Viola. 2015. "A Child Cannot Be Bought? Economies of Hope and Failure When Using ARTs in Mali." In *Assisted Reproductive Technologies in the Third Phase,* ed. Kate Hampshire and Bob Simpson, 152–170. New York: Berghahn Books.

Hunt, Nancy Rose. 1999. *A Colonial Lexicon of Birth Ritual, Medicalization, and Mobility in the Congo.* Durham, N.C.: Duke University Press.

Idrissa, Abdourahmane, and Samuel Decalo. 2012. *Historical Dictionary of Niger.* Lanham, Md.: Scarecrow Press.

Inhorn, Marcia C. 2003. "Global Infertility and the Globalization of New Reproductive Technologies: Illustrations from Egypt." *Social Science and Medicine* 56 (9): 1837–1851.

———. 2007. *Reproductive Disruptions: Gender, Technology and Biopolitics in the New Millennium.* New York: Berghahn Books.

Institut National de la Statistique (INS) and ICF International. 2013. *Enquête démographique et de santé et à indicateurs multiples du Niger 2012.* Calverton, Md.: INS and ICF International, https://dhsprogram.com/pubs/pdf/FR277/FR277.pdf.

International Women's Health Program (IWHP). 2009. "Obstetric Fistula: A Labour of Loss." Society of Obstetricians and Gynaecologists of Canada, http://iwhp.sogc.org/index.php?page=obstetric-fistula.

IRIN Staff. 2007a. "Niger: Botched Birth Survivors Battle Fistula." *IRIN News,* December 21, http://www.irinnews.org/report/75970/niger-botched-birth-survivors-battle-fistula.

———. 2007b. "Niger: Why Are So Many Mothers Dying?" IRIN News, December 14, http://www.irinnews.org/report/75869/niger-why-are-so-many-mothers-dying.

———. 2009. "Fistula—Two-Hour Operation Corrects Decades-Long Affliction." April 7, http://www.irinnews.org/report/83840/cote-d-ivoire-fistula-two-hour-operation-corrects-decades-long-affliction.

Issoufou, Elh, and M Tassiou. 2013. "Etats des lieux sur la stratégie de traitement de la fistule obstétricale au Niger." UNFPA Atelier de Réflexion Stratégique sur la Fistule Obstétricale au Niger/Conference on a Strategic Reflection on Obstetric Fistula in Niger. Grand Hotel, Niamey, Niger. October 8, 2013.

Izugbara, Chimaraoke, and Alex Ezeh. 2010. "Women and High Fertility in Islamic Northern Nigeria." *Studies in Family Planning* 41 (3): 193–204.

Jaffré, Yannick, and Jean-Pierre Olivier de Sardan. 2002. *Une médecine inhospitalière: Les difficiles relations entre soignants et soignés dans cinq capitales d'Afrique de l'Ouest.* Collection Hommes et Sociétés. Marseille: APAD.

Jaffré, Yannick, and Alain Prual. 1994. "Midwives in Niger: An Uncomfortable Position between Social Behaviours and Health Care Constraints." *Social Science and Medicine* 38 (3): 1069–1073.

James, Erica. 2010. *Democratic Insecurities: Violence, Trauma, and Intervention in Haiti.* Berkeley: University of California Press.

Janevic, Teresa, Pooja Sripad, Elizabeth Bradley, and Vera Dimitrievska. 2011. "'There's No Kind of Respect Here.' A Qualitative Study of Racism and Access to Maternal Health Care among Romani Women in the Balkans." *International Journal for Equity in Health* 10 (1): 1–12.

Jankowiak, William, Monika Sudakov, and Benjamin C. Wilreker. 2005. "Co-wife Conflict and Co-operation." *Ethnology* 44 (1): 81–98.

Janssen, Gertie. 2007. "10-Solitary Births in Téra, Niger: A Local Quest for Safety." In *Strength beyond Structure*, ed. Mirjam de Bruijn, Rijk van Dijk, and Jan-Bart Gewald, 240–262. Boston: Brill.

Jenkins, Janis H., and Elizabeth A. Carpenter-Song. 2008. "Stigma Despite Recovery: Strategies from Living in the Aftermath of Psychosis." *Medical Anthropology Quarterly* 22 (4): 381–409.

Johnson, Susan. 2003. *A Better Woman: A Memoir of Motherhood*. New York: Simon & Schuster.

Jones, E. E., A. Farina, A. H. Hastorf, H. Markus, D. T. Miller, and R. Scott. 1984. *Social Stigma: The Psychology of Marked Relationships*. New York: W. H. Freeman.

Kabir, M., Z. Iliyasu, I. Abubakar, and U. Umar. 2003. "Medico-Social Problems of Patients with Vesico-Vaginal Fistula in Murtala Mohammed Specialist Hospital, Kano." *Annals of African Medicine* 2 (2): 54–57.

Kammerer, Béatrice. 2017. "L'Expression Abdominal Existe Encore et c'est Dramatique." *Slate*, June 17, http://www.slate.fr/story/147183/mensonge-maltraitances-gynecologiques-abdominale.

Kapur, Ratna. 2002. "The Tragedy of Victimization Rhetoric: Resurrecting the 'Native' Subject in International/Post-colonial Feminist Legal Politics." *Harvard Human Rights Journal* 15 (Spring): 1–38.

Karateke, Ates, Cetin Cam, Arman Ozdemir, Buhara Guney, Dogan Vatansever, and Cem Celik. 2010. "Characteristics of Obstetric Fistula and the Need for a Prognostic Classification System." *Archives of Medical Science* 6 (2): 253–256.

Kardas-Nelson, Mara. 2013. "Women in Uganda Dismantle Stigma of Fistula." *Mail & Guardian*, August 8, http://mg.co.za/article/2013-08-08-00-women-dismantle-stigma-of-fistula.

Klein, Naomi. 2007. *The Shock Doctrine: The Rise of Disaster Capitalism*. New York: Metropolitan Books.

Kleinman, Arthur. 2006. *What Really Matters: Living a Moral Life amidst Uncertainty and Danger*. Oxford: Oxford University Press.

Kleinman, Arthur, Veena Das, and Margaret Lock. 1997. *Social Suffering*. Berkeley: University of California Press.

Kleinman, Arthur, and Joan Kleinman. 1996. "The Appeal of Experience; the Dismay of Images: Cultural Appropriations of Suffering in our Times." *Daedalus* 125 (1): 1–23.

Körling, Gabriella. 2011. "In Search of the State: An Ethnography of Public Service Provision in Urban Niger." PhD diss., Uppsala University (Sweden). Republished as Uppsala Studies in Cultural Anthropology, vol. 51 (Uppsala: Acta Universitatis Upsaliensis, 2011).

Kristof, Nicholas D. 2003. "Alone and Ashamed." *New York Times*, May 16, https://www.nytimes.com/2003/05/16/opinion/alone-and-ashamed.html.

———. 2005. "The Illiterate Surgeon." *New York Times*, June 12, https://www.nytimes.com/2005/06/12/opinion/the-illiterate-surgeon.html.

———. 2009. "New Life for the Pariahs." *New York Times*, October 31, https://www.nytimes.com/2009/11/01/opinion/01kristof.html.

———. 2013. "Where Young Women Find Healing and Hope." *New York Times*, July 13, https://www.nytimes.com/2013/07/14/opinion/sunday/kristof-where-young-women-find-healing-and-hope.html.

———. 2016. "The World's Modern-Day Lepers: Women with Fistulas." *New York Times*, March 19, https://www.nytimes.com/2016/03/20/opinion/sunday/the-worlds-modern-day-lepers-women-with-fistulas.html.

Kristof, Nicholas, and Sheryl WuDunn. 2010. *Half the Sky: Turing Oppression into Opportunity for Women Worldwide*. New York: Vintage Books.

LaFraniere, Sharon. 2005. "Nightmare for African Women: Birthing Injury and Little Help." *New York Times*, September 28, https://www.nytimes.com/2016/03/20/opinion/sunday/the-worlds-modern-day-lepers-women-with-fistulas.html.

Lagro-Janssen, Toine, Anton Smits, and Chris Van Weel. 1992. "Urinary Incontinence in Women and the Effects on their Lives." *Scandinavian Journal of Primary Health Care* 10 (3): 211–216.

Landry, Evelyn, Vera Frajzyngier, Joseph Ruminjo, Frank Asiimwe, Thierno Hamidou Barry, Abubakar Bello, Dantani Danladi, et al. 2013. "Profiles and Experiences of Women Undergoing Genital Fistula Repair: Findings from Five Countries." *Global Public Health* 8 (8): 926–942.

Lavender, T., S. Wakasiaka, L. McGowan, M. Moraa, J. Omari, and W. Khisa. 2016. "Secrecy Inhibits Support: A Grounded Theory of Community Perspectives of Women Suffering from Obstetric Fistula, in Kenya." *Midwifery* 42: 54–60.

Lazareva, Inna. 2017. "Africa Fights Fistula with Mobile Money and Community Ambassadors." *Reuters*, July 17, https://www.reuters.com/article/us-africa-women-health-fistula/africa-fights-fistula-with-mobile-money-and-community-ambassadors-idUSKBN1A22CP.

Lewis, Gwyneth, Luc De Bernis, and World Health Organization (WHO). 2006. "Obstetric Fistula: Guiding Principles for Clinical Management and Programme Development." Geneva: Department of Reproductive Health and Research, World Health Organization, http://www.who.int/iris/handle/10665/43343.

Li, Florence Ling Wai, Lisa Pau Le Low, and Diana Tze Fan Lee. 2007. "Chinese Women's Experiences in Coping with Urinary Incontinence." *Journal of Clinical Nursing* 16 (3): 610–612.

Link, Bruce G., and Jo C. Phelan. 2001. "Conceptualizing Stigma." *Annual Review of Sociology* 27: 363–385.

Link, Bruce, Q. H. Yang, Jo C. Phelan, and Pamela Y. Collins. 2004. "Measuring Mental Illness Stigma." *Schizophrenia Bulletin* 30 (3): 511–542.

Livingston, Julie. 2012. *Improvising Medicine: An African Oncology Ward in an Emerging Cancer Epidemic*. Durham, N.C.: Duke University Press.

Lombard, Ladeisha, Jenna de St. Jorre, Rosemary Geddes, Alison M. El Ayadi, and Liz Grant. 2015. "Rehabilitation Experiences after Obstetric Fistula Repair: Systematic Review of Qualitative Studies." *Tropical Medicine and International Health* 20 (5): 554–568.

Lose, Gunnar. 2005. "The Burden of Stress Urinary Incontinence." *European Urology Supplements* 4: 5–10.

Lyotard, Jean-François. 1984. *The Postmodern Condition: A Report on Knowledge*. Minneapolis: Minnesota University Press.

Madhavan, S. 2002. "Best of Friends and Worst of Enemies: Competition and Collaboration in Polygyny." *Ethnology* 41 (1): 69–84.

Major, Brenda, and Laurie T. O'Brien. 2005. "The Social Psychology of Stigma." *Annual Review of Psychology* 56: 393–421.

Malkki, Liisa. 1996. "Speechless Emissaries: Refugees, Humanitarianism, and Dehistoricization." *Cultural Anthropology* 11 (3): 377–404.

Manderson, Lenore. 2011. *Surface Tensions: Surgery, Bodily Boundaries, and the Social Self*. Walnut Creek, Calif.: Left Coast Press.

Manderson, Lenore, and Carolyn Smith-Morris. 2010. *Chronic Conditions, Fluid States: Chronicity and the Anthropology of Illness*. New Brunswick, N.J.: Rutgers University Press.

Manvell, Adam. 2006. "Sahelian Action Spaces: An Examination of Livelihood Configurations in a Rural Hausa Community." *Journal of International Development* 18 (6): 803–818.

Manzo, Kate. 2008. "Imaging Humanitarianism: NGO Identity and the Iconography of Childhood." *Antipode* 40 (4): 632–657.

Marcus, George. 1998. *Ethnography through Thick and Thin*. Princeton, N.J.: Princeton University Press.

Marris, Emma. 2013. "Charismatic Mammals Can Help Guide Conservation." *Nature,* December 24, https://www.nature.com/news/charismatic-mammals-can-help-guide-conservation -1.14396.

Mascarenhas, Maya, S. R. Flaxman, T. Boerma, S. Vanderpoel, and G. A. Stevens. 2012. "National, Regional, and Global Trends in Infertility Prevalence since 1990: A Systematic Analysis of 277 Health Surveys." *PLoS Medicine* 9 (12): e1001356.

Masquelier, Adeline Marie. 2001a. "Behind the Dispensary's Prosperous Facade: Imagining the State in Rural Niger." *Public Culture* 13 (2): 267–291.

———. 2001b. *Prayer Has Spoiled Everything: Possession, Power, and Identity in an Islamic Town of Niger.* Durham, N.C.: Duke University Press.

———. 2005. "The Scorpion's Sting: Youth, Marriage and the Struggle for Social Maturity in Niger." *Journal of the Royal Anthropological Institute* 11 (1): 59–83.

———. 2009. *Women and Islamic Revival in a West African Town.* Bloomington: Indiana University Press.

Matsuo, Koji, Yasuhiko Shiki, Masato Yamasaki, and Koichiro Shimoya. 2009. "Use of Uterine Fundal Pressure Maneuver at Vaginal Delivery and Risk of Severe Perineal Laceration." *Archives of Gynecology and Obstetrics* 280 (5): 781–786.

Mattingly, Cheryl, and Linda C. Garro, eds. 2000. *Narrative and the Cultural Construction of Illness and Healing.* Berkeley: University of California Press.

Maulet, Nathalie, Abdramane Berthé, Salamatou Traoré, and Jean Macq. 2015. "Obstetric Fistula 'Disease' and Ensuing Care: Patients' Views in West-Africa." *African Journal of Reproductive Health* 19 (1): 112–123.

Maulet, Nathalie, Mahamoudou Keita, and Jean Macq. 2013. "Medico-social Pathways of Obstetric Fistula Patients in Mali and Niger: An 18-Month Cohort Follow-up." *Tropical Medicine and International Health* 18 (5): 524–533.

Mauss, Marcel. Mauss, Marcel. 1925/2016. *The Gift.* Trans. Jane I. Guyer. Chicago: HAU Books.

———. 1935/1973. "Techniques of the Body." *Economy and Society* 2 (1): 70–88.

Menard-Freeman, Lindsay. 2013. "Celebrate Solutions: Video Series Combats Fistula Stigma." Women Deliver [website], November 25, https://web.archive.org/web/20140821045853/ http://www.womendeliver.org/updates/entry/celebrate-solutions-video-series-com bats-fistula-stigma.

Meyer, Larissa, Charles J. Ascher-Walsh, Rachael Norman, Abdoulaye Idrissa, Hadley Herbert, Oumou Kimso, and Jeffrey Wilkinson. 2007. "Commonalities among Women Who Developed Vesicovaginal Fistulae as a Result of Obstetric Trauma in Niger: Results from a Survey Given at the National Hospital Fistula Center, Niamey, Niger." *American Journal of Obstetrics and Gynecology* 197 (90): e1–e4.

Michaelson, Bryony. 2018. "Oprah: Time's Up for Sexual Abuse." Operation Fistula, January 10, https://www.opfistula.org/obstetric-fistula/Oprah.

Miles, William. 1994. *Hausaland Divided: Colonialism and Independence in Nigeria and Niger.* Ithaca, N.Y.: Cornell University Press.

Miller, S., F. Lester, M. Webster, and B. Cowan. 2005. "Obstetric Fistula: A Preventable Tragedy." *Journal of Midwifery and Women's Health* 50 (4): 286–294.

Miller, Susan Gilson. 2006. "Sleeping Fetus." In *Encyclopedia of Women and Islamic Cultures,* volume 3, ed. Suad Joseph, 421–424. Leiden, Netherlands: Brill.

Moeller, Susan. 2002. "A Hierarchy of Innocence: The Media's Use of Children in the Telling of International News." *Harvard International Journal of Press/Politics* 7 (1): 36–56.

Mohammad, R. H. 2007. "A Community Program for Women's Health and Development: Implications for the Long-Term Care of Women with Fistulas." *International Journal of Gynecology and Obstetrics* 99 (Suppl. 1): S137–S142.

Mohanty, Chandra. 1991. "Under Western Eyes: Feminist Scholarship and Colonial Discourses." In *Third World Women and the Politics of Feminism*, ed. Chandra Mohanty, Ann Russo, and Lourdes Torres. Bloomington: Indiana University Press.

Mosher W. D., A. Chandra, and J. Jones. 2002. "Sexual Behavior and Selected Health Measures: Men and Women 15–44 Years of Age, United States, 2002." Advance Data from Vital and Health Statistics, no. 362. Hyattsville, Md.: National Center for Health Statistics.

Mosse, David. 2005. *Cultivating Development: An Ethnography of Aid Policy and Practice*. London: Pluto Press.

Moyer, Cheryl A., Philip B. Adongo, Raymond A. Aborigo, Abraham Hodgson, and Cyril M. Engmann. 2014. "'They Treat You Like You Are Not a Human Being': Maltreatment during Labour and Delivery in Rural Northern Ghana." *Midwifery* 30 (2): 262–268.

Moylan, Danielle. 2016. "Fistula: The Affliction Destroying Afghan Women's Lives." *Al Jazeera*, 27 July, http://www.aljazeera.com/indepth/features/2016/05/affliction-destroying-afghan-women-lives-160516104239351.html.

Mselle, Lilian, and Thecla Kohi. 2015. "Perceived Health System Causes of Obstetric Fistula from Accounts of Affected Women in Rural Tanzania: A Qualitative Study." *African Journal of Reproductive Health* 19 (1): 124.

Mselle, Lilian, Karen Marie Moland, Bjorg Evjen-Olsen, Abu Mvungi, and Thecla Kohi. 2011. "'I Am Nothing': Experiences of Loss among Women Suffering from Severe Birth Injuries in Tanzania." *BMC Health Services Research* 11 (49), DOI: 10.1186/1472-6874-11-49.

Munir, Sarah. 2014. "Inside Pakistan's Only Fistula Hospital." *Al Jazeera*, March 8, http://www.aljazeera.com/indepth/features/2014/03/inside-pakistan-only-fistula-hospital-2014369361327715.html.

Murray, Christine, Judith T. Goh, Michelle Fynes, and Marcus P. Carey. 2002. "Urinary and Faecal Incontinence following Delayed Primary Repair of Obstetric Genital Fistula." *BJOG* 109 (7): 828–832.

Mwini-Nyaledzigbor, Prudence P., Alice A. Agana, and F. Beryl Pilkington. 2013. "Lived Experiences of Ghanaian Women with Obstetric Fistula." *Health Care for Women International* 34 (6): 440–460.

Nafiou, I., A. Idrissa, A. K. Ghaichatou, M. L. Roenneburg, C. R. Wheeless, and R. R. Genadry. 2007. "Obstetric Vesico-Vaginal Fistulas at the National Hospital of Niamey, Niger." *International Journal of Gynecology and Obstetrics* 99 (Suppl. 1): S71–S74.

Nathan, Lisa M., Charles H. Rochat, Bogdan Grigorescu, and Erika Banks. 2009. "Obstetric Fistulae in West Africa: Patient Perspectives." *American Journal of Obstetrics and Gynecology* 200 (5): e40–e42.

Ndiaye, P., G. Amoul Kini, Idrissa Abdoulaye, Camara Diagne, and A. Tal-Dia. 2009. "Parcours de la Femme Souffrant de Fistule Obstétricale au Niger." *Médecine Tropicale* 69 (1): 61–65.

Nguyen, Vinh-Kim. 2010. *The Republic of Therapy: Triage and Sovereignty in West Africa's Time of AIDS*. Durham, N.C.: Duke University Press.

Nussbaum, Martha. 1999. *Sex and Social Justice*. New York: Oxford University Press.

"Obstetric Fistula." 2014. Wikipedia, https://web.archive.org/web/20140908013102/http://en.wikipedia.org/wiki/Obstetric_fistula.

Okafor, Innocent I., Emmanuel O. Ugwu, and Samuel N. Obi. 2015. "Disrespect and Abuse during Facility-Based Childbirth in a Low-Income Country." *International Journal of Gynecology and Obstetrics* 128 (2): 110–113.

O'Kane, Maggie. 1998. "An African Tragedy; Death Stalks Each Birth in Niger." *The Guardian*, June 23.

Okoye, Uzoma O., Nkechi Emma-Echiegu, and Perpetua L. Tanyi. 2014. "Living with Vesico-Vaginal Fistula: Experiences of Women Awaiting Repairs in Ebonyi State, Nigeria." *Tanzania Journal of Health Research* 16 (4): 322–328.

Olivier de Sardan, Jean-Pierre. 1999. "A Moral Economy of Corruption in Africa?" *Journal of Modern African Studies* 37 (1): 25–52.

———. 2001. "La sage-femme et le douanier: Cultures professionnelles locales et culture bureaucratique privatisée en Afrique de l'Ouest." *Autrepart* 20 (4): 61–73.

———. 2002. "Pourquoi le malade anonyme est-il si 'mal traité'? Culture bureaucratique commune et culture professionnelle de la santé." In *Une médecine inhospitalière: Les difficiles relations entre soignants et soignés dans cinq capitales d'Afrique de l'Ouest,* ed. Yannick Jaffré and Jean-Pierre Olivier de Sardan, 165–184. Collection Hommes et Sociétés. Marseille: APAD.

Oni-Orisan, Adeola. 2016. "The Obligation to Count: The Politics of Monitoring." In *Metrics: What Counts in Global Health,* ed. Vincanne Adams, 82–101. Durham, N.C.: Duke University Press.

Onsrud, Mathias, Solbjorg Sjoveian, and Denis Mukwege. 2011. "Cesarean Delivery-Related Fistulae in the Democratic Republic of Congo." *International Journal of Gynecology and Obstetrics* 114 (1): 10–14.

Oprah.com. 2005. "Inside the Fistula Hospital." Oprah.com, www.oprah.com/spirit/inside-the-fistula-hospital.

Østergaard, Lise Rosendal. 2015. "Maternal Healthcare in Context: A Qualitative Study of Women's Tactics to Improve Their Experience of Public Healthcare in Rural Burkina Faso." *Social Science and Medicine* 147: 98–104.

Ousseni, Abdoulaye. 2011. "Une politique publique de santé au Niger: La mise en place d'exemptions de paiement des soins en faveur des femmes et des enfants." *Etudes & Travaux,* no. 91. Niamy, Niger: Laboratoire d'Etudes et de Recherches sur le Dynamiques Sociales et le Développement Local (LASEL).

Parker, R., and P. Aggleton. 2003. "HIV and AIDS Related Sigma and Discrimination: A Conceptual Framework and Implications for Action." *Social Science and Medicine* 57: 13–24.

Phillips, Beth S., Dorothy N. Ononokpono, and Nsikanabasi W. Udofia. 2016. "Complicating Causality: Patient and Professional Perspectives on Obstetric Fistula in Nigeria." *Culture, Health and Sexuality* 18 (9): 996–1009.

Pierce, Steven. 2007. "Identity, Performance, and Secrecy: Gendered Life and the 'Modern' in Northern Nigeria." *Feminist Studies* 33 (3): 539–565.

Prost, André. 1970. "Statut de la femme songhay." *Bulletin de l'Institut Fondamental d'Afrique Noire, Série B: Sciences Humaines* 32 (2): 486–517.

Prual, Alain, Dominique Huguet, Olivier Garbin, and Gomna Rabé. 1998. "Severe Obstetric Morbidity of the Third Trimester, Delivery and Early Puerperium in Niamey (Niger)." *African Journal of Reproductive Health* 2 (1): 10–19.

Rasmussen, Susan. 1994. "Female Sexuality, Social Reproduction, and the Politics of Medical Intervention in Niger: Kel Ewey Tuareg Perspectives." *Culture, Medicine and Psychiatry* 18 (4): 433–462.

———. 2004. "Tuareg." In *Cultures,* vol. 2 of *Encyclopedia of Medical Anthropology,* ed C. R. Ember and M. Ember, 1001–1009. New York: Kluwer Academic/Plenum.

Rathee, S., and S. Nanda. 1995. "Vesicovaginal Fistulae: A 12-Year Study." *Journal of the Indian Medical Association* 93 (3): 93–4.

Redfield, Peter. 2006. "A Less Modest Witness: Collective Advocacy and Motivated Truth in a Medical Humanitarian Movement." *American Ethnologist* 33 (1): 3–26.

———. 2013. *Life in Crisis: The Ethical Journey of Doctors without Borders.* Berkeley: University of California Press.

République du Niger. 2017. "Annuaire des Statistiques Sanitaires du Niger, Année 2016." Ministère de la Sante Publique Secrétariat General Direction Des Statistiques. http://www.stat-niger.org/statistique/file/Annuaires_Statistiques/snis/Annuaire_statistiques_2016.pdf.

Reuters Staff. 2013. "Niger Arrests Doctors after Graft Probe by Bill Gates Charity." *Reuters,* February 26, http://www.reuters.com/article/niger-doctors-idUSL6N0BP8NX20130226.

Rhine, Kathryn. 2009. "Support Groups, Marriage, and the Management of Ambiguity among HIV-Positive Women in Northern Nigeria." *Anthropological Quarterly* 82 (2): 369–400.

Ridde, Valéry. 2015. "From Institutionalization of User Fees to Their Abolition in West Africa: A Story of Pilot Projects and Public Policies." *BMC Health Services Research* 15 (Suppl. 3): S6.

Riesman, Paul. 1992. *First Find Your Child a Good Mother: The Construction of Self in Two African Communities.* Rutgers, N.J.: Rutgers University Press.

Rispler-Chaim, Vardit. 2006. *Disability in Islamic Law.* Vol. 32. Dordrecht, Netherlands: Springer Science & Business Media.

Rohy, V. 1996. "Displacing Desire: Passing, Nostalgia and Giovanni's Room." In *Passing and the Fictions of Identity,* ed. E. K. Ginsberg, 218–233. Durham, N.C.: Duke University Press.

Ruder, Bonnie, Melissa Cheyney, and Alice Aturo Emasu. 2018. "Too Long to Wait: Obstetric Fistula and the Sociopolitical Dynamics of the Fourth Delay in Soroti, Uganda." *Qualitative Health Research* 28 (5): 721–732.

Russell, Katie W., Ryan E. Robinson, Mary C. Mone, and Courtney L. Scaife. 2016. "Enterovaginal or Vesicovaginal Fistula Control Using a Silicone Cup." *Obstetrics and Gynecology* 128 (6): 1365–1368.

Salgo, Steven, dir. 2010. *Lighting a Candle: A Midwife for Every Mother.* Canberra, Australia: Ronin Films.

Samsky, Ari. 2012. "Scientific Sovereignty: How International Drug Donation Programs Reshape Health, Disease, and the State." *Cultural Anthropology* 27 (2): 310–332.

Sange, Chandbi, Lois Thomas, Christina Lyons, and Simon Hill. 2008. "Urinary Incontinence in Muslim Women." *Nursing Times* 104 (25): 49–52.

Sargent, Carolyn. 1989. *Maternity, Medicine and Power: Reproductive Decisions in Urban Benin.* Berkeley: University of California.

Save the Children. 2012. "2012 Mothers' Index Rankings." In *Nutrition in the First 1,000 Days: State of the World's Mothers 2012,* ed. Tracy Geoghegan, 47. Westport, Conn.: Save the Children, https://web.archive.org/web/20130910112606/http://www.savethechildren.org:80/site/c.8rKLIXMGIpI4E/b.8050465/k.CC42/Save_the_Children__State_of_the_Worlds_Mothers_2012__Downloads.htm.

Scheper-Hughes, Nancy. 1992. *Death without Weeping: The Violence of Everyday Life in Brazil.* Berkeley: University of California Press.

Schoepf, Brooke. 2001. "International AIDS Research in Anthropology: Taking a Critical Perspective on the Crisis." *Annual Review of Anthropology* 30: 335–361.

Sedgh, Gilda, Lori Ashford, and Rubina Hussain. 2016. *Unmet Need for Contraception in Developing Countries: Examining Women's Reasons for Not Using a Method.* New York: Guttmacher Institute, https://www.guttmacher.org/report/unmet-need-for-contraception-in-developing-countries.

Semere, Luwam, and Nawal M. Nour. 2008. "Obstetric Fistula: Living with Incontinence and Shame." *Reviews in Obstetrics and Gynecology* 1 (4): 193–197.

Sermrittirong, S., and W. H. Van Brakel. 2014. "Stigma in Leprosy: Concepts, Causes and Determinants." *Leprosy Review* 85 (1): 36–47.

Shankar, Shobana. 2006. "The Social Dimensions of Christian Leprosy Work among Muslims: American Missionaries and Young Patients in Colonial Northern Nigeria, 1920–40." In *Healing Bodies, Saving Souls: Medical Missions in Asia and Africa,* ed. David Hardiman, 281–305. New York: Rodopi.

Shepard, L. D. 2013. "The Impact of Polygamy on Women's Mental Health: A Systematic Review." *Epidemiology and Psychiatric Sciences* 22: 47–62.

Shih, Margaret. 2004. "Positive Stigma: Examining Resilience and Empowerment in Overcoming Stigma." *Annals of the American Academy of Political and Social Science* 591 (1): 175–185.

Shrime, Mark, Ambereen Sleemi, and Thulasiraj Ravilla. 2015. "Charitable Platforms in Global Surgery: A Systematic Review of Their Effectiveness, Cost-Effectiveness, Sustainability, and Role in Training." *World Journal of Surgery* 39 (1): 10–20.

Siddle, Kathryn, Liesbeth Vieren, and Alison Fiander. 2014. "Characterizing Women with Obstetric Fistula and Urogenital Tract Injuries in Tanzania." *International Urogynecology Journal* 25 (2): 249–255.

SIM Niger. 2013. CSFL Danja. Accessed 02/2014: http://www.sim.ne/index.php/en/whatwedo/ministries/cslfdanja.

Smith, Daniel Jordan. 2007. *A Culture of Corruption: Everyday Deception and Popular Discontent in Nigeria.* Princeton, N.J.: Princeton University Press.

Smith, Mary Felice. 1954. *Baba of Karo, A Woman of the Muslim Hausa.* New Haven, Conn.: Yale University Press.

Smith, Mary Olive, dir. 2007. *A Walk to Beautiful.* New York: Engel Entertainment.

Solivetti, Luigi. 1994. "Family, Marriage and Divorce in a Hausa Community: A Sociological Model." *Africa: Journal of the International African Institute* 64 (2): 252–271.

Sontag, Susan. 1988. *Illness as Metaphor and AIDS and its Metaphors.* New York, N.Y.: Anchor Books Doubleday.

Soumana, Assane. 2017. "Amani Abdou, ministre du Développement Communautaire et de L'Aménagement du Territoire." *Le Sahel.* http://www.lesahel.org/index.php/societe/item/14653.

Spivak, Gayatri Chakravorty. 1993. "Can the Subaltern Speak?" In *Colonial Discourse and Post-Colonial Theory: A Reader,* ed. Patrick Williams and Laura Chrisman, 66–111. Hemel Hempstead, United Kingdom: Harvester Wheatsheaf.

Stanton, C., S. A. Holtz, and S. Ahmed. 2007. "Challenges in Measuring Obstetric Fistula." *International Journal of Gynecology and Obstetrics* 99 (Suppl. 1): S4–S9.

Stoller, Paul. 2016. "The Power of Public Scholarship." *Huffington Post,* June 12, https://www.huffingtonpost.com/paul-stoller/the-power-of-public-schol_b_10409082.html.

Street, Alice. 2014. *Biomedicine in an Unstable Place: Infrastructure and Personhood in a Papua New Guinean Hospital.* Durham, N.C.: Duke University Press.

Sullivan, Ginger, Beverley O'Brien, and Prudence Mwini-Nyaledzigbor. 2016. "Sources of Support for Women Experiencing Obstetric Fistula in Northern Ghana: A Focused Ethnography." *Midwifery* 40: 162–168.

Summers, Carol. 1991. "Intimate Colonialism: The Imperial Production of Reproduction in Uganda, 1907–1925." *Signs: Journal of Women in Culture and Society* 16 (4): 787–807.

Sutton, Rebecca, Darshan Vigneswaran, and Harry Wels. 2011. "Waiting in Liminal Space: Migrants' Queuing for Home Affairs in South Africa." *Anthropology Southern Africa* 34 (1–2): 30–37.

Tabi, Marian M., C. Doster, and T. Cheney. 2010. "A Qualitative Study of Women in Polygynous Marriages." *International Nursing Review* 57 (1): 121–127.

Tebu, Pierre Marie, Luc de Bernis, Anderson Sama Doh, Charles Henry Rochat, and Therese Delvaux. 2009. "Risk Factors for Obstetric Fistula in the Far North Province of Cameroon." *International Journal of Gynecology and Obstetrics* 107: 12–15.

Thaddeus, Sereen, and Deborah Maine. 1994. "Too Far to Walk: Maternal Mortality in Context." *Social Science and Medicine* 38: 1091–1110.

Thom, D. H., and Rortveit, G. 2010. "Prevalence of Postpartum Urinary Incontinence: A Systematic Review." *Acta Obstetricia et Gynecologica Scandinavica* 89: 1511–1522.

Ticktin, Miriam. 2011. *Casualties of Care: Immigration and the Politics of Humanitarianism in France*. Berkeley: University of California Press.

———. 2017. "A World without Innocence." *American Ethnologist* 44 (4): 577–590.

Treister-Goltzman, Yula, and Roni Peleg. 2018. "Urinary Incontinence among Muslim Women in Israel: Risk Factors and Help-Seeking Behavior." *International Urogynecology Journal* 29 (4): 539–546.

United Nations Development Programme. 2014. "Human Development Report 2014." https:// web.archive.org/web/20141221143254/http://hdr.undp.org/en/content/table-1-human -development-index-and-its-components.

Van Balen, F., and T. Gerrits. 2001. "Quality of Infertility Care in Poor-Resource Areas and the Introduction of New Reproductive Technologies." *Human Reproduction* 16 (2): 215–219.

Van Brakel, Wim H., Alison M. Anderson, R. K. Mutatkar, Zoica Bakirtzief, Peter G. Nicholls, M. S. Raju, and Robert K. Das-Pattanayak. 2006. "The Participation Scale: Measuring a Key Concept in Public Health." *Disability and Rehabilitation* 28 (4): 193–203.

Van Hollen, Cecilia Coale. 2003. *Birth on the Threshold: Childbirth and Modernity in South India*. Berkeley: University of California Press.

———. 2018. "Handle with Care: Rethinking the Rights versus Culture Dichotomy in Cancer Disclosure in India." *Medical Anthropology Quarterly* 32 (1): 59–84.

Vaughan, Meghan. 1991. *Curing Their Ills: Colonial Power and African Illness*. Cambridge, United Kingdom: Polity Press.

Velez, A., K. Ramsey, and K. Tell. 2007. "The Campaign to End Fistula: What Have We Learned? Findings of Facility and Community Needs Assessments." *International Journal of Gynaecology and Obstetrics* 99 (Suppl. 1): S143–S150.

Verghese, Abraham. 2012. *Cutting for Stone*. New York: Random House.

Vongsathorn, Kathleen. 2012. "Gnawing Pains, Festering Ulcers, and Nightmare Suffering: Selling Leprosy as a Humanitarian Cause in the British Empire, c. 1890–1960." *Journal of Imperial and Commonwealth History* 40 (5): 863–878.

Waaldijk, K., and Y. D. Armiya'u. 1993. "The Obstetric Fistula: A Major Public Health Problem Still Unsolved." *International Urogynecology Journal* 4 (2): 126–128.

Walker, Alice. 1992. *Possessing the Secret of Joy*. New York: Harcourt Brace Jovanovich.

Walker, Alice, and Pratibha Parmar. 1993. *Warrior Marks: Female Genital Mutilation and the Sexual Blinding of Women*. New York: Harcourt Brace.

Wall, L. Lewis. 1988. *Hausa Medicine: Illness and Well-Being in a West African Culture*. Durham, N.C.: Duke University Press.

———. 1998. "Dead Mothers and Injured Wives: The Social Context of Maternal Morbidity and Mortality among the Hausa of Northern Nigeria." *Studies in Family Planning* 29 (4): 341–359.

———. 2002. "*Fitsari 'dan Duniya:* An African (Hausa) Praise Song about Vesicovaginal Fistulas." *Obstetrics and Gynecology* 100 (6): 1328–1232.

———. 2006. "Obstetric Vesicovaginal Fistula as an International Public-Health Problem." *Lancet* 368: 1201–1209.

———. 2012. "Preventing Obstetric Fistulas in Low-Resource Countries: Insights from a Haddon Matrix." *Obstetrical and Gynecological Survey* 67 (2): 111–121.

———. 2014. "A Bill of Rights for Patients with Obstetric Fistula." *International Journal of Gynecology and Obstetrics* 127: 301–304.

———. 2016. "Residual Incontinence after Obstetric Fistula Repair." *Obstetrics and Gynecology* 128 (5): 943–944.

Wall, L. Lewis, and Steven D. Arrowsmith. 2007. "The "Continence Gap": A Critical Concept in Obstetric Fistula Repair." *International Urogynecology Journal* 18 (8): 843–844.

Walraven, Gijs, Caroline Scherf, Beryl West, Gloria Ekpo, Katie Paine, Rosalind Coleman, Robin Bailey, and Linda Morison. 2001. "The Burden of Reproductive-Organ Disease in Rural Women in the Gambia, West Africa." *The Lancet* 357 (9263): 1161–1167.

Ware, Helen. 1979. "Polygyny: Women's Views in a Transitional Society, Nigeria 1975." *Journal of Marriage and the Family* 41 (1): 185–195.

Wark, McKenzie. 1995. "Fresh Maimed Babies." *Transition* 65: 36–47.

Warner, Gregory. 2014. "Moved by Emotion: This Story Changed a Photographer's Lens." *NPR News: All Things Considered,* January 2, https://www.npr.org/2014/01/02/259121412/moved -by-emotion-this-story-changed-a-photographer-s-lens.

Watt, Melissa, Sarah Wilson, Mercykutty Joseph, Gileard Masenga, Jessica MacFarlane, Olola Oneko, and Kathleen Sikkema. 2014. "Religious Coping among Women with Obstetric Fistula in Tanzania." *Global Public Health* 9 (5): 516–527.

Wendland, Claire. 2010. *A Heart for the Work: Journeys through an African Medical School.* Chicago: University of Chicago Press.

———. 2012. "Moral Maps and Medical Imaginaries: Clinical Tourism at Malawi's College of Medicine." *American Anthropologist* 114 (1): 108–122.

———. 2016. "Estimating Death: A Close Reading of Maternal Mortality Metrics in Malawi." In *Metrics: What Counts in Global Health,* ed. Vincanne Adams, 57–81. Durham, N.C.: Duke University Press.

Wilson, Kalpana. 2008. "Reclaiming 'Agency,' Reasserting Resistance." *IDS Bulletin* 39 (6): 83–91.

Winsor, Morgan. 2013. "A Fate Worse Than Death for Scores of African Women." *CNN,* May 23, http://www.cnn.com/2013/05/23/health/end-obstetric-fistula-day.

Wittrup, Inge. 1990. "Me and My Husband's Wife: An Analysis of Polygyny among Mandinka in the Gambia." *Folk* 32: 117–142.

World Bank. 2013. *Republic of Niger: 2012 Public Expenditure Review.* Washington, DC.

———. 2018. World Bank Open Data: Indicators [search page]. Accessed January 5, 2018. http://data.worldbank.org/indicator.

Wright, Jeremy, Fekade Ayenachew, and Karen D. Ballard. 2016. "The Changing Face of Obstetric Fistula Surgery in Ethiopia." *International Journal of Women's Health* 2016 (8): 243–248.

Yang, Lawrence Hsin, Arthur Kleinman, Bruce G. Link, Jo C. Phelan, Sing Lee, and Byron Good. 2007. "Culture and Stigma: Adding Moral Experience to Stigma Theory." *Social Science and Medicine* 64 (7): 1524–1535.

Yeakey, Marissa Pine, Effice Chipeta, Frank Taulo, and May Tsui. 2009. "The Lived Experience of Malawian Women with Obstetric Fistula." *Culture, Health and Sexuality* 11 (5): 499–513.

Yunus, Muhammad. 1994. *Banking on the Poor.* Dhaka, Bangladesh: Grameen Bank.

INDEX

Page numbers followed by "t" indicates tables; followed by "f" indicates figures; followed by "n" indicates notes.

ABOUT THE AUTHOR

ALISON HELLER is an assistant professor of anthropology at the University of Maryland. Her research, focusing on reproductive health and humanitarianism in West Africa, has been funded by the Fulbright-Hays Program, the National Science Foundation, the Wenner-Gren Foundation, and the School for Advanced Research. You can follow her at http://ali-heller.com.

Printed and bound by CPI Group (UK) Ltd, Croydon, CR0 4YY

16/04/2025

14658332-0003